Post-Covid Rehabilitation

Editor

MONICA VERDUZCO-GUTIERREZ

PHYSICAL MEDICINE AND REHABILITATION CLINICS OF NORTH AMERICA

www.pmr.theclinics.com

Consulting Editor
BLESSEN C. EAPEN

August 2023 • Volume 34 • Number 3

ELSEVIER

1600 John F. Kennedy Boulevard ● Suite 1800 ● Philadelphia, Pennsylvania, 19103-2899

http://www.theclinics.com

**PHYSICAL MEDICINE AND REHABILITATION CLINICS OF NORTH AMERICA Volume 34, Number 3
August 2023 ISSN 1047-9651, 978-0-443-12947-6**

Editor: Megan Ashdown
Developmental Editor: Malvika Shah

Reprints. For copies of 100 or more of articles in this publication, please contact the Commercial Reprints Department, Elsevier Inc., 360 Park Avenue South, New York, NY 10010-1710. Tel.: 212-633-3874; Fax: 212-633-3820; E-mail: reprints@elsevier.com.

Physical Medicine and Rehabilitation Clinics of North America (ISSN 1047-9651) is published quarterly by Elsevier Inc., 360 Park Avenue South, New York, NY 10010-1710. Months of issue are February, May, August, and November. Business and Editorial Offices: 1600 John F. Kennedy Blvd., Suite 1800, Philadelphia, PA 19103-2899. Customer Service Office: 3251 Riverport Lane, Maryland Heights, MO 63043. Periodicals postage paid at New York, NY and additional mailing offices. Subscription price per year is $342.00 (US individuals), $722.00 (US institutions), $100.00 (US students), $388.00 (Canadian individuals), $950.00 (Canadian institutions), $100.00 (Canadian students), $491.00 (foreign individuals), $950.00 (foreign institutions), and $210.00 (foreign students). Foreign air speed delivery is included in all *Clinics* subscription prices. All prices are subject to change without notice. **POSTMASTER:** Send address changes to *Physical Medicine and Rehabilitation Clinics of North America,* Customer Service Office: Elsevier Health Sciences Division, Subscription Customer Service, 3251 Riverport Lane, Maryland Heights, MO 63043. **Customer Service: 1-800-654-2452 (US). From outside of the United States, call 314-447-8871. Fax: 314-447-8029.** E-mail: JournalsCustomer Service-usa@elsevier.com **(for print support);** JournalsOnlineSupport-usa@elsevier.com **(for online support).**

Physical Medicine and Rehabilitation Clinics of North America is indexed in *Excerpta Medica, MEDLINE/ PubMed (Index Medicus), Cinahl,* and *Cumulative Index to Nursing and Allied Health Literature.*

Contributors

CONSULTING EDITOR

BLESSEN C. EAPEN, MD
Chief, Physical Medicine and Rehabilitation, VA Greater Los Angeles Health Care System, Health Sciences Clinical Associate Professor, Department of Medicine, Division of Physical Medicine and Rehabilitation, David Geffen School of Medicine at UCLA, Los Angeles, California

EDITOR

MONICA VERDUZCO-GUTIERREZ, MD
Professor and Distinguished Chair, Department of Rehabilitation Medicine, Joe R. and Teresa Lozano Long School of Medicine, University of Texas Health Science Center at San Antonio, San Antonio, Texas

AUTHORS

ZACHARY ABBOTT, DO
Resident Physician, Department of Physical Medicine and Rehabilitation, University of Colorado School of Medicine, Aurora, Colorado

PAULA ACKERMAN, DO
Associate Professor, Department of Physical Medicine and Rehabilitation, University of Florida College of Medicine, Gainesville, Florida

SURENDRA BARSHIKAR, MD, MBA
Associate Professor, Vice Chair of Clinical Operations, Medical Director of UTSW and Parkland PMR Clinics, Physical Medicine and Rehabilitation, UT Southwestern Medical Center, Dallas, Texas

RATNA BHAVARAJU-SANKA, MD
Associate Professor, Department of Neurology, The University of Texas Health Science Center at San Antonio, San Antonio, Texas

W. MICHAEL BRODE, MD
Department of Internal Medicine, Dell Medical School, The University of Texas at Austin, Austin, Texas

JUSTIN M. BURTON, MD
Division of Pediatric Rehabilitation Medicine, Children's National Health System, Washington, DC

ERIN Y. CHEN, BS
Johns Hopkins School of Medicine, Baltimore, Maryland

MICHELLE COPLEY, MD
Department of Rehabilitation Medicine, University of Washington, Seattle, Washington

MIGUEL X. ESCALON, MD, MPH
Associate Professor, Department of Rehabilitation and Human Performance, Icahn School of Medicine at Mount Sinai, New York, New York

RACHEL ESPARZA, MD
Resident Physician, Department of Physical Medicine and Rehabilitation, McGaw Medical Center, Northwestern University Feinberg School of Medicine, Shirley Ryan Ability Lab (Formerly the Rehabilitation Institute of Chicago), Chicago, Illinois

IRENE M. ESTORES, MD
Associate Professor, Department of Physical Medicine and Rehabilitation, Director, Integrative Medicine Program, University of Florida College of Medicine, Gainesville, Florida

LAURA E. FLORES, PhD
Medical Student, College of Allied Health Professions, University of Nebraska Medical Center, Omaha, Nebraska

JANNA FRIEDLY, MD, MPH
Department of Rehabilitation Medicine, University of Washington, Seattle, Washington

NICOLE GENTILE, MD, PhD
Department of Family Medicine, Department of Laboratory Medicine and Pathology, University of Washington, Seattle, Washington

RACHEL GEYER, MPH
Department of Family Medicine, University of Washington, Seattle, Washington

PATRICIA GORDON, MSN, MPH, APRN, FNP-BC
Nurse Practitioner, Physical Medicine and Rehabilitation, UT Southwestern Medical Center, Dallas, Texas

JUSTIN HALOOT, DO, MS
Chief Resident of Research and Education, Department of Internal Medicine, The University of Texas Health Science Center at San Antonio, San Antonio, Texas

TRACEY L. HUNTER, MD
Resident Physician, Department of Physical Medicine and Rehabilitation, Harvard Medical School, Boston, Massachusetts; Spaulding Rehabilitation Hospital, Charlestown, Massachusetts

ALICIA JOHNSTON, MD
Division of Infectious Disease, Boston Children's Hospital, Boston, Massachusetts

ORANICHA JUMREORNVONG, MD
Resident Physician, Department of Physical Medicine and Rehabilitation, Icahn School of Medicine at Mount Sinai, New York, New York

NICOLE B. KATZ, MD
Resident Physician, Department of Physical Medicine and Rehabilitation, Harvard Medical School, Boston, Massachusetts; Spaulding Rehabilitation Hospital, Charlestown, Massachusetts

AMANDA A. KELLY, MD
Department of Rehabilitation and Human Performance, Icahn School of Medicine at Mount Sinai, New York, New York

BARBARA KOZMINSKI, MD
Department of Rehabilitation Medicine, University of Washington, Seattle, Washington

MARTIN LAGUERRE, MD
Resident Physician, Physical Medicine and Rehabilitation, UT Southwestern Medical Center, Dallas, Texas

CAROLINE A. LEWIS, MD
Department of Rehabilitation and Human Performance, Icahn School of Medicine at Mount Sinai, New York, New York

CAROL LI, MD
Department of Rehabilitation Medicine, Joe R. and Teresa Lozano Long School of Medicine, The University of Texas Health Science Center at San Antonio, Polytrauma Outpatient Neurorehabilitation Services, Audie L. Murphy VA Medical Center, Polytrauma Rehabilitation Center, San Antonio, Texas

MARIELISA LOPEZ, MD
Assistant Professor, Physical Medicine and Rehabilitation, UT Southwestern Medical Center, Dallas, Texas

LAURA A. MALONE, MD, PhD
Kennedy Krieger Institute, Department of Physical Medicine and Rehabilitation, Department of Neurology, Johns Hopkins School of Medicine, Baltimore, Maryland

BETSY J. MEDINA-INOJOSA, MD
Division of Preventive Cardiology, Department of Cardiovascular Medicine, Mayo Clinic, Rochester, Minnesota

ESTHER MELAMED, MD, PhD
Assistant Professor, Department of Neurology, Dell Medical School, The University of Texas at Austin, Austin, Texas

AMANDA K. MORROW, MD
Kennedy Krieger Institute, Department of Physical Medicine and Rehabilitation, Johns Hopkins School of Medicine, Baltimore, Maryland

ERIC NICOLAU, DO, MS
West Virginia School of Osteopathic Medicine, Austin, Texas

WILLIAM NIEHAUS, MD
Outpatient Medical Director and Associate Residency Program Director, Department of Physical Medicine and Rehabilitation, University of Colorado School of Medicine, Aurora, Colorado

JAYASREE PILLARISETTI, MD, MSc
Associate Professor of Cardiac Electrophysiology, Department of Medicine, The University of Texas Health Science Center at San Antonio, San Antonio, Texas

DAVID PUTRINO, PhD
Department of Rehabilitation and Human Performance, Icahn School of Medicine at Mount Sinai, New York, New York

AKSHARA RAMASAMY
Department of Neurology, Dell Medical School, The University of Texas at Austin, Austin, Texas

ANDREW RIVERA, MS
Tulane University School of Medicine, New Orleans, Louisiana

DANIELLE L. SARNO, MD
Instructor, Department of Physical Medicine and Rehabilitation, Harvard Medical School, Massachusetts General Hospital, Brigham and Women's Hospital, Boston, Massachusetts; Spaulding Rehabilitation Hospital, Charlestown, Massachusetts

JULIE K. SILVER, MD
Associate Professor and Associate Chair, Department of Physical Medicine and Rehabilitation, Harvard Medical School, Massachusetts General Hospital, Brigham and Women's Hospital, Boston, Massachusetts; Spaulding Rehabilitation Hospital, Charlestown, Massachusetts

WILLIAM SUMMERS, MD
Resident Physician, Department of Physical Medicine and Rehabilitation, University of Colorado School of Medicine, Aurora, Colorado

LAURA TABACOF, MD
Department of Rehabilitation and Human Performance, Icahn School of Medicine at Mount Sinai, New York, New York

CARMEN M. TERZIC, MD, PhD
Professor, Department of Physical Medicine and Rehabilitation, Director, Cardiovascular Rehabilitation, Co-Director, Rehabilitation Medicine Research Center, Division of Preventive Cardiology, Department of Cardiovascular Medicine, Mayo Clinic, Rochester, Minnesota

MONICA VERDUZCO-GUTIERREZ, MD
Professor and Distinguished Chair, Department of Rehabilitation Medicine, Joe R. and Teresa Lozano Long School of Medicine, University of Texas Health Science Center at San Antonio, San Antonio, Texas

CHUMENG WANG, BS
Department of Neurology, Dell Medical School, The University of Texas at Austin, Austin, Texas

JONATHAN H. WHITESON, MD
Medical Director, Cardiac and Pulmonary Rehabilitation, Co-Director, NYU Langone Health Post COVID Care Program, Vice Chair, Clinical Operations, Rusk Rehabilitation, NYU Langone Medical Center, Associate Professor, Physical Medicine and Rehabilitation, Associate Professor, Medicine, NYU Grossman School of Medicine, New York, New York

ALEXANDRA B. YONTS, MD
Division of Infectious Diseases, Children's National Health System, Washington, DC

Contents

Post-COVID condition (PCC), also known as long COVID, is a multi-systemic illness estimated to affect 10% to 20% of those infected, regardless of age, baseline health status, or initial symptom severity. PCC has affected millions of lives, with long-lasting debilitating effects, but unfortunately it remains an underrecognized and therefore poorly documented condition. Defining and disseminating the burden of PCC is essential for developing effective public health strategies to address this issue in the long term.

Patients who are hospitalized due to COVID-19 are predisposed to requiring acute inpatient rehabilitation. Multiple factors have posed challenges to inpatient rehabilitation during the COVID-19 pandemic, such as staff shortages, restrictions with therapy, and barriers to discharge. Despite these challenges, data have shown that inpatient rehabilitation plays a key role in functional gains for this patient population. There remains a need for more data on the current challenges that are faced in the inpatient rehabilitation setting, as well as better understanding of long-term functional outcomes following COVID-19.

The challenging circumstances of the COVID-19 pandemic caused a regression in baseline health of disadvantaged populations, including individuals with frail syndrome, older age, disability, and racial-ethnic minority status. These patients often have more comorbidities and are associated with increased risk of poor postoperative complications, hospital readmissions, longer length of stay, nonhome discharges, poor patient satisfaction, and mortality. There is critical need to advance frailty assessments to improve preoperative health in older populations. Establishing a gold standard for measuring frailty will improve identification of vulnerable, older patients, and subsequently direct designs for population-specific,

in cellular and organ function. This can result in multiple symptoms and associated functional limitations. Respiratory symptoms in acute COVID-19 and in post-acute sequelae of COVID-19 (PASC) are common and can range from mild and intermittent to severe and persistent, correlating with functional limitations. Although the long-term pulmonary sequelae of COVID-19 infection and PASC are not known, a considered rehabilitative approach is recommended to yield optimal functional outcomes with a return to pre-morbid functional, avocational, and vocational status.

Musculoskeletal and pain sequelae of COVID-19 are common in both the acute infection and patients experiencing longer term symptoms associated with recovery, known as postacute sequelae of COVID-19 (PASC). Patients with PASC may experience multiple manifestations of pain and other concurrent symptoms that complicate their experience of pain. In this review, the authors explore what is currently known about PASC-related pain and its pathophysiology as well as strategies for diagnosis and management.

Fatigue from post-acute sequelae of coronavirus disease 2019 is a complex constellation of symptoms that could be driven by a wide spectrum of underlying etiologies. Despite this, there seems to be hope for treatment plans that focus on addressing possible etiologies and creating a path to improving quality of life and a paced return to activity.

The COVID-19 pandemic has resulted in a significant number of people developing long-term health effects of postacute sequelae SARS-CoV-2 infection (PASC). Both acute COVID-19 and PASC are now recognized as multiorgan diseases with multiple symptoms and disease causes. The development of immune dysregulation during acute COVID-19 and PASC is of high epidemiologic concern. Both conditions may also be influenced by comorbid conditions such as pulmonary dysfunction, cardiovascular disease, neuropsychiatric conditions, prior autoimmune conditions and cancer. This review discusses the clinical symptoms, pathophysiology, and risk factors that affect both acute COVID-19 and PASC.

Pediatric post-acute sequelae of SARS-CoV-2 (PASC) or "long COVID" are a complex multisystemic disease that affects children's physical, social, and mental health. PASC has a variable presentation, time course, and severity and can affect children even with mild or asymptomatic acute COVID-19 symptoms. Screening for PASC in children with a history of SARS-CoV-2 infection is important for early detection and intervention. A multifaceted treatment approach and utilization of multidisciplinary care, if available, are beneficial in managing the complexities of PASC. Lifestyle interventions, physical rehabilitation, and mental health management are important treatment approaches to improve pediatric PASC patients' quality of life.

The coronavirus disease-2019 pandemic exposed and expanded upon preexisting health care disparities. Individuals with disabilities and those who identify with racial/ethnic minority groups have been disproportionately adversely impacted. These inequities are likely present in the proportions of individuals impacted by post-acute sequelae of severe acute respiratory syndrome coronavirus 2 infection requiring specialized rehabilitation. Specific populations including, but not limited to pregnant, pediatric, and older individuals, may also necessitate tailored medical care during acute infection and beyond. Telemedicine may reduce the care gap. Further research and clinical guidance are needed to provide equitable, culturally competent, and individualized care to these historically or socially marginalized and underrepresented populations.

Physiatry and Integrative Medicine practice approaches the care of patients holistically to achieve recovery and optimal function. The current lack of knowledge on proven treatments for long COVID has resulted in a surge in both demand and use of complementary and integrative health (CIH) treatments. This overview summarizes CIH therapies using the framework of the United States National Center for Complementary and Integrative Health, divided into nutritional, psychological, physical, and combinations of these categories. Representative therapies selected based on the availability of published and ongoing research for post-COVID conditions are described.

Professional or governmental agencies and organizations have developed guidelines to define the problem and evaluate and manage patients with Post-Acute Sequelae of SARS CoV-2 (PASC). Multidisciplinary models largely exist in academic centers and larger cities; however, most care for PASC patients is provided by the primary care providers. The American Academy of Physical Medicine and Rehabilitation has been in the forefront in releasing consensus statements as a part of the long COVID collaborative.

PHYSICAL MEDICINE AND REHABILITATION CLINICS OF NORTH AMERICA

VISIT THE CLINICS ONLINE!
Access your subscription at:
www.theclinics.com

Clinical Management and Rehabilitation of Post-COVID-19 Sequalae

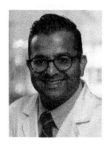

Blessen C. Eapen, MD
Consulting Editor

The COVID-19 global pandemic is caused by an infectious agent transmitted by the highly contagious severe acute respiratory corona virus 2 (SARS-CoV-2) and has infected over 700 million people worldwide and over 100 million individuals in the United States.

The COVID-19 infection can present with a variety of symptoms, with the most reported symptoms being fatigue, fever, cough, shortness of breath, and symptoms exacerbated by mental and physical exertion. In addition, the COVID-19 infection can also affect multiple organ systems and present with an array of symptoms, such as, neurologic symptoms (eg, concentrating, headaches, insomnia, taste changes), cardiac (eg, tachycardia, chest pain), gastrointestinal issues, vascular, mental health (eg, depression, anxiety), and pain (eg, joint pain, musculoskeletal pain, neuropathic pain). While most cases of COVID-19 infection are typically mild and recover within the first several weeks, there are some cases that may present with severe illness, requiring acute hospitalization and subsequent inpatient acute rehabilitation.

In addition, there is a subset of individuals that may continue to have symptoms beyond the typical recovery period and can experience long-lasting effects of their infection, which is commonly referred to as Long-Covid or Post-Covid Condition. While there are currently no comprehensive clinical practice guidelines for the rehabilitation management of this evolving disease process, we lean heavily on our previous experiences, as we continue to grow and refine our treatment paradigms, to meet the needs of this unique population. The current mainstay of treatment includes a physiatrist-led, multidisciplinary team approach to the improving physical, cognitive, emotional, and overall well-being of individuals with Long-Covid.

We hope this timely special issue provides guidance on the management of post-COVID-19 sequalae and provides insight into current rehabilitation programming, while highlighting the health care disparities related to the COVID-19 pandemic. We want to

Phys Med Rehabil Clin N Am 34 (2023) xiii–xiv
https://doi.org/10.1016/j.pmr.2023.04.009
1047-9651/23/© 2023 Published by Elsevier Inc.

pmr.theclinics.com

thank Dr Monica Verduzco-Gutierrez and colleagues for leading this special issue and for sharing their valuable experience and expertise with the physical medicine and rehabilitation community!

Blessen C. Eapen, MD
Physical Medicine and Rehabiltion Service
VA Greater Los Angeles Healthcare System
Divsion of Physical Medicine and Rehabilitation
David Geffen School of Medicine at UCLA
11301 Wilshire Boulevard
Los Angeles, CA 90073, USA

E-mail address:
blessen.Eapen2@va.gov

Preface

Sequelae of COVID-19 and the Need for Post-COVID Rehabilitation

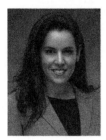

Monica Verduzco-Gutierrez, MD
Editor

The COVID-19 pandemic is defining for our generation. The pandemic has had an unprecedented impact on every aspect of our lives. It not only has affected patients, particularly those from marginalized communities, highlighting health care disparities, but also has had long-lasting effects on the health care workforce for generations to come.

One area that has emerged as a significant concern is the growing number of persons who are acquiring new disabilities, and therefore, there is a need for care from a multidisciplinary team, inclusive of Physical Medicine and Rehabilitation specialists, to address those needs throughout the health care continuum.

This issue of *Physical Medicine and Rehabilitation Clinics of North America* explores the various ways in which the pandemic has led to the emergence of new disabilities and how these challenges have been addressed by physical medicine and rehabilitation specialists and their colleagues via post-COVID rehabilitation. We address the impacts of SARS-CoV-2 infection on a person's health in this issue of *Physical Medicine and Rehabilitation Clinics of North America*. These impacts range from acute tissue damage and critical illness polyneuromyopathy in hospitalized patients to the development of long COVID or postacute sequelae of SARS-CoV-2 (PASC) in individuals with mild disease. The pandemic also disrupted health care services and rehabilitation programs, often making it more difficult for patients to access health care, and this will be addressed as well. The pandemic also showed us the need for prehabilitation services, and this is also discussed.

A comprehensive understanding of the impact of COVID-19 on individuals who are acquiring new disabilities and have a need for post-COVID rehabilitation is provided by a series of expert authors who have delivered quality care on the front lines, in clinics,

Phys Med Rehabil Clin N Am 34 (2023) xv–xvi
https://doi.org/10.1016/j.pmr.2023.03.001
1047-9651/23/© 2023 Published by Elsevier Inc.

pmr.theclinics.com

and in rehabilitation centers. Long COVID, thought to impact 10% to 20% of those who had COVID-19, will be the defining illness of our generation. This series offers guidance and recommendations for health care professionals to care for persons who may have new challenges and disabilities due to PASC, and ensure the patients have the necessary support and resources to adapt and thrive.

Monica Verduzco-Gutierrez, MD
Department of Rehabilitation Medicine
Joe R. and Teresa Lozano Long School of Medicine
University of Texas Health Science Center at San Antonio
7703 Floyd Curl Drive, Mail Code 7798
San Antonio, TX 78229, USA

E-mail address:
Gutierrezm19@uthscsa.edu

Post-COVID Conditions and Burden of Disease

Laura Tabacof, MD[a],*, Eric Nicolau, DO, MS[b], Andrew Rivera, MS[c], David Putrino, PhD[a]

KEYWORDS

• Long COVID • Post COVID condition • Disability • Burden of disease

KEY POINTS

- Post-COVID Condition describes a multi-systemic illness that affects multiple organs and encompasses dysautonomia, ME/CFS and other vascular and neurological conditions.
- PCC is estimated to affect 10-20% of COVID-19 survivors, with long-lasting and debilitating effects on function, employment, and quality of life.
- At present, diagnostic and treatment options for PCC still need further validation.
- Recognizing PCC as an entity and quantifying its functional impacts is pivotal to accurately quantify burden of disease, and guide social, economic, and public health strategies.

WHAT ARE POST-COVID CONDITIONS
Epidemiology

As of March 2023, over 761 million confirmed cases of coronavirus disease 2019 (COVID-19) have been confirmed worldwide, leading to more than 6.8 million deaths.[1] Although most epidemiologic reports have focused on the number of severe acute respiratory syndrome coronavirus 2 (SARS-CoV-2) infections, hospitalizations, and deaths, the number of COVID-19 individuals suffering persistent, long-lasting symptoms has been rapidly growing.

In October 2021, the World Health Organization (WHO) released a clinical case definition for the post-COVID condition (PCC) as the continuation or development of new symptoms 3 months after the initial SARS-CoV-2 infection, with symptoms lasting for at least 2 months and not explained by an alternative diagnosis.[2] PCC is the term used by the WHO, and it is interchangeable with long COVID or long-haul COVID (the patient-derived term) and post-acute sequelae of COVID-19 (or PASC, term used by the Center for Disease Control [CDC]).

[a] Department of Rehabilitation and Human Performance, Icahn School of Medicine at Mount Sinai, 5 East 98th Street SB-18, 10029, New York, NY, USA; [b] West Virginia School of Osteopathic Medicine, 5718 Merrywing Circle, Austin, TX 78730, USA; [c] Tulane University School of Medicine, 1430 Tulane Avenue, New Orleans, LA 70130, USA
* Corresponding author.
E-mail address: laura.tabacof@mountsinai.org

Phys Med Rehabil Clin N Am 34 (2023) 499–511
https://doi.org/10.1016/j.pmr.2023.04.007
1047-9651/23/© 2023 Elsevier Inc. All rights reserved.
pmr.theclinics.com

PCC affects individuals of all ages and acute disease severity levels, though it is most diagnosed in individuals between the ages of 36 and 50 years who had mild acute SARS-CoV-2 infections. Overall, the incidence is estimated at 10% to 30% of non-hospitalized cases, 50% to 70% of hospitalized cases, and 10% to 12% of vaccinated cases.[3] Around 16 million working-age Americans are currently living with PCC. Of those, 2 to 4 million are out of work due to PCC-related disability.[4]

Clinical Presentation

The breadth of impact COVID-19 has on the body was not initially recognized, and as PCC becomes more prevalent, it is increasingly evident that the clinical presentation can vary significantly, affecting virtually any organ system. Although common symptoms of PCC can include fatigue, shortness of breath, and cognitive dysfunction, over 200 different symptoms have been reported that can have an impact on everyday functioning.[3,5] Symptoms and impairments might present as either clusters or isolated symptoms, limiting daily activities and restricting social participation, and may be present for prolonged time frames and/or relapse over time.

Cardiovascular and pulmonary symptoms are common in PCC, which can significantly impact quality of life.[6,7] Chest pain and palpitations are frequently cited despite no prior history of cardiovascular disease or comorbidities.[7,8] There have also been findings of right ventricular dysfunction, acute myocardial infarction, and stroke.[9] Pulmonary symptoms vary, although chronic cough and dyspnea are most common.[10] The severity of lung disease and abnormalities in pulmonary function may depend on the severity of the acute COVID-19 episode. Individuals who initially had mild COVID-19 are less likely to have post-acute pulmonary function or imaging abnormalities,[11,12] whereas more severe initial infections have demonstrated evidence of lung injury on testing. However, shortness of breath and breathing discomfort are still common in patients with initial mild acute COVID-19 and should be evaluated closely.

Post-exertional malaise (PEM) is commonly reported by patients with PCC. PEM is the worsening of symptoms after physical exertion that would not have caused a problem before an illness. It is also a hallmark feature of another post-acute infectious syndrome known as myalgic encephalomyelitis/chronic fatigue syndrome (ME/CFS).[13] Studies have found that approximately 50% of patients with PCC meet criteria for ME/CFS.[14] Identifying PEM or ME/CFS in patients with PCC is of clinical importance to provide appropriate treatment (eg, physical therapy and exercise recommendations may vary). A better understanding of the relationship between PEM and ME/CFS in PCC patients is crucial to improving patient care.

Autonomic dysfunction (AD, or dysautonomia) is a term that broadly refers to symptoms and conditions that result from abnormal functioning of processes regulated by the autonomic nervous system. As such, it also considered a category of conditions including postural orthostatic tachycardia syndrome, neurocardiogenic syncope (also known as vasovagal syncope), orthostatic hypotension, inappropriate sinus tachycardia, among others.[15] Patients with PCC frequently report AD symptoms with orthostatic intolerance being the most common.[6,13,16] Of note, approximately 66% of individuals with mild COVID-19, who did not require hospitalization, reported experiencing moderate-to-severe symptoms of AD.[17,18] The prevalence of AD in PCC highlights the need for further research that seeks to understand the relationship of PCC and the autonomic nervous system and the underlying pathophysiology.

Pathobiological Causes/Hypotheses

Currently, the primary disease hypotheses for the pathogenesis of PCC include viral persistence (infectious virus or viral components, ie, RNA or proteins), autoimmunity triggered by viral infection, reactivation of latent viruses (i.e., herpes and Epstein-Barr virus), and inflammation-triggered alterations causing injury or dysfunction of tissues and organs.[19] Individuals with PCC have exhibited various pathologic changes, such as the development of microclots and platelet activation, reduced cortisol levels, and mitochondrial dysfunction.[20–22]

Another proposed mechanism suggests that due to its strong affinity for the human angiotensin-converting enzyme 2 receptor, SARS-CoV-2 might directly infect the nervous system, as this receptor is also present in neuronal and glial cells. Neuroradiologic imaging studies have found that more than 66% of patients with PCC exhibit neuronal hypometabolism on cerebral PET.[23] Areas of involvement include the bilateral orbital gyrus (including olfactory gyrus), right parahippocampal gyrus, right temporal lobe (including the amygdala, hippocampus, and thalamus), bilateral cerebellum, and bilateral pons/medulla brainstem.[24–26] No imaging findings are specific for PCC, and there is significant overlap with other neurologic illnesses.

The search for biomarkers of PCC has provided insight into possible mechanisms involved in the disease. Studies have shown that patients with nonspecific symptoms of PCC may have increased levels of circulating SARS-CoV-2 spike protein[27] to upregulated cytokines/chemokines and acute phase proteins, such as elevated interleukin 6, C-reactive protein, and tumor necrosis factor α.[28] Those with neurologic symptoms may have higher levels of neurofilament light chain and glial fibrillary acidic protein, while those with pulmonary symptoms may have elevated transforming growth factor β. The significant presence of fibrin amyloid microclots and platelet hyperactivation have also led some researchers to postulate that cellular hypoxia could be a key component to PCC.[20] It is important to note that while individual biomarkers lack specificity for a PCC diagnosis, certain patterns of biomarkers may be associated with PCC-specific symptoms. The current findings set the stage for future research on biological assays that could help define distinct types of PCC, which can help in selecting appropriate therapeutic approaches.

Patient-Reported Outcomes

Although clinical reporting and past medical history are sufficient to confirm a diagnosis, patient-reported outcomes (PROs) are instrumental to quantify symptom range and severity, as well as to provide meaningful information pertaining to the burden of disease (BD) and disability. Combined with biomedical research, these data inform disease mechanisms and phenotypes, which can ultimately inform resource allocation, inform policymakers, and improve delivery of care.

Examples of well-validated PROs commonly used in PCC include the EuroQOL EQ-5D-5 L,[29] the Fatigue Severity Scale,[30] Patient Health Questionnaires,[31] the COMPASS-31,[32] as well as PROMIS and NeuroQOL[33] instruments. Analysis of PRO results in individuals with PCC has confirmed prolonged multisystem effects (mainly debilitating fatigue, cognitive dysfunction, and PEM), regardless of hospitalization status, with significant disability, and alarming effects on ability to work.[5,6,34]

Unfortunately, different countries and institutions use different sets of PROs, which ultimately limits our ability to combine findings for more robust clinical conclusions. Another limitation regarding the use of PRO in PCC is the fact that these instruments have been validated in different populations but not specifically PCC. Therefore, to increase specificity, PCC-specific PROs have been developed including the COVID-19 Yorkshire Rehabilitation Scale, the Post-COVID-19 Functional Status scale,[35] and the Symptom Burden Questionnaire for Long COVID.[36]

Current Treatments

Treating the complex symptomatology of PCC can present a considerable challenge. The American Academy of Physical Medicine and Rehabilitation[37] (AAPM&R) provides clinical guidelines for assessment and management of specific PCC-related issues such as AD, fatigue, cognitive symptoms, and cardiovascular and pulmonary symptoms.[38] It is important to note that if specific etiologies of PCC-related symptoms are identified, they should be addressed appropriately.

The decision to utilize pharmaceuticals is usually made on a case-by-case basis with careful consideration of patient comorbidities, adherence to guidelines, out-of-pocket cost, possible risks and side effects, and correspondence with patient's providers. In general, treatments address the most disabling symptoms that the patient is experiencing. Patients with breathing discomfort might be given inhaled therapies as a trial of treatment, including short-acting beta-agonists and inhaled corticosteroids. However, these therapies do not always improve symptoms or pulmonary function and may have side effects, and their use should be guided by objective assessment. For pain, analgesics such as acetaminophen and nonsteroidal anti-inflammatory drugs are often used.[6] Beta blockers, such as propranolol or atenolol, are helpful in the management of postural or resting tachycardia in the absence of significant orthostatic hypotension. Midodrine or fludrocortisone may be considered for patients with significant orthostatic intolerance accompanied by low blood pressure, while pyridostigmine may be utilized for orthostatic intolerance in the setting of normal or elevated blood pressure.

Non-pharmaceutical strategies that focus on inflammatory and immunologic processes show promise in reducing PCC symptoms. One emerging therapy is noninvasive transcutaneous auricular vagus nerve stimulation (tVNS), which indirectly targets inflammatory pathways by regulating the hypersympathetic state in PCC-related dysautonomia. Animal models have validated the anti-inflammatory effects of vagal stimulation.[39,40] Recently, handheld tVNS devices that can be self-administered have been developed for human use. In an early double-blind study, a specific set of PCC symptoms, including anxiety, depression, vertigo, anosmia, ageusia, headaches, fatigue, irritability, and brain fog, were monitored. The study results indicated that tVNS might provide mild to moderate improvement in mental fatigue, without causing bradycardia or any serious adverse events.[41] However, it should be noted that the study had a small sample size (n = 12), and participants endorsed a heterogeneity of PCC symptoms. Pilot randomized controlled trials investigating the efficacy of tVNS for PCC-related dysautonomia are currently underway.[42]

Other approaches, such as acupuncture[43] and osteopathic manipulative treatment (OMT),[44] may serve as safe and synergistic interventions to complement the treatment of PCC. For example, craniosacral and ligamentous articular strain are types of OMT that may improve symptoms of AD by normalizing autonomic function. Although promising, most of the current research on non-pharmaceutical therapies consists of small-scale pilot studies, and further further research is needed to determine the extent of their efficacy in treating PCC.

As a complex multisystemic disease, effective management often requires a comprehensive and coordinated effort by a multidisciplinary rehabilitation team, as recommended by the National Institute for Health and Care Excellence[45] and the AAPM&R.[37] For individuals experiencing chronic symptoms and functional limitations, an accurate assessment of physical and cognitive impairments, pain, mood disorders, and performance in activities of daily living should be conducted. Furthermore, the

WHO has released guidelines for the rehabilitation of patients recovering from COVID-19.[46]

1. In hospitalized patients, during the acute phase of illness, rehabilitation professionals may provide interventions that relieve respiratory distress, prevent complications, and support communication.
2. Prior to hospital discharge, patients with COVID-19 should be screened for rehabilitation needs to facilitate onward referral.
3. Patients with COVID-19, should be provided with education and support for the self-management of breathlessness and resumption of activities, both in a hospitalized and a non-hospitalized setting caring for COVID-19.
4. For patients who have been discharged from the hospital or patients who have been managed at home and experience persistent symptoms and/or limitations in functioning; screen for physical, cognitive, and mental impairments; and manage accordingly.
5. Provide individualized rehabilitation programs from subacute to long term according to patient needs. The prescription and provision of rehabilitation programs should be guided by persistent symptoms (especially the presence and severity of post-exertional symptom exacerbation) and functional limitations.

Rehabilitation outcomes for PCC is limited although emerging data have been encouraging. For example, patients with functional impairments with pulmonary symptoms have notable functional improvement and relief from respiratory symptoms following outpatient resistance and strength training programs. [28,47,48] However, owing to the prominence of PEM in a majority of patients with PCC, such pulmonary rehabilitation programs are not always appropriate and may run the risk of significantly worsening symptoms.[49] This underpins a critical need to properly evaluate all PCC patients for PEM prior to initiating care and approach rehabilitation with significant caution, as advancing therapies too quickly or with excessive intensity may worsen symptoms. Although evidence on specific rehabilitation interventions is still limited,[50] further research is necessary to investigate the effectiveness of rehabilitation protocols, particularly for patients who may have limited access to care. Developing inclusive and equitable guidelines for the assessment and management for patients with PCC is imperative.

BURDEN OF DISEASE
What Is Burden of Disease?

Understanding the diseases that pose the greatest threats to health and well-being is essential for public health practitioners and policymakers. Such knowledge helps to allocate limited resources effectively for maximum benefit for all. It leads to interventions and services to prevent disease, control its spread, improve outcomes, and reduce health disparities. To evaluate the health of a population, mortality can be used, but this approach fails to consider the suffering caused by diseases to those who live with them. To gain a comprehensive view, it may be appropriate to evaluate health outcomes based on both the morbidity and mortality rates of prevalent diseases. The term BD (or disease burden) refers to the impact that disease, including its health, social, and economic consequences has on a population. BD can be conceptualized as the disparity between an ideal scenario in which everyone is free of disease and disability, and the current cumulative health status.[51]

Commonly used metrics of BD are *disability-adjusted life years* (DALYs) and *quality-adjusted life years* (QALYs). One DALY represents 1 year of healthy life lost due to *premature death* or *disease* or *disability*. The practice of interpreting BD via DALYs is particularly helpful when analyzing how certain diseases can differentially impact populations across geographic regions, ages, and other variables. For global insight on BD, the Institute of Health Metrics and Evaluation and the 'Disease Burden Unit' at the WHO publish the 'Global BD' study, producing extensive data on the BD using DALYs. QALYs, another metric, is similar but accounts for quality of life during the years lived with a disease.[52,53] Epidemiologists and public health officials regularly estimate and monitor BD through data mining prospective clinical studies, retrospective research of electronic health records, case reports, and patient surveys. The outcome of BD research has been instrumental to the implementation of public health interventions and policies that have saved countless lives, improving health and quality of life worldwide.

The Burden of Post-COVID Condition

PCC poses a significant burden of symptomatology impacting physical function, quality of life, and well-being. An estimated 96 million people worldwide have reported symptoms of PCC with fatigue, dyspnea, and exercise intolerance consistently noted.[54,55] While measures of BD (ie, DALYs) due to PCC have not yet been published, research has suggested that PCC has a greater burden of long-term sequelae than influenza. The epidemiologic data of PCC not only implicate the threat of the condition on the ability to work, but overall quality of life.[5]

In addition to the physical toll of PCC, patients are facing significant financial burdens due to health care costs and the impact on their employment. Anywhere from 10% to 22% of individuals stop working within 6 to 8 months after SARS-CoV-2 infection.[7,54] In fact, of the 16 million working-age Americans who have PCC, 2 to 4 million are out of work as a result of the condition.[4] The estimated annual health care cost for PCC is $17,776 per person,[56] with many patients struggling to get medical coverage leading them to apply for disability insurance. The condition has affected their lives and livelihood: an analysis of people with PCC who filed workers' compensation claims in New York State between January 1, 2020 and March 31, 2022 found that 18% of them had still not returned to work more than a year after SARS-CoV-2 infection.[57] There is still a lack of information on the number of people who applied for disability insurance because of PCC, as well as the number of those who were either approved or denied coverage for this chronic condition. Additionally, individuals with PCC have a lower likelihood of having full time employment and a higher likelihood of being unemployed.[58,59] To address these challenges, it is crucial that patients with PCC receive adequate health care coverage for diagnosis and treatment. Further research is needed to better understand the full scope of the burden of PCC to further develop public health strategies focused on helping patients regain the ability to work and improve their overall function and quality of life.

Health Disparity Considerations

Included in the national call to action regarding PCC from Congress is ensuring that there is equitable access to care for all.[37] As such, we must recognize and address inequities in the U.S. health care system that result in diminished access to sustained quality care because of racial, ethnic, or socioeconomic factors.

During the first waves of the pandemic, access to polymerase chain reaction (PCR) and antigen tests was limited, and the results varied in accuracy. Unfortunately, owing to lack of confirmatory laboratory tests, understanding, and clinical guidance for PCC, patients have reported feeling dismissed and stigmatized by medical professionals leading to a lack of care and treatment options for such a disabling condition.[60] Interestingly, one study found a higher prevalence of reported health care stigma (external and internalized) in patients with a PCC diagnosis than in those without a diagnosis.[61] This finding highlights the unfortunate reality that individuals with medical conditions lacking clear pathobiological basis often face stigmatization from health care providers, such as the perception that the disease is psychosomatic. Historically, individuals who suffer from conditions such as ME/CFS and fibromyalgia have reported experiencing stigma, which could lead to difficulty navigating care for their illness.[62,63] Stigma related to PCC may be hindering public health by negatively impacting the mental health of patients and their willingness to engage with the health care system.

PCC and its burden disproportionately affect certain populations from racial and ethnic minority groups to people with preexisting disabilities. Racial and ethnic minority groups are at higher risk of PCC, with significantly higher adjusted odds of being diagnosed.[64] Black and Latino individuals have been found to be more likely to report PCC symptoms than White individuals, even after adjusting for factors such as age, sex, and comorbidities.[65] Access to medical care may also play a role, as individuals who report difficulty accessing care are more likely to experience PCC. People with disabilities are also at higher risk for PCC.[66,67] Addressing PCC requires consideration of how health disparities may be exacerbated for individuals at the intersection of multiple marginalized identities, such as race, ethnicity, and disability. Therefore, inclusive interdisciplinary interventions are critical for making progress.

FUTURE DIRECTIONS AND CONCLUSION
Future Directions

PCC has not received the same level of attention or resources from the governments, international organizations, pharmaceutical companies, and general population as the acute months of COVID-19 pandemic have.[68] Therefore, it is critical to provide quality data to adequately inform these entities to provide resources to mitigate the social, economic, and public health impact of PCC.

Research

The National Institutes of Health (NIH) has launched the Researching COVID to Enhance Recovery initiative, a collaborative effort that brings together patients, caregivers, clinicians, community leaders, and scientists from across the country to comprehensively understand, prevent, and treat PASC.[69] This ongoing initiative is aimed at addressing the multifaceted challenges posed by COVID-19. In addition, the CDC has allocated a significant $46 million toward researching the long-term effects of COVID-19.[70] Together, the NIH and CDC's combined efforts demonstrate a sustained commitment to combating the far-reaching impacts of this global health crisis.

Proposed Bills

The Comprehensive Access to Resources and Education for Long COVID Act (the CARE for Long COVID Act) was introduced to the Senate on March 02, 2022, to help address the social, economic, and public health impact of the PCC. In part, the bill is designed to identify health care strategies that help mitigate disparities in COVID-19 infection rates, hospitalizations, severity and length of symptoms, and outcomes, and to provide recommendations on ensuring equity in diagnosis and access to quality post-infectious treatments.[71] Although the bill was not enacted, its provisions have the potential to be implemented by being incorporated into a new bill in subsequent Congress sessions. As an important milestone, PCC was recognized as a disability under the Americans with Disabilities Act[72] (ADA—Section 504 and Section

1557) in July 2021. Unfortunately, because this has not been sufficiently reinforced, several individuals with PCC continue to face discrimination.

Telerehabilitation

Telerehabilitation has the potential of being a promising approach to care for patients with PCC. A systematic review investigated the effectiveness of telerehabilitation using six articles that provided information on 140 patients with persistent PCC. The review details the symptomology manifested, the assessment, the telerehabilitation intervention applied and monitoring. This review concludes that telerehabilitation exercise program and therapeutic patient education are proving to be good alternative treatment methods for patients with PCC; however, there still remains a need for more to provide more reliable data for future use.[73]

Employment

Employers have a legal obligation to provide effective accommodations for employees with PCC, which may qualify as a disability under the ADA. Examples of accommodations may include workplace flexibility, such as telework and flexible scheduling. Providing workplace flexibility can help all employees balance personal and workplace demands but can be especially beneficial to employees with PCC. Importantly, PCC has been identified as a contributing factor to the current and national labor shortage in the United States.[74] Thus, it is critical to implement new strategies to retain employees who are affected by PCC.

One study in the United Kingdom aimed to understand the factors that impacted workability of workers following COVID-19, to better guide sustainable workplace accommodations. An online survey was disseminated to workers. The respondents (n = 145) provided various suggestions such as improving line manager competencies which would include regular meetings, a shared return-to-work plan, managing peer expectations, improved access to health care and utility, improving occupational health, creating more COVID-centric sickness absence policies and normalizing COVID-19.[75]

SUMMARY

PCC is a complex and debilitating illness that affects multiple bodily systems, causes dysautonomia, and can present similarly to ME/CFS. In addition, it can lead to vascular and clotting abnormalities. This illness has already impacted millions of people worldwide, and unfortunately, the numbers continue to rise and therefore, a significant number of people with PCC will develop permanent disabilities if appropriate medical interventions are not taken. However, because of the varying symptomology and lack of diagnostic tests, many patients struggle to find a definitive diagnosis and as a result, are dismissed as a psychosomatic condition.[68] While diagnostic and treatment options remain under validation, there is a critical need to address the devastating implications of PCC. Accurately identifying PCC and PCC-related burden is instrumental to inform health care policy and drive public health care resource allocations.

Governments and health care systems must prioritize the establishment of comprehensive data systems that can accurately capture crucial information on the broader impacts of PCC, encompassing education, employment, disability, and health-related quality of life. This information will be invaluable in guiding health care policies, treatment, and prevention strategies. Furthermore, it is essential to conduct clinical trials to evaluate potential therapies that target underlying biological mechanisms such as viral persistence, neuroinflammation, thrombosis, and autoimmunity.

CLINICS CARE POINTS

- PCC or long COVID describes a multi-systemic illness that affects multiple organs and encompasses dysautonomia, ME/CFS, and other vascular and neurologic conditions.
- PCC can develop in patients regardless of age, baseline health status, or initial symptom severity.
- PCC is estimated to affect 10% to 20% of COVID-19 survivors, with long-lasting debilitating effects on function, employment, and quality of life.
- Main pathobiological etiologies hypothesized include viral persistence, neuroinflammation, auto-immunity, and blood clotting.
- At present, diagnostic and treatment options for PCC still need further validation. Although clinical trials are urgently needed to address underlying pathobiological causes, rehabilitation management is instrumental to mitigate the disabilities of PCC.
- Recognizing PCC as an entity and quantifying its functional impacts is pivotal to accurately quantify BD, and guide social, economic, and public health strategies.

DISCLOSURE

The authors have nothing to disclose.

REFERENCES

1. World Health Organization (WHO). Coronavirus (COVID-19) Dashboard. Published 2023. Available at: https://covid19.who.int/. Accessed March 28, 2023.
2. Soriano JB, Murthy S, Marshall JC, et al. A clinical case definition of post-COVID-19 condition by a Delphi consensus. Lancet Infect Dis 2022;22(4):e102–7.
3. Davis HE, McCorkell L, Vogel JM, et al. Long COVID: major findings, mechanisms and recommendations. Nat Rev Microbiol 2023. https://doi.org/10.1038/s41579-022-00846-2.
4. Bach K. New Data Shows Long Covid Is Keeping as Many as 4 Million People out of Work. Brookings.edu. Published 2022. Available at: https://www.brookings.edu/research/new-data-shows-long-covid-is-keeping-as-many-as-4-million-people-out-of-work/. Accessed March 28, 2023.
5. Tabacof L, Tosto-Mancuso J, Wood J, et al. Post-acute COVID-19 Syndrome Negatively Impacts Physical Function, Cognitive Function, Health-Related Quality of Life, and Participation. Am J Phys Med Rehabil 2022;101(1). Available at: https://journals.lww.com/ajpmr/Fulltext/2022/01000/Post_acute_COVID_19_Syndrome_Negatively_Impacts.8.aspx.
6. Davis HE, Assaf GS, McCorkell L, et al. Characterizing long COVID in an international cohort: 7 months of symptoms and their impact. EClinicalMedicine 2021;38:101019.
7. Nalbandian A, Sehgal K, Gupta A, et al. Post-acute COVID-19 syndrome. Nat Med 2021;27(4):601–15.
8. Puntmann VO, Carerj ML, Wieters I, et al. Outcomes of Cardiovascular Magnetic Resonance Imaging in Patients Recently Recovered From Coronavirus Disease 2019 (COVID-19). JAMA Cardiol 2020;5(11):1265–73.
9. Raman B, Bluemke DA, Lüscher TF, et al. Long COVID: post-acute sequelae of COVID-19 with a cardiovascular focus. Eur Heart J 2022;43(11):1157–72.

10. Maley JH, Alba GA, Barry JT, et al. Multi-disciplinary collaborative consensus guidance statement on the assessment and treatment of breathing discomfort and respiratory sequelae in patients with post-acute sequelae of SARS-CoV-2 infection (PASC). Pharm Manag PM R 2022;14(1):77–95.

11. Abdallah SJ, Voduc N, Corrales-Medina VF, et al. Symptoms, Pulmonary Function, and Functional Capacity Four Months after COVID-19. Ann Am Thorac Soc 2021;18(11):1912–7.

12. Beyond Myalgic Encephalomyelitis/Chronic Fatigue Syndrome: Redefining an Illness. Mil Med 2015. https://doi.org/10.17226/19012.

13. Radin JM, Quer G, Ramos E, et al. Assessment of Prolonged Physiological and Behavioral Changes Associated With COVID-19 Infection. JAMA Netw Open 2021;4(7):e2115959.

14. Wong TL, Weitzer DJ. Long COVID and Myalgic Encephalomyelitis/Chronic Fatigue Syndrome (ME/CFS)—A Systemic Review and Comparison of Clinical Presentation and Symptomatology. Medicina (Kaunas) 2021;57(5):418.

15. Dani M, Dirksen A, Taraborrelli P, et al. Autonomic dysfunction in "long COVID": rationale, physiology and management strategies. Clin Med 2021;21(1):e63–7.

16. Stute NL, Stickford JL, Province VM, et al. COVID-19 is getting on our nerves: sympathetic neural activity and haemodynamics in young adults recovering from SARS-CoV-2. J Physiol 2021;599(18):4269–85.

17. Larsen NW, Stiles LE, Shaik R, et al. Characterization of autonomic symptom burden in long COVID: A global survey of 2,314 adults. Front Neurol 2022;13: 1012668.

18. Sivan M, Taylor S. NICE guideline on long covid. BMJ 2020;371:m4938.

19. Iwasaki A, Putrino D. Why we need a deeper understanding of the pathophysiology of long COVID. Lancet Infect Dis 2023;23(4):393–5.

20. Pretorius E, Venter C, Laubscher GJ, et al. Prevalence of symptoms, comorbidities, fibrin amyloid microclots and platelet pathology in individuals with Long COVID/Post-Acute Sequelae of COVID-19 (PASC). Cardiovasc Diabetol 2022; 21(1):148.

21. Klein J, Wood J, Jaycox J, et al. Distinguishing features of Long COVID identified through immune profiling. medRxiv : the preprint server for health sciences 2022. https://doi.org/10.1101/2022.08.09.22278592.

22. Guntur VP, Nemkov T, de Boer E, et al. Signatures of Mitochondrial Dysfunction and Impaired Fatty Acid Metabolism in Plasma of Patients with Post-Acute Sequelae of COVID-19 (PASC). Metabolites 2022;12(11). https://doi.org/10.3390/metabo12111026.

23. Hosp JA, Dressing A, Blazhenets G, et al. Cognitive impairment and altered cerebral glucose metabolism in the subacute stage of COVID-19. Brain 2021; 144(4):1263–76.

24. Guedj E, Campion JY, Dudouet P, et al. 18)F-FDG brain PET hypometabolism in patients with long COVID. Eur J Nucl Med Mol Imag 2021;48(9):2823–33.

25. Sollini M, Morbelli S, Ciccarelli M, et al. Long COVID hallmarks on [18F]FDG-PET/CT: a case-control study. Eur J Nucl Med Mol Imag 2021;48(10):3187–97.

26. Verger A, Barthel H, Tolboom N, et al. 2-[(18)F]-FDG PET for imaging brain involvement in patients with long COVID: perspective of the EANM Neuroimaging Committee. Eur J Nucl Med Mol Imag 2022;49(11):3599–606.

27. Swank Z, Senussi Y, Manickas-Hill Z, et al. Persistent Circulating Severe Acute Respiratory Syndrome Coronavirus 2 Spike Is Associated With Post-acute Coronavirus Disease 2019 Sequelae. Clin Infect Dis 2023;76(3):e487–90.

28. Lai YJ, Liu SH, Manachevakul S, et al. Biomarkers in long COVID-19: A systematic review. Front Med 2023;10:1085988.
29. Balestroni G, Bertolotti G. [EuroQol-5D (EQ-5D): an instrument for measuring quality of life]. Monaldi Arch Chest Dis 2012;78(3):155–9.
30. Krupp LB, LaRocca NG, Muir-Nash J, et al. The fatigue severity scale. Application to patients with multiple sclerosis and systemic lupus erythematosus. Arch Neurol 1989;46(10):1121–3.
31. Arroll B, Goodyear-Smith F, Crengle S, et al. Validation of PHQ-2 and PHQ-9 to screen for major depression in the primary care population. Ann Fam Med 2010;8(4):348–53.
32. Sletten DM, Suarez GA, Low PA, et al. COMPASS 31: a refined and abbreviated Composite Autonomic Symptom Score. Mayo Clin Proc 2012;87(12):1196–201.
33. Cella D, Lai JS, Nowinski CJ, et al. Neuro-QOL: brief measures of health-related quality of life for clinical research in neurology. Neurology 2012;78(23):1860–7.
34. Johns T. The Sequential Evaluation Process. Published online February 23, 2009. Available at: https://www.ssa.gov/oidap/Documents/Social%20Security%20Administration.%20%20SSAs%20Sequential%20Evaluation.pdf. Accessed April 7, 2023.
35. Klok FA, Boon GJAM, Barco S, et al. The Post-COVID-19 Functional Status scale: a tool to measure functional status over time after COVID-19. Eur Respir J 2020; 56(1). https://doi.org/10.1183/13993003.01494-2020.
36. National Institute for Health Research. Symptom Burden QuestionnaireTM for Long COVID. Published 2023. Available at: https://www.birmingham.ac.uk/research/applied-health/research/symptom-burden-questionnaire/index.aspx. Accessed March 31, 2023.
37. The American Academy of Physical Medicine and Rehabilitation. PASC Consensus Guidance. Published 2022. Available at: https://www.aapmr.org/members-publications/covid-19/pasc-guidance. Accessed April 1, 2023.
38. The American Academy of Physical Medicine and Rehabilitation. March 18 News Release Regarding Long COVID. Published March 18, 2023. Available at: https://www.aapmr.org/docs/default-source/news-and-publications/covid/news-release-march-18-2021.pdf?sfvrsn=e028207c_3. Accessed April 1, 2023.
39. Deng J, Li H, Guo Y, et al. Transcutaneous vagus nerve stimulation attenuates autoantibody-mediated cardiovagal dysfunction and inflammation in a rabbit model of postural tachycardia syndrome. J Interv Card Electrophysiol 2023; 66(2):291–300.
40. Azabou E., Bao G., Bounab R., et al., Vagus Nerve Stimulation: A Potential Adjunct Therapy for COVID-19. Frontiers in Medicine. Published 2021. Available at: https://www.frontiersin.org/articles/10.3389/fmed.2021.625836. Accessed April 2, 2023.
41. Badran BW, Huffman SM, Dancy M, et al. A pilot randomized controlled trial of supervised, at-home, self-administered transcutaneous auricular vagus nerve stimulation (taVNS) to manage long COVID symptoms. Research square 2022. https://doi.org/10.21203/rs.3.rs-1716096/v1. rs.3.rs-1716096.
42. Tornero C, Pastor E, Garzando MDM, et al. Non-invasive Vagus Nerve Stimulation for COVID-19: Results From a Randomized Controlled Trial (SAVIOR I). Front Neurol 2022;13:820864.
43. Williams JE, Moramarco J. The Role of Acupuncture for Long COVID: Mechanisms and Models. Med Acupunct 2022;34(3):159–66.
44. Certain Curi AC, Antunes Ferreira AP, Calazans Nogueira LA, et al. Osteopathy and physiotherapy compared to physiotherapy alone on fatigue in long COVID:

Study protocol for a pragmatic randomized controlled superiority trial. Int J Osteopath Med 2022;44:22–8.

45. National Institute for Health and Care Excellence. COVID-19 Rapid Guideline: Managing the Long-Term Effects of COVID-19. 2020.

46. World Health Organization (WHO). Clinical Management of COVID-19: Living Guideline. Published September 15, 2022. Available at: https://apps.who.int/iris/handle/10665/362783. Accessed April 2, 2023.

47. Grosbois JM, Gephine S, Le Rouzic O, et al. Feasibility, safety and effectiveness of remote pulmonary rehabilitation during COVID-19 pandemic. Respir Med Res 2021;80:100846.

48. Gloeckl R, Leitl D, Jarosch I, et al. Benefits of pulmonary rehabilitation in COVID-19: a prospective observational cohort study. ERJ Open Res 2021;7(2): 00108–2021.

49. Blitshteyn S, Whiteson JH, Abramoff B, et al. Multi-disciplinary collaborative consensus guidance statement on the assessment and treatment of autonomic dysfunction in patients with post-acute sequelae of SARS-CoV-2 infection (PASC). Pharm Manag PM R 2022;14(10):1270–91.

50. Fugazzaro S, Contri A, Esseroukh O, et al. Rehabilitation Interventions for Post-Acute COVID-19 Syndrome: A Systematic Review. IJERPH 2022;19(9):5185.

51. Hessel F. Burden of DiseaseBurdenof disease(s). In: Kirch W, editor. Encyclopedia of public health. Springer Netherlands; 2008. p. 94–6.

52. Murray C.J.L., Lopez A.D., World Health Organization, World Bank, Harvard School of Public Health. The Global burden of disease: a comprehensive assessment of mortality and disability from diseases, injuries, and risk factors in 1990 and projected to 2020. Published 1996. Available at: https://apps.who.int/iris/handle/10665/41864. Accessed March 29, 2023.

53. Institute for Health Metrics and Evaluation. Global Burden of Disease Study. Published 2020. Available at: https://www.healthdata.org/gbd. Accessed March 24, 2023.

54. Office of National Statistics (ONS). Self-reported long COVID and labour market outcomes, UK: 2022. Self-reported long COVID and labour market outcomes, UK: 2022. Published December 5, 2022. Available at: https://www.ons.gov.uk/peoplepopulationandcommunity/healthandsocialcare/conditionsanddiseases/bulletins/selfreportedlongcovidandlabourmarketoutcomesuk2022/selfreportedlongcovidandlabourmarketoutcomesuk2022#main-points. Accessed April 7, 2023.

55. Global Burden of Disease Long COVID Collaborators. Estimated Global Proportions of Individuals With Persistent Fatigue, Cognitive, and Respiratory Symptom Clusters Following Symptomatic COVID-19 in 2020 and 2021. JAMA 2022; 328(16):1604–15.

56. COVID-19 Longhaulers & Their Families Call for the Immediate Formation of Long COVID Assistance Programs and a Long COVID Task Force.

57. NYSIF Releases Report on Long-Term Impacts of Covid-19. Published 2023. Available at: https://ww3.nysif.com/en/FooterPages/Column1/AboutNYSIF/NYSIF_News/2023/20230124LongCovid. Accessed April 1, 2023

58. Perlis RH, Lunz Trujillo K, Safarpour A, et al. Association of Post–COVID-19 Condition Symptoms and Employment Status. JAMA Netw Open 2023;6(2): e2256152.

59. National Center for Health Statistics. U.S. Census Bureau, Household Pulse Survey, 2022–2023, Long COVID. Available at: https://www.cdc.gov/nchs/covid19/pulse/long-covid.htm. Accessed April 2, 2023.

60. Au L, Capotescu C, Eyal G, et al. Long covid and medical gaslighting: Dismissal, delayed diagnosis, and deferred treatment. SSM Qual Res Health 2022;2: 100167.
61. Pantelic M, Ziauddeen N, Boyes M, et al. Long Covid stigma: Estimating burden and validating scale in a UK-based sample. PLoS One 2022;17(11):e0277317.
62. Froehlich L, Hattesohl DB, Cotler J, et al. Causal attributions and perceived stigma for myalgic encephalomyelitis/chronic fatigue syndrome. J Health Psychol 2022;27(10):2291–304.
63. Gustafsson M, Ekholm J, Ohman A. From shame to respect: musculoskeletal pain patients' experience of a rehabilitation programme, a qualitative study. J Rehabil Med 2004;36(3):97–103.
64. Khullar D, Zhang Y, Zang C, et al. Racial/Ethnic Disparities in Post-acute Sequelae of SARS-CoV-2 Infection in New York: an EHR-Based Cohort Study from the RECOVER Program. J Gen Intern Med 2023;1–10.
65. Magesh S, John D, Li WT, et al. Disparities in COVID-19 Outcomes by Race, Ethnicity, and Socioeconomic Status: A Systematic Review and Meta-analysis. JAMA Netw Open 2021;4(11):e2134147.
66. Zhang Y, Hu H, Fokaidis V, et al. Identifying environmental risk factors for post-acute sequelae of SARS-CoV-2 infection: An EHR-based cohort study from the recover program. Environmental Advances 2023;11:100352.
67. Burns A. Will Long COVID Exacerbate Existing Disparities in Health and Employment? KFF (Kaiser Family Foundation). Published 2023. Available at: https://www.kff.org/policy-watch/will-long-covid-exacerbate-existing-disparities-in-health-and-employment/. Accessed April 3, 2023.
68. The Lancet. Long COVID: 3 years in. Lancet 2023;401(10379):795.
69. Collins F. NIH Launches New Initiative to Study "Long COVID". Published 2021. Available at: https://www.nih.gov/about-nih/who-we-are/nih-director/statements/nih-launches-new-initiative-study-long-covid. Accessed April 2, 2023.
70. Saydah S. Understanding Long COVID: CDC Current Projects & Collaborations.
71. GovTrack. S. 3726 — 117th Congress: CARE for Long COVID Act. 2022. Available at: https://www.govtrack.us/congress/bills/117/s3726. Accessed April 1, 2023.
72. U.S. Department of Health & Human Services. Discrimination on the Basis of Disability. Published 2023. Available at: https://www.hhs.gov/civil-rights/for-individuals/disability/index.html. Accessed March 31, 2023.
73. Valverde-Martínez MÁ, López-Liria R, Martínez-Cal J, et al. A Viable Option in Patients with Persistent Post-COVID Syndrome: A Systematic Review. Healthcare 2023;11(2):187.
74. U.S. Department of Labor. Supporting Employees With Long Covid: A Guide for Employers. Published 2022. Available at: https://www.dol.gov/sites/dolgov/files/ODEP/topics/pdf/long-covid-report-v2-accessibilized.pdf. Accessed April 1, 2023.
75. Lunt J, Hemming S, Burton K, et al. What workers can tell us about post-COVID workability. Occup Med 2022. https://doi.org/10.1093/occmed/kqac086. kqac086.

Inpatient Rehabilitation Issues Related to COVID-19

Amanda A. Kelly, MD*, Caroline A. Lewis, MD[1],
Miguel X. Escalon, MD, MPH

KEYWORDS

- Rehabilitation • COVID-19 • Inpatient • PICS

KEY POINTS

- Patients who are hospitalized due to COVID-19 are likely to require acute inpatient rehabilitation.
- Multiple factors have posed challenges to inpatient rehabilitation during the COVID-19 pandemic.
- Studies have shown lower rates of transfer to acute care, higher rates of discharge home, and equal or more functional gains in survivors of COVID-19 following acute rehabilitation.

INTRODUCTION

Patients hospitalized due to COVID-19 can develop neurologic, neuromuscular, cardiovascular, pulmonary, musculoskeletal, cognitive, and psychiatric impairments that predispose them to require acute inpatient rehabilitation. Preliminary studies have shown that up to 50% of patients diagnosed with COVID-19, developed neurologic pathologies including stroke, disorders of consciousness, encephalopathy, and polyneuropathy. Amputations of digits and/or limbs, dysphagia, pressure injuries, and dysautonomia were also observed in this population.[1] Additionally, containment measures imposed on patients with COVID-19 to reduce the spread of the virus lead to severe limitations in mobility. As a result, immobilization syndrome was observed in patients even with mild COVID-19 symptoms such as fever, fatigue, and muscle pain.[2]

Patients who require prolonged stay in an intensive care unit (ICU) due to acute respiratory distress syndrome (ARDS), are at risk of ICU acquired (ICUAW) resulting in functional impairment. One study showed that patients with ICUAW had increased mortality and significantly decreased strength, function, and quality of life up to 5 years later.[1] Approximately 50% of patients with ICUAW were unable to return to work 1 year

---

Department of Rehabilitation and Human Performance, Icahn School of Medicine at Mount Sinai (Mount Sinai), One Gustave L Levy Place, Box 1240B, New York, NY 10029, USA
[1] Present address: 1677 Lexington Avenue, Apartment 6A, New York, NY 10029.
* Corresponding author. One Gustave L Levy Place, Box 1240B, New York, NY 10029
E-mail address: DrAmandaAKelly@gmail.com

Phys Med Rehabil Clin N Am 34 (2023) 513–522
https://doi.org/10.1016/j.pmr.2023.04.001
1047-9651/23/© 2023 Elsevier Inc. All rights reserved.
pmr.theclinics.com

after hospital discharge due to functional deficits.[1] Although data on long-term outcomes of survivors of severe COVID-19 are not currently available, it is clear that many persons suffering from COVID-19 have had prolonged ICU lengths of stay with ARDS, and any person in that situation is at high risk of ICUAW and its long-term deleterious effects.

One of the unique challenges for ICU survivors from severe COVID-19 acute respiratory distress syndrome (CARDS) versus patients with ARDS is the need for higher amounts of analgesics and sedation while on mechanical ventilation.[3] This is thought, in part, to be due to the need for deeper sedation to avoid patient–ventilator dyssynchrony in the setting of high respiratory drive, as well as to avoid self-inflicted lung injury.[3] One study evaluated the effects of early rehabilitation and weaning from mechanical ventilation in patients with CARDS, and its results showed significant improvement in physical and mental recovery, with functionality and frailty scores comparable to pre-ICU admission.[4] These data suggest that early ICU respiratory rehabilitation in CARDS patients could prevent post-intensive care syndrome (PICS), and improve the 1-year outcome of survivors.[4] This is in line with studies of other ICU populations showing that early and continued rehabilitation is crucial to functional outcomes and independence.[5–7]

Despite the higher medical acuity and complications of many patients with COVID-19, studies have shown significant improvements in functionality and better ability to perform activities of daily living (ADLs) following acute rehabilitation.[2] Although multiple factors posed and continue to pose challenges to inpatient rehabilitation for survivors of COVID-19, rehabilitation plays a key role for this patient population.

DEMOGRAPHICS

The leading comorbidities in patients with COVID-19 include hypertension (55%), coronary artery disease and stroke (32%), and diabetes (31%).[8] In a case series involving patients admitted with COVID-19 to New York hospitals, 6% were discharged to facilities, such as skilled nursing facilities, other than their homes.[9] Studies suggest that men 50 to 70 years of age have a higher prevalence of severe COVID-19 infection.[1]

A study comparing the demographics between patients that were COVID-19 positive (those who tested positive within 3 months of admission to rehabilitation) and COVID-19 negative admitted to a rehabilitation facility noted that patients with COVID-19 were younger (mean age 59.4 years vs 62.9 years; $P = .04$) and had a higher mean body mass index (BMI) (32 vs 28; $P < .01$).[10] Another study analyzing persons with COVID-19 admitted to acute inpatient rehabilitation facilities in New Jersey and New York reported that patients were mostly men and White (41%), with an average age of 61.9 years. Most of these institutions admitted significantly younger patients during the height of the pandemic (May and June 2020) compared to pre-pandemic times. The average length of acute hospital stay was 24.5 days and the mean length of stay in acute inpatient rehabilitation was 15.2 days.[1]

Additionally, a retrospective cohort study involving 132 academic medical centers found that adults hospitalized with COVID-19 discharged to inpatient rehabilitation facilities were more likely to have received intensive care and mechanical ventilation while hospitalized ($P < .001$), be more medically complex, and have longer lengths of stay ($P < .0001$). Even so, those discharged to inpatient rehabilitation facilities showed 1.4 times lower odds of readmission within 30 days of hospital discharge compared to those discharged to skilled nursing facilities.[11]

COMMON PRESENTATIONS

There are several ICU-associated sequelae seen in survivors of COVID-19 after a prolonged stay and immobilization in the ICU. One study showed that 4% to 11% of all patients with COVID-19 required admission to the ICU, with the most severely ill of those patients developing ARDS.[12] In another study, 14% of patients hospitalized with COVID-19 were treated in the ICU and 12% required mechanical ventilation.[9]

In a study, 46% of patients who were admitted to the ICU with ARDS due to any underlying diagnosis presented with critical illness polyneuropathy (CIP), which is a mixed sensorimotor neuropathy that results in axonal degeneration.[12,13] Patients with CIP can have significant functional limitations. It can present with generalized, symmetric weakness affecting the distal more than proximal extremities, as well as distal sensory loss, atrophy, and decreased/absent deep tendon reflexes. It can also result in diaphragmatic weakness resulting in difficulty weaning from mechanical ventilation.[13] Another ICU-related condition that has been seen in patients with COVID-19 is critical illness myopathy (CIM), which is a diffuse myopathy associated with fatty degeneration, fiber atrophy, and fibrosis, and is associated with exposure to corticosteroids, paralytics, and sepsis.[13] CIM presents similarly to CIP, however, CIM typically results in more proximal than distal weakness and sensory preservation and has a quicker recovery. Similar to CIP, CIM can result in poor endurance that may persist for up to 2 years or longer.[13] The decreased strength, sensation, and endurance associated with ICU sequelae result in functional impairments necessitating inpatient physical rehabilitation to promote functional recovery and independence.

Additionally, PICS is commonly seen after COVID-19 infection. PICS is a collection of symptoms that persist once a patient leaves the ICU. It is characterized by the possession of any impairment in the physical, psychiatric, or cognitive domains due to a critical illness. In patients with a critical illness related to COVID-19 infection requiring an ICU stay of 7 days or more, 91% fit the diagnostic criteria for PICS with 87%, 48%, and 8% of patients having impairments in the physical, psychiatric, and/or cognitive domains, respectively.[14] Psychiatric conditions affecting survivors of ARDS due to any cause include anxiety (38%), depression (32%), and PTSD (23%), with 52% having prolonged psychiatric morbidity in one of the three areas with a mean total duration of 33 to 39 months in one study.[15] PICS is associated with decreased pulmonary function, decreased inspiratory muscle strength, decreased range of motion, strength, and endurance.[13] Other ICU-related presentations include entrapment neuropathies related to prone positioning with the majority affecting peripheral nerves of the upper limb. The most common presentations include hyposthenia, hypoesthesia, and paresthesia along the affected nerve distributions.[16] The most frequent injury sites include the ulnar nerve, radial nerve, sciatic nerve, brachial plexus, and median nerve.[17]

Furthermore, many patients with COVID-19 also present with malnutrition due to a hyper-catabolic state. The prevalence of malnutrition is greater than 50% in severe COVID-19 infections. In one study involving 37 patients admitted to a rehabilitation facility following admission to reanimation or intensive care units for COVID-19, 81% of patients presented with severe malnutrition and 11% presented with moderate malnutrition. This study also showed that malnutrition had a significantly negative correlation with functional independence (P <.05).[18] Malnutrition can also lead to weight loss, and when it is observed to be $\geq$ 5% with noted functional impairment and metabolic derangement, cachexia in patients with COVID-19 can be diagnosed. In a study that evaluated weight loss and cachexia in patients with COVID-19, the frequency of cachexia was revealed to be 37%. Contributing factors to body wasting associated with COVID-19 are thought to include loss of appetite, loss of taste and smell, fever, immobilization, general malnutrition, catabolic–anabolic imbalance, and endocrine, cardiac, and renal dysfunction related to COVID-19 complications.[19]

Many patients also present with tachypnea, oxygen desaturation with exertion, and tachycardia, which can make mobilization difficult.[1] Additionally, patients may exhibit other cardiovascular, autonomic, pulmonary, neurologic, cognitive, immunologic sequelae, and post-exertional fatigue, which will be further described in more detail in subsequent articles.

Lastly, patients with COVID-19, particularly those with prolonged stays in the ICU, are susceptible to pressure injuries given inactivity, use of artificial airways, and prone positioning. Pressure injuries must be closely monitored and treated as they cause 60,000 deaths annually in the United States. One study in Iran involving pressure injuries in patients with COVID-19 with a Braden score of less than 14 admitted to the ICU, showed an incidence ratio of 47% and prevalence of 80%.[20] A United Kingdom retrospective study involving patients admitted to the ICU with COVID-19 showed that the incidence of developing a pressure injury was 76%, and that 71% of patients were put in prone positioning for ARDS; 88% of anterior surface ulcers were located on the head and neck, with the remaining percentage on the genitalia, fingers, and anterior torso. The most common site for pressure injuries was oral commissures (35%) related to endotracheal tube placement. Other facial pressure injuries included the nose (12%), central lip (9%), ear (7%), cheek (5%), and periorbital area (3%).[21]

Patients with COVID-19 are predisposed to numerous complications and sequelae that lead to poor endurance, decreased strength, and severe functional limitations. Acute inpatient rehabilitation facilities have the ability to address these issues with multidisciplinary teams including physiatrists, therapists, neuropsychologists, nutritionists, and wound care teams. Despite the obstacles faced at the start of the pandemic and the unique functional demands of this patient population, rehabilitation facilities have become accustomed to treating the challenging conditions that patients with COVID-19 present with, which will better equip facilities in the event of similar circumstances.

ADMISSION CRITERIA

Discharge from acute care hospitals with admission to acute rehabilitation facilities was initially dependent on state and centers for disease control and prevention (CDC) guidelines, which were constantly changing at the start of the pandemic. Obtaining insurance authorization was a barrier to timely discharge to inpatient acute rehabilitation given that evaluations from several disciplines were required. During the pandemic, the centers for medicare & medicaid services (CMS) 1135 rule waiver declared a public health emergency and waived the normal insurance authorization process. This allowed for faster transfers from acute care hospitals to inpatient rehabilitation facilities, thus increasing bed availability and turnover.[1] Institutions developed their own set of admission criteria with consideration of factors such as the number of days since initial symptom onset, number of days since resolution of fever, negative COVID-19 testing, infection control clearance, and oxygen requirements.

Though facilities have their own unique admission criteria, it is reasonable to outline certain acceptance guidelines based on current practices.[1,10] A recommendation of admission criteria can include.

- Patients admitted to inpatient rehabilitation with a primary diagnosis unrelated to COVID-19 should test negative for COVID-19 within 72 hours of admission.
- Patients admitted to inpatient rehabilitation with a primary diagnosis related to COVID-19 should meet the following criteria:

- At least 7 days since initial symptom onset
- Afebrile for at least 3 days without the use of antipyretics
- Exhibit clinical improvement in symptoms
- Cleared by infection control at the acute care hospital before transfer
- Require less than or equal to 5 L of oxygen via nasal cannula or stable on current ventilatory settings if tracheostomy is in place

CHALLENGES TO INPATIENT REHAB

At the start of the pandemic, numerous inpatient rehabilitation facilities were temporarily closed to allow for reallocation of beds and staff to COVID-19 units.[22] Those that remained open were forced to address challenges specific to the pandemic. Utilization of physical space was adjusted to comply with constantly evolving social distancing and infection prevention guidelines, and some facilities needed to rapidly create new therapy gyms and units to treat patients on precautions.

There was also a considerable shift from frequent socialization of patients and staff to isolation when not in therapies as well as the use of personal protective equipment (PPE) to minimize the spread of infection.[1] Because staff and patients were required to wear PPE covering most of the face, and time spent face-to-face was limited to decrease infection risk, communication became more difficult and impersonal.[23]

Units were also faced with staffing shortages from sickness and reassignment to medical units. Physicians were deployed to acute care teams and physical and occupational therapists were reallocated to prone teams. To combat staffing shortages and limit unnecessary infectious exposure, CMS 1135 rule waiver temporarily lifted the normal therapy requirement of 15 hours per week of inpatient therapy for patients admitted to inpatient rehabilitation facilities and authorized the use of telehealth in place of traditional in-person therapies.[1]

One of the other challenges faced by acute inpatient rehabilitation facilities was the risk of COVID-19 outbreaks. One study focused on the impact a COVID-19 outbreak had within a 27-person neuromusculoskeletal rehabilitation unit, in which patients were exposed to an asymptomatic health care professional. Because patients who tested positive were transferred to isolation rooms, therapy mainly took place in the patient's rooms, and many were given instructions on self-training with smaller therapy devices. Furthermore, exposed patients on average received 2.5 therapy sessions/day and 81.9 therapy minutes/day during isolation compared to 3.5 sessions/day and 132.3 minutes/day before COVID-19 exposure. Ten of the affected patients (37%) required supplemental oxygen and two patients (7%) had to be transferred to the acute hospital secondary to respiratory failure, leading to one death. Overall, patients who were exposed to COVID-19 during inpatient rehabilitation received less frequent therapy, with less intensity, and limited resources with a significantly longer length of stay compared to non-COVID patients.[24]

The staff also experienced anxiety and uncertainty related to COVID-19 and burnout. They faced numerous obstacles including increased workload caused by staff shortages related to hospital outbreaks, fear of infection of oneself and loved ones in the setting of limited information regarding a novel disease, staying informed of frequently changing guidelines, shortages of PPE, caring for patients who can deteriorate quickly, and social isolation. The staff may have also felt culpable for preventing patients' family and friends from visiting the hospital setting. Health care workers who were exposed to and/or infected with COVID-19 were forced to quarantine and may have felt guilty about leaving the frontlines understaffed.[23]

Currently, challenges such as oxygen requirements, pressure injuries, and malnutrition continue to be prevalent in acute rehabilitation facilities for patients with COVID-19, especially those post-ICU. Close monitoring of oxygen saturations during therapy sessions is essential and the involvement of auxiliary teams such as wound care, nutrition, and neuropsychology for behavioral and social challenges continue to be utilized during the rehabilitation course for this population. To help address anxiety and burnout of staff at the start of the pandemic, facilities provided food, mental health services, and recharge/respite rooms which continue to be resources offered today. It is vital for institutions to continue to collaborate to discuss the challenges faced during the pandemic, share experiences, and introduce adaptations and solutions for providing rehabilitation services for patients with COVID-19.[1]

MULTIDISCIPLINARY SERVICES

Many team members were forced to adapt to new roles. Rehabilitation physicians needed to adjust to a new patient population with different symptoms. They were required to stay up to date on the latest COVID-19 presentations and treatment. Given the various COVID-19 sequelae affecting various body systems such as pulmonary, cardiovascular, cognitive, neurologic, psychiatric, musculoskeletal, etc. rehabilitation physicians needed to coordinate care between a larger variety of team members.

Physical and occupational therapists addressed significant weaknesses from CIM, CIP, vital sign derangements for autonomic dysfunction, limitations in positioning due to pressure injuries, and more limited interaction with family members and caregivers due to isolation guidelines. Speech therapists were essential in addressing swallowing deficits related to ventilator use, communication with speaking valves in patients with tracheostomies, and cognitive deficits related to COVID-19. Psychologists were important in treating anxiety, depression, adjustment disorder, and other psychiatric issues related to prolonged hospital stay and immobilization seen in patients with COVID-19. Respiratory therapists were essential in managing ventilatory status, and nutritionists were necessary for the management of malnutrition commonly seen in this patient population.

Nurses carefully monitored vital signs and respiratory status, played important roles in caring for pressure injuries, including pressure relief positioning for patients debilitated with significant weakness, and assisting in ADLs such as eating, bathing, and dressing. Recreational therapists were also useful in providing relaxing and entertaining activities during a time when patients often felt bored and isolated. Lastly, social workers were crucial in addressing discharge needs, often having to communicate with family members virtually, and keeping note of which home services remained available to patients during the pandemic.

DISCHARGE PLANNING

Planning for safe discharge proved to be difficult during the pandemic. Family training plays a significant role in arranging appropriate care, supervision, and support when patients are discharged home. However, during the height of the pandemic, most facilities instituted a "no visitor policy" to minimize infectious exposure. Instead, there was a reliance on telehealth for communication and education by physicians, therapists, social workers, and off-site family education. There was also a lack of resources, such as oxygen, which were necessary for discharge home. Family members of patients with prolonged lengths of stay were also more anxious about caring for their loved ones and were fearful for their own safety, necessitating education, counseling, and access to PPE. Numerous home health care agencies required negative COVID-

19 tests before allowing staff to enter patients' homes, further adding to caregiver anxiety and delaying discharge home.

Patients who were unable to be safely discharged home were recommended for subacute rehabilitation (SAR), however, family members were apprehensive given the high COVID-19 infection rates and mortality. This may have led to an increased length of stay.[1] A retrospective observational study using US Medicare claims and Minimum Data Set 3.0 compared skilled nursing facilities with at least one active COVID-19 case in 2020 to their pre-pandemic baselines and reported that mortality increased by about 2%. Furthermore, patients required assistance with an additional 0.36 ADLs, lost 3.1 pounds more weight, and were 4% more likely to have worsened symptoms of depression.[25] The regulation of SAR admission also served as another obstacle. For example, in New York, SARs were prohibited from accepting patients with COVID-19 and then instructed to refuse admissions simply based on patients' COVID-19 status.[1]

As COVID-19 guidelines continue to change, hospitals at this time have lifted the "no visitor policy," making it easier for family training to take place for safe discharge planning. There is also more abundance in resources such as oxygen and PPE, compared to during the height of the pandemic, making the transition home for survivors of COVID-19 smoother and less taxing for families. Additionally, the rollout of COVID-19 vaccines and boosters has provided families and caregivers with greater peace of mind at the time of discharge home for this patient population. As more family members return to work, however, there may be less help available at home at the time of discharge, leading to greater need for home attendants. Lastly, most SAR facilities still require a negative COVID test, which will likely continue to increase the length of stay for patients who are unable to be safely discharged home.

OUTCOMES

Studies showed that survivors of COVID-19 who underwent inpatient rehabilitation had great functional gains with home discharge rates that were similar to that of the pre-pandemic inpatient rehabilitation period and these persons had low complication rates. Some inpatient rehabilitation facilities had higher rates of patients discharged home during the pandemic compared to the prior period. Possible reasons include increased caregiver availability as family members were able to work from home, hesitancy of family members discharging loved ones to SAR, as well as SAR admission regulations, decreased amounts of physical assistance needed as compared to patients who suffered a brain or spinal cord injury, and different admission criteria.[1]

Furthermore, a study involving several acute rehabilitation facilities reported higher GG scores for mobility and self-care in patients with COVID-19, with each patient gaining two levels on functional and self-care outcomes. A GG score is a measure of functional status that replaced the Functional Independence Measure in inpatient rehabilitation facilities and is based on the US Centers for Medicare and Medicaid Services (CMS) mandated section GG Functional Abilities and Goals of the Improving Post-Acute Care Transformation Act, with a greater change in GG score indicating increased improvement in functional independence. In context, this gain is equivalent to improving from maximal assistance to supervision levels. This accomplishment increases the probability of patients discharging home and illustrates the significance of providing rehabilitation for patients with COVID-19.[1] Another study demonstrated that patients with COVID-19 had equivalent or increased improvements in functional ability measures in self-care (FA-SC), mobility (FA-Mob), functional change efficiency, length of stay, and rate of return to the community when compared to patients without

COVID-19.[10] This further shows that patients with COVID-19 who qualify for inpatient rehabilitation can benefit at least as much from inpatient rehabilitation as patients without COVID-19. With regard to hospital readmission rates, the overall acute care transfer rate across seven New York and New Jersey inpatient rehabilitation facilities was about 8% (27/320 patients) among patients with COVID-19, with the range of individual institution rates being 0% to 25%, overall lower compared to 17% from the Uniform Data System and 12% from the eRehabData during 2019 (pre-pandemic).[1] This suggests that acute inpatient rehabilitation provides a safe disposition option for survivors of COVID-19.

Most studies to date have discussed outcomes in these patients during earlier stages of the pandemic; however, there is a need for data on the current challenges, measures of mobility, length of stay, and return to community for patients with COVID-19. Despite the vast amount of complications and higher medical acuity of many patients with COVID-19, studies have shown the significant role acute rehabilitation has played during the pandemic for this population. These patients not only had higher rates of discharge home, but equal or more functional gains compared to patients without COVID-19, with a lower rate of transfer. It is essential to continue to encourage acute rehabilitation for survivors of COVID-19, to optimize the recovery, functionality, and safe discharge for this patient population.

CLINICS CARE POINTS

- Patients hospitalized due to COVID-19 are at risk of multisystem impairments that predispose them to require acute inpatient rehabilitation.
- Challenges to inpatient rehabilitation facilities during the pandemic included temporary closure, social distancing and isolation of patients, staffing shortages, anxiety and burnout, COVID-19 outbreaks, and adaptation of new roles by team members.
- Multidisciplinary teams in acute inpatient rehabilitation facilities, such as physiatrists, therapists, neuropsychologists, nutritionists, and wound care teams, can address the numerous complications and sequelae of patients with COVID-19.
- Studies showed that survivors of COVID-19 who underwent inpatient rehabilitation had great functional gains and can benefit at least as much from inpatient rehabilitation as patients without COVID-19.
- It is essential to continue to encourage acute rehabilitation for survivors of COVID-19 to optimize recovery, functionality, and safe discharge.

DISCLOSURE

The authors have nothing to disclose.

REFERENCES

1. Maltser S, Trovato E, Fusco HN, et al. Challenges and lessons learned for acute inpatient rehabilitation of persons with COVID-19: clinical presentation, assessment, needs, and services utilization. Am J Phys Med Rehabil 2021;100(12): 1115–23.
2. Puchner B, Sahanic S, Kirchmair R, et al. Beneficial effects of multi-disciplinary rehabilitation in postacute COVID-19: an observational cohort study. Eur J Phys Rehabil Med 2021;57(2):189–98.

3. Kapp CM, Zaeh S, Niedermeyer S, et al. The use of analgesia and sedation in mechanically ventilated patients with covid-19 acute respiratory distress syndrome. Anesth Analg 2020;131(4):e198–200.

4. Lemyze M, Komorowski M, Mallat J, et al. Early intensive physical rehabilitation combined with a protocolized decannulation process in tracheostomized survivors from severe COVID-19 pneumonia with chronic critical illness. J Clin Med 2022;(13):11. https://doi.org/10.3390/jcm11133921.

5. Marra A, Ely EW, Pandharipande PP, et al. The ABCDEF bundle in critical care. Crit Care Clin 2017;33(2):225–43.

6. Herridge MS, Tansey CM, Matte A, et al. Functional disability 5 years after acute respiratory distress syndrome. N Engl J Med 2011;364(14):1293–304.

7. Escalon MX, Lichtenstein AH, Posner E, et al. The effects of early mobilization on patients requiring extended mechanical ventilation across multiple ICUs. Crit Care Explor 2020;2(6):e0119.

8. Kakodkar P, Kaka N, Baig MN. A comprehensive literature review on the clinical presentation, and management of the pandemic coronavirus disease 2019 (COVID-19). Cureus 2020;12(4):e7560.

9. Richardson S, Hirsch JS, Narasimhan M, et al. Presenting characteristics, comorbidities, and outcomes among 5700 patients hospitalized with COVID-19 in the New York City Area. JAMA 2020;323(20):2052–9.

10. Groah SL, Pham CT, Rounds AK, et al. Outcomes of patients with COVID-19 after inpatient rehabilitation. Pharm Manag PM R 2022;14(2):202–9.

11. Valbuena Valecillos AD, Gober J, Palermo A, et al. A comparison of patients discharged to skilled nursing and inpatient rehabilitation facilities following hospitalization for COVID-19: a retrospective study. Am J Phys Med Rehabil 2022. https://doi.org/10.1097/PHM.0000000000002162.

12. Sun T, Guo L, Tian F, et al. Rehabilitation of patients with COVID-19. Expet Rev Respir Med 2020;14(12):1249–56.

13. Sheehy LM. Considerations for postacute rehabilitation for survivors of COVID-19. JMIR Public Health Surveill 2020;6(2):e19462.

14. Martillo MA, Dangayach NS, Tabacof L, et al. Postintensive care syndrome in survivors of critical illness related to coronavirus disease 2019: cohort study from a New York City critical care recovery clinic. Crit Care Med 2021;49(9):1427–38.

15. Bienvenu OJ, Friedman LA, Colantuoni E, et al. Psychiatric symptoms after acute respiratory distress syndrome: a 5-year longitudinal study. Intensive Care Med 2018;44(1):38–47.

16. Brugliera L, Filippi M, Del Carro U, et al. Nerve compression injuries after prolonged prone position ventilation in patients with sars-cov-2: a case series. Arch Phys Med Rehabil 2021;102(3):359–62.

17. Malik GR, Wolfe AR, Soriano R, et al. Injury-prone: peripheral nerve injuries associated with prone positioning for COVID-19-related acute respiratory distress syndrome. Br J Anaesth 2020;125(6):e478–80.

18. Ghanem J, Passadori A, Severac F, et al. Effects of rehabilitation on long-covid-19 patient's autonomy, symptoms and nutritional observance. Nutrients 2022;(15):14. https://doi.org/10.3390/nu14153027.

19. Anker MS, Landmesser U, von Haehling S, et al. Weight loss, malnutrition, and cachexia in COVID-19: facts and numbers. J Cachexia Sarcopenia Muscle 2021;12(1):9–13.

20. Amini M, Mansouri F, Vafaee K, et al. Factors affecting the incidence and prevalence of pressure ulcers in COVID-19 patients admitted with a Braden scale

below 14 in the intensive care unit: Retrospective cohort study. Int Wound J 2022. https://doi.org/10.1111/iwj.13804.

21. Challoner T, Vesel T, Dosanjh A, et al. The risk of pressure ulcers in a proned COVID population. Surgeon 2022;20(4):e144–8.

22. Escalon MX, Herrera J. Adapting to the coronavirus disease 2019 pandemic in New York City. Am J Phys Med Rehabil 2020;99(6):453–8.

23. Walton M, Murray E, Christian MD. Mental health care for medical staff and affiliated healthcare workers during the COVID-19 pandemic. Eur Heart J Acute Cardiovasc Care 2020;9(3):241–7.

24. Spielmanns M, Pekacka-Egli AM, Cecon M, et al. COVID-19 outbreak during inpatient rehabilitation: impact on settings and clinical course of neuromusculoskeletal rehabilitation patients. Am J Phys Med Rehabil 2021;100(3):203–8.

25. Barnett ML, Waken RJ, Zheng J, et al. Changes in health and quality of life in us skilled nursing facilities by covid-19 exposure status in 2020. JAMA 2022. https://doi.org/10.1001/jama.2022.15071.

The Role of Surgical Prehabilitation During the COVID-19 Pandemic and Beyond

Tracey L. Hunter, MD[a,b,c,d],*, Danielle L. Sarno, MD[a,b,c,d],
Oranicha Jumreornvong, MD[e,f], Rachel Esparza, MD[g,h],
Laura E. Flores, PhD[i], Julie K. Silver, MD[a,b,c,d]

KEYWORDS

- Rehabilitation • Prehabilitation • Surgery • Disability • COVID-19 • Long COVID
- Postacute sequelae SARS CoV2 • Pandemic

KEY POINTS

- Comorbid, older populations including individuals with frail syndrome, disability, or racial-ethnic minority status are associated with higher rates of postoperative complications, hospital readmissions, longer length of stay, nonhome discharges, mortality, and poor patient satisfaction.
- Surgical prehabilitation may improve poor postoperative outcomes of acute and nonacute surgery for high-risk surgical candidates within older patients.
- Standardization of frailty tools and multimodal prehabilitation programs can enhance identification of comorbid, older patients and reduce postoperative risks and mortality.
- Use of the GRADE (Grading of Recommendations, Assessment, Development and Evaluations) approach could help establish clinical guidelines for prehabilitation.

[a] Department of Physical Medicine and Rehabilitation, Harvard Medical School, 25 Shattuck Street, Boston, MA 02115, USA; [b] Spaulding Rehabilitation Hospital, 300 First Avenue, Charlestown, MA 02129, USA; [c] Massachusetts General Hospital, 55 Fruit Street, Boston, MA 02114, USA; [d] Brigham and Women's Hospital, 75 Francis Street, Boston, MA 02115, USA; [e] Department of Physical Medicine and Rehabilitation, Icahn School of Medicine at Mount Sinai, New York, NY, USA; [f] Mount Sinai Hospital, 1468 Madison Avenue, New York, NY 10029, USA; [g] Department of Physical Medicine and Rehabilitation, McGaw Medical Center, Northwestern University Feinberg School of Medicine, Chicago, IL, USA; [h] Shirley Ryan Ability Lab (Formerly the Rehabilitation Institute of Chicago), 355 East Erie Street, Chicago, IL 60611, USA; [i] College of Allied Health Professions, University of Nebraska Medical Center, 42nd and Emile, Omaha, NE 68198, USA
* Corresponding author. Department of Physical Medicine and Rehabilitation, Harvard Medical School, Boston, MA, USA; Spaulding Rehabilitation Hospital, 300 First Avenue, Charlestown, MA 02129.
E-mail address: thunter@mgh.harvard.edu
Twitter: @TraceyHunterMD (T.L.H.); @DanielleSarnoMD (D.L.S.); @RachelEsparzaMD (R.E.); @LauraFlowersE (L.E.F.); @JulieSilverMD (J.K.S.)

Phys Med Rehabil Clin N Am 34 (2023) 523–538
https://doi.org/10.1016/j.pmr.2023.03.002
1047-9651/23/© 2023 Elsevier Inc. All rights reserved.

INTRODUCTION

The COVID-19 pandemic, beginning in late 2019, led to significant changes in surgical care. Profound delays in timing of operations, along with a confluence of unprecedented conditions contributed to the deteriorating health of many individuals across various populations. Despite unforeseen adverse outcomes, the cancellations and postponements of elective surgeries were part of heightened efforts to prioritize safety concerns. Simultaneously, mandates were enforced for home isolation and social distancing in public places, such as gyms, parks, and local schools, resulting in an increase in sedentary lifestyles. Widespread shortages in products combined with the collapse of the prepandemic transportation infrastructure has also limited access to nutritious food for some individuals; whereas, consumption of alcohol has increased.[1] The plethora of pandemic-related issues have exacerbated a situation in which surgical outcomes may be negatively impacted beyond known factors, such as frailty, older age, disability, and minority race/ethnicity status (**Fig. 1**).

Prehabilitation may be an antidote to decreasing surgical risk, especially for vulnerable populations, such as people who are older, frail, or disabled. Those with comorbidities, such as diabetes, chronic obstructive pulmonary disease, or other medical conditions that may affect surgical outcomes, might also benefit. High morbidity and mortality during or after surgery is an important concern, particularly in vulnerable populations. For example, a study by Shinall and colleagues[2] examined veterans who underwent a noncardiac surgical procedures at Veterans Health Administration Hospitals and found that patients with higher levels of frailty had higher mortality at 30, 90, and 180 days after surgery. Mortality increased as frailty, time, and operative stress increased. Another study assessed patients undergoing noncardiac procedures and found that frailty was associated with higher mortality at 30 and 180 days for all noncardiac surgical specialties regardless of operative stress.[3]

Individuals with disabilities may also benefit from prehabilitation. Multiple studies have suggested that higher preoperative level of disability is associated with worse surgical outcomes.[4–6] For instance, Mazzola and colleagues[7] compared individuals between age 85 and 89 years with those greater than 90 years that underwent hip fracture surgery. Prefracture disability was found to be a predictor of higher rates of

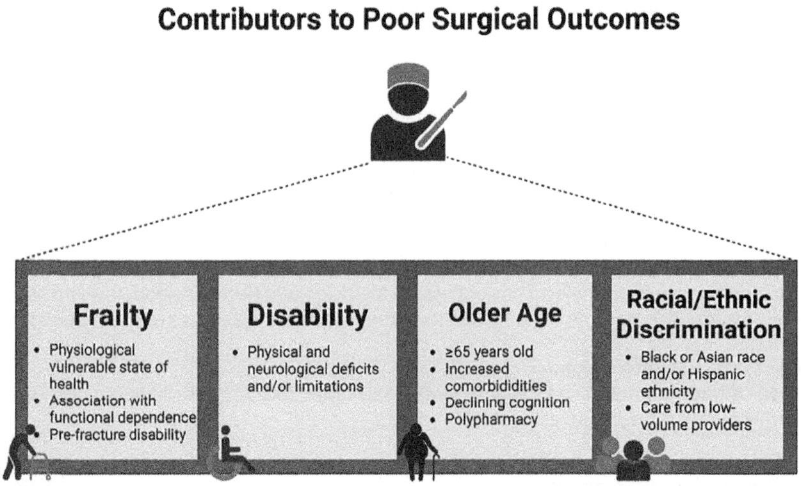

Contributors to Poor Surgical Outcomes

Frailty	Disability	Older Age	Racial/Ethnic Discrimination
• Physiological vulnerable state of health • Association with functional dependence • Pre-fracture disability	• Physical and neurological deficits and/or limitations	• ≥65 years old • Increased comorbididities • Declining cognition • Polypharmacy	• Black or Asian race and/or Hispanic ethnicity • Care from low-volume providers

Fig. 1. Contributors to poor surgical outcomes in acute and nonacute surgery.

mortality in those greater than 90 years old. Afilalo and colleagues[4] found that the addition of disability and frailty to cardiac surgery risk scores improved model discrimination of individuals at higher risk for cardiac surgery. Outcomes in spine surgery have been tied to disability-related issues (**Table 1**). In one study, higher preoperative disability was a risk factor for worsening postoperative disability after surgery for lumbar spinal stenosis.[5] However, individuals with higher preoperative disability were also more likely to have clinically significant improvement in disability after surgery. In a cohort of patients undergoing minimally invasive transforaminal lumbar interbody fusion, patients with preoperative disability were more likely to report worse postoperative outcomes and patient satisfaction.[6]

Individuals who identify with racial or ethnic minority groups are also known to have worse surgical outcomes (see **Table 1**). For example, a recent systematic review examining 63 studies in total joint arthroplasty (TJA) reported that despite being less likely to undergo TJA, Black patients had higher rates of complications, readmissions, mortality, nonhome discharges, and longer lengths of stay (LOS) compared with White patients.[8] Hispanic patients also used TJA less but had higher rates of complications, prolonged LOS, and nonhome discharges. Asian patients had longer LOS but fewer readmissions. Cardinal and colleagues[9] focused on disparities in the surgical treatment of adult spine conditions. In this systematic review, the authors noted that despite individuals from minority groups having lower spinal surgery utilization rates, they were more likely to undergo surgery from low-volume providers, and had greater LOS and more complications. Black patients had higher rates of mortality and reported lower outcomes at discharge than White patients. Individuals from certain racial and ethnic minority groups often have more comorbidities, such as obesity, diabetes, and heart disease, which may make surgeons concerned about the potential risks of surgery in these patients. Prehabilitation might help to reduce their risk profile and support more access to operative interventions.

DISCUSSION

Prehabilitation improves patients' physical and mental function, through buffering the deconditioning between the time of diagnosis and recovery. Such mechanisms as accessibility, motivation, role of health care professionals and organizations, acceptability, and prioritization have been shown to improve physical fitness, reduce LOS, reduce delay for surgery, reduce postoperative complications, and improve quality of life.[10] In order for health care professionals to deliver and engage in prehabilitation,

Table 1
Disparities in outcomes after spinal surgery[9]

Factor/Outcome Measure	Disparity
Spinal surgery utilization	Lower rates of surgery in Black, Hispanic, and non-White patients
Length of stay	Increased intensive care unit and overall length of stay in Black, Hispanic, and Asian patients
In-hospital mortality	Higher in non-White patients and Black patients
Complication rates	Increased in Black patients after spinal surgery, including higherrates of bleeding and infection

Data from [Cardinal T, Bonney PA, Strickland BA, et al. Disparities in the Surgical Treatment of Adult Spine Diseases: A Systematic Review. *World Neurosurgery.* 2022;158:290-304.e1. https://doi.org/10.1016/j.wneu.2021.10.121].

there needs to be strong evidence-based protocols for implementation and clinical practice in a multidisciplinary system that provides specific guidance for screening and triage of patients. Numerous studies have investigated unimodal prehabilitation intervention, with exercise being the most studied (**Fig. 2**). Other interventions have included nutritional, educational, psychological, or clinical components.[10–12] However, a single prehabilitation literature review on nutrition within oncology research revealed a lack of standardization and validation of nutritional assessment. Investigation of this model frequently revealed inadequate evidence-based intervention that failed to include monitoring or evaluation of its outcome.[13] Development of core outcomes could improve the quality of unimodal prehabilitation studies to enable pooling of evidence and address research gaps. Although unimodal prehabilitation, such as exercise, can improve functional capacity and reduce complication rates, the evidence of effectiveness ranges from very low to moderate because of relegating serious risk of bias, imprecision, and inconsistency.[12]

More recent studies have assessed multimodal prehabilitation programs, which include multiple preoperative interventions to prepare patients for surgery with the goal of improving resilience and postoperative outcomes (see **Fig. 2**). Although a single prehabilitation intervention, such as nutrition alone (oral nutritional supplements with and without counseling) has been shown to significantly decrease LOS, evidence of multimodal prehabilitation combining exercise (oral nutritional supplements with and without counseling and with exercise) suggests an accelerated return to presurgical functional capacity.[14] Because there is often a waiting period before elective surgical procedures, multimodal prehabilitation provides an opportunity to intervene in a targeted fashion to improve postoperative recovery. Active engagement of the patient in the multimodal prehabilitation including exercise, nutrition, and psychological well-being may alleviate the physical and emotional distress presurgery and postsurgery.[15] A meta-analysis study on colorectal cancer surgery reveals that multimodal prehabilitation comprising at least two preoperative interventions shows improvement in functional capacity and postoperative outcomes.[12]

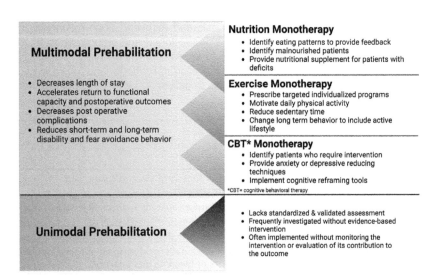

Fig. 2. Describes prehabilitation program designs and potential benefits and disadvantages of multimodal versus unimodal prehabilitation. These are general comments based on the available research. Further investigation is needed. CBT, cognitive behavioral therapy.

However, the included studies did not report a difference between groups for health-related quality of life and LOS. Nevertheless, multimodal programs also increase perioperative functional capacity and potentially decrease postoperative complications in older adults undergoing major abdominal surgery.[11] Studies also suggest that multimodal rehabilitation, including exercise and cognitive-based therapy, reduces short- and long-term disability and fear-avoidance behavior following a lumbar fusion surgery. High-quality research that assesses study outcomes is required to confirm the effectiveness of multimodal prehabilitation programs. Furthermore, use of the GRADE (Grading of Recommendations, Assessment, Development and Evaluations) approach, including critique of bias risk and quality of evidence, could help establish clinical guidelines from prehabilitation research, especially for older adults (**Box 1**).[11,16]

PRESURGICAL FRAILTY AND OUTCOMES

As the aging population continues to grow with increasing life expectancy, older adults are predicted to account for 23% of the US population by 2050, with potential to outnumber the percent of children.[17,18] Unfortunately, hospitalizations are three times as high among older adults (eg, $\geq$65 years) considering health profiles of increased comorbidities, which are greater in quantity and severity than younger populations.[17,18] However, the unidimensional clinical use of comorbidity is an inadequate measure of health status because it excludes significant factors, such as functionality, physical endurance, and cognition. The multifactorial components of health are known to impact medical management and surgery.

Numerous studies including systematic reviews and meta-analyses have demonstrated that frailty is a valuable predictor of poor outcomes in surgical patients (**Fig. 1**).[17,19–21] Frailty is defined as a weakened state of physical function, cognition, and physiologic capacity that precedes disability and vulnerability to stressors (eg, surgery, anesthesia).[17,22–24] Frailty has been associated with older adults, dependent status, metabolic syndrome, greater hospitalization rates and intensive care unit admissions, surgical complications and readmissions, and higher mortality.[17,22,23,25] Frailty, in addition to comorbidities, has also been associated with severe COVID-19

Box 1
The methodology of the GRADE (Grading of Recommendations, Assessment, Development and Evaluations) approach and its advantages for establishing clinical guidelines

GRADE Approach for Establishing Clinical Guidelines[16]
- Use explicit definitions and judgments to reduce strategy error or bias
- Systematically assess study designs and confirm a direct relationship to quality of evidence
- Consider data precision, confounders, and strength of outcomes and associations
- Identify the weakest outcomes to represent the overall quality of evidence for clinical decision-making because this reduces overestimation of data power
- Determine relative importance of outcomes (critical vs noncritical vs ignored) to support the quality and strength of clinical recommendations
- Pay direct attention to the relationship of health benefits and harms to ensure transparency of net positive health outcomes
- Establish summaries of evidence and findings that can provide consistent information for research evaluations
- Incorporate international collaborations with a wide spectrum of organizations to develop a sensible, reliable, and generalizable system

Data from [Atkins D, Best D, Briss PA, et al. Grading quality of evidence and strength of recommendations. *BMJ*. 2004;328(7454):1490. https://doi.org/10.1136/bmj.328.7454.1490].

disease that may prolong recovery and worsen functional decline.[26,27] The vulnerable physiologic state of frail persons may be a corollary of an aged and weakened immune system that has poor defense mechanisms from pathogens.[26,27] Accurate measurement and application of frailty may be essential for establishing effective presurgical interventions that can improve surgical outcomes, reduce postoperative complications (eg, delirium and long-term cognitive dysfunction), identify candidates for surgical revision, and decrease mortality.[17,23,28,29]

Greater than 50 frailty instruments currently exist (Appendix 1); however, research shows lack of clinical standardization necessary to create treatment guidelines or predict surgical outcomes.[18,30] In a 7-year prospective study by Kapadia and colleagues,[17] frailty was used to assess outcomes of acute care surgery in older patients. The analysis included 1045 patients, 65 years or older, who were divided into frail and nonfrail groups. The Emergency General Surgery Frailty Index and the Trauma-Specific Frailty Index were used to measure frailty and its impact on emergency and trauma-specific surgeries. Both indices were based on a 15-variable questionnaire that included patient comorbidities, activities of daily living, nutrition status, and health habits. Hypertension and diabetes were the most common comorbidities among the study population. The analysis of all patients measured by both frailty indices revealed significantly greater risks for the frail group in comparison with nonfrail group for inpatient complications, disposition to rehabilitation or skilled-nursing facilities, and mortality. The secondary outcome of implementation of routine frailty assessment was independently associated with a lower adjusted risk for major complications, and a higher adjusted risk for rehabilitation/skilled-nursing facilities disposition. When analysis of the frail group was stratified by frailty index, results for the trauma and emergency patients independently revealed significantly higher outcomes in complications, disposition, and mortality, and LOS in the intensive care unit and overall hospital LOS.

Frailty measurements have also been used in various types of nonacute surgery. A systematic review conducted by Shaw and colleagues[24] focused on frailty and cancer surgery outcomes. This included 71 studies worldwide on older patients who underwent various types of oncologic surgery, most commonly abdominopelvic. The meta-analysis found that frailty increased the likelihood of 30-day mortality, adverse discharge disposition, postoperative complications, long-term mortality, and LOS. Nevertheless, there is still inadequate research about the effects of frailty in cancer surgery, including relationships specific to tumor type, cancer stage, and metastasis, and use of adjunctive therapies.[24]

The clinical value of frailty in orthopedic surgery is also generally inconclusive; however, it has potential based on the findings of available research.[18] A cohort study by Schuijt and colleagues revealed that a higher frailty index was associated with a higher risk of 90-day mortality.[31,32] Additionally, Bai and colleagues[33] published a large systematic review revealing the association of frailty with higher mortality risk in total knee arthroplasty and total hip arthroplasty. However, Lemos and colleagues[18] and Kitamura and colleagues[32] conducted reviews, each including more than 80 orthopedic studies, that emphasize major knowledge discrepancies because of the lack of substantial prospective research and homogeneous use of frailty indices.

PREHABILITATION IN THE CONTEXT OF PRESURGICAL FRAILTY

As the general demand for surgery continues to rise with the aging population, there is critical need to better qualify frailty and enhance preoperative health of older patients.[34] Emerging use of multimodal prehabilitation, incorporating exercise, nutrition, and/or psychosocial components, may potentially improve surgical outcomes in frail patients (see **Fig. 3**).[29,34–36] The exercise component may include such activities as walking capacity (eg, 6-minute-walking test), balance and strength exercises, and inspiratory muscle training.[34,35] Nutrition programs may involve monitoring of dietary intake and weight changes and preoperative carbohydrate loading.[34,35] The psychosocial portion typically focuses on behavioral management and mental health screening.[1,34] When used for surgical candidates, prehabilitation has been shown to optimize mind-body fitness to endure the physiologic stress of surgery while also improving various postoperative outcomes.[34,35]

Prehabilitation also has potential in optimizing the functional capacity of frail persons. Baimas-George and colleagues[34] conducted a systematic review comparing five studies about prehabilitation for frail patients undergoing nonacute surgeries. One of two studies measuring mortality showed a remarkably decreased rate within 30-days and 3-month periods. One of two other studies demonstrated a significant improvement in LOS by 3 days, whereas the other study displayed a trend toward reduced LOS. Yet another study found that improvement in the 6-minute-walking test was associated with shorter LOS. Three of the studies demonstrated that preoperative exercise improved physical functionality. However, there was no difference found in the two studies that analyzed postoperative discharge disposition. Despite some evidence of promising results, this systematic review revealed major inconsistencies in frailty assessments and lack of heterogeneity of prehabilitation programs. Therefore, making comparisons between the studies is limited and simply reinforces the need for standardization of prehabilitation.

The preoperative health of frail individuals may be positively impacted by prehabilitation. This is evidenced by Milder and colleagues,[35] who performed a systematic review evaluating prehabilitation in frail patients. Two of several studies assessed prehabilitation in patients undergoing oncologic surgical resections. One of these two studies, which included all frail patients, incorporated prehabilitation via incentive deep breathing exercises at a minimum of three times daily along with nutritional supplementation 5 to 14 days preoperatively depending on malnutrition risk. In comparison with the retrospective control group, the prehabilitation group showed significant

Potential Contributors to Improved Surgical Outcomes

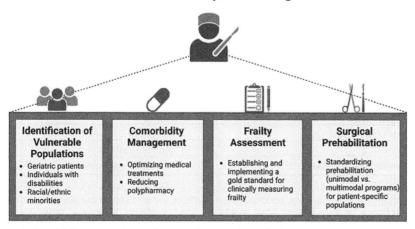

Identification of Vulnerable Populations	Comorbidity Management	Frailty Assessment	Surgical Prehabilitation
• Geriatric patients • Individuals with disabilities • Racial/ethnic minorities	• Optimizing medical treatments • Reducing polypharmacy	• Establishing and implementing a gold standard for clinically measuring frailty	• Standardizing prehabilitation (unimodal vs. multimodal programs) for patient-specific populations

Fig. 3. Potential factors that contribute to improved surgical outcomes in acute and nonacute surgery.

reduction in 30-day and 3-month mortality by 14% and 28%, respectively. Additionally, severe complications decreased by 26% and the overall complication rate decreased by 33%. The second study included a prospective analysis of exercise and nutritional prehabilitation conducted remotely at home or in a rehabilitation center for a 2-week period. Most of the patients, however, were classified as nonfrail (73.6%). The outcomes for mortality, postoperative complications, and functional recovery revealed no significant differences between the control and interventional groups. Despite design limitations, comparison of both studies may support that surgical prehabilitation has a greater impact for frail patients.

MEASURING FRAILTY BEFORE ELECTIVE SURGERY

It is important to explore how frailty is measured given its correlation with negative surgical outcomes. Multiple reviews have found that no single tool has been identified as a gold standard for gauging frailty.[18,23] It has been conceptualized by two models: a phenotype, proposed by Fried and colleagues, which describes frailty as a clinical presentation including at least three of the five features of weakness, slow gait speed, low physical activity, exhaustion, and unintentional weight loss; or an accumulation of age-related deficits, described by Rockwood and colleagues, which uses a multidimensional score based on the total of health deficits across various domains (**Table 2**).[18,19,23]

Several instruments assessing frailty have stemmed from these two models (**Table 3**). Based on the multidimensional risk state model, the Frailty Index (FI) developed by Rockwood and colleagues, has been used to calculate a score based on the quantity of deficits, with the severity of frailty determined by the number of deficits rather than the nature of each deficit.[19] The FI signifies a continuum of frailty, but the index may be trichotomized to indicate low, intermediate, and high level of frailty.[23] However, Obeid and colleagues proposed the modified Frailty Index (mFI), originally consisting of 11 preoperative risk factors (mFI-11); alterative versions later emerged and reduced measurements to five risk factors (mFI-5).[18] In a systematic review by Panayi and colleagues,[19] most of the studies used the mFI because the patient characteristics are easily determined clinically through medical history and physical examination. Similarly, a review on the orthopedic surgery population by Lemos and colleagues also used the "cumulative deficit" model (eg, mFI) most frequently; however, there was no consensus on defining and evaluating frailty.

Table 2 Frailty models[18,19,23]	
Phenotype Model (Frailty as a Clinical Presentation of ≥3 Features)	**Cumulative Deficit Model (Frailty as a Multidimensional Risk State)**
Weakness	Functional deficits
Slow gait speed	Comorbidities[a]
Minimal physical activity	Cognitive dysfunction
Exhaustion	Psychosocial risk factors
Unintended weight loss	Geriatrics syndromes[b]

[a] Comorbidities may include diabetes mellitus, angina, congestive heart failure, cerebrovascular accident, myocardial infarction, transient ischemic attack, chronic obstructive pulmonary disease, peripheral vascular disease, diminished sensorium, and functionally dependent status.[17]
[b] Geriatrics syndromes are multifactorial conditions that may include falls, polypharmacy, depression, cognitive impairment, and/or delirium.[23]
    Data from Refs.[17–19,23]

Table 3
Tests that measure frailty in surgical patients[a,23]

	Measurements	Comments
Clinical Tests that Measure Frailty[28]		
Fried phenotype	≥3 of 5 features: muscle weakness, slow gait speed, low level of physical activity, poor endurance/exhaustion, and unintentional weight loss/loss of muscle mass.[36] Modified Fried criteria: Fried + cognitive impairment + depressed mood.	Across studies, frailty based on the Fried phenotype was associated with mortality.
Clinical Frailty Scale	7 levels of frailty based on visual observation combined with a condensed medical record review.	After the Fried phenotype, this was the next most studied instrument per Aucoin et al[30]; also associated with mortality and with the largest effect size of any instrument.
Frailty Index	An index between 0 and 1 equal to the number of deficits present divided by the deficits measured. Denominator ranges from 30–71 from various domains including comorbidities, polypharmacy, physical and cognitive impairments, psychosocial risk factors, and common geriatric syndromes.	
Modified Frailty Index	5, 11, or 19 items. mFI-11: 11 deficits in the domains of functional status, cardiovascular comorbidities, chronic obstructive pulmonary disease, pneumonia, and reduced sensorium.	mFI-11 was the most frequently used frailty instrument per multiple systematic reviews.[18,19,34]
Edmonton Frailty Scale	Includes cognitive impairment, dependence in instrumental ADLs, recent burden of illnesses, self-perceived health, depression, weight loss, medication issues, incontinence, inadequate social support, and mobility difficulties.	

(*continued on next page*)

Table 3
(continued)

	Measurements	Comments
Emergency General Surgery Frailty Index[17]	15-variable questionnaire including patient comorbidities, activities of daily living, nutrition status, and health attitude. 0 = nonfrail status, 1 = severely frail status, with frailty defined as ≥0.325.	
Trauma-Specific Frailty Index[17]	15 variables from the modified Rockwood frailty questionnaire <0.27 = nonfrail, ≥0.27 = frail.	
Fatigue, Resistance, Ambulation, Illnesses, and Loss of Weight (FRAIL) Scale	A 5-point system based on fatigue, mobility, comorbidities, and weight loss.[22]	
Reported Edmonton Frail Scale-Thai	Gait speed substituted with "In the last 2 wk, were you able to (i) climb one flight of stairs (ii) walk 1 km"	
Comprehensive geriatric assessment	Cumulative score from 11 different frailty measures: • Fall in the last 6 mo • Requiring assistance with any ADLs • Body mass index or unintentional weight loss • Self-reported exhaustion • Self-reported low physical activity • Serum albumin • Hematocrit • Serum creatinine • 5-min-walk time • Chair rise time • Grip strength	
Adult spinal deformity frailty index	Based on comorbidities and patient-reported motility, ADL, independence, cognitive function, and mood.	
Cervical deformity frailty index	Based on comorbidities (eg, the mFI-11 and the mFI-5) with the addition of emergent admission and anterior/combined surgical approach.[21]	Contains components that are specific to metastatic spine disease (less generalizable to other pathologies).

(continued on next page)

Table 3 *(continued)*		
	Measurements	**Comments**
Hospital frailty risk score	Based on an ICD-10 code algorithm to identify diagnoses associated with frailty.	
Psoas size[21]	Measured on preoperative computed tomography psoas muscle index: cross-sectional area of bilateral psoas muscle/height^{2}.[37]	Used as a measure of sarcopenia as a proxy for frailty. Between studies, there is variation in how psoas size is calculated and some studies report that the psoas muscle is not representative of total human skeletal muscle mass, and therefore, not representative of whole-body sarcopenia.[21,37,38] In the review by Chan et al,[21] psoas size was the measure reporting no association with outcomes most commonly.
Comprehensive Assessment of Frailty	Fried phenotype without unintentional weight loss, plus balance assessment, albumin, creatinine, brain natriuretic peptide, forced expiratory volume in 1 s, and Clinical Frailty Scale.	
Blood Tests That Measure Frailty[38]		
FI from routine blood and urine tests[39–42]	White blood cell count, hemoglobin, sodium, potassium, creatinine, and albumin; and standard physical measures including blood pressure and/or pulse.	
Proinflammatory cytokines, such as interleukin-6 and tumor necrosis factor-α		Elevated levels are associated with frailty and worse outcomes.
Insulin-like growth factor 1		IGF-1 is involved with maintaining muscle mass, assisting with injury recovery, and is a marker of metabolism. Lower levels of IGF-1 are associated with frailty.

(continued on next page)

	Measurements	Comments
Table 3 **(continued)**		
Imaging Tests That Measure Frailty		
Computed tomography and ultrasonography[38]	Because these tests often are performed preoperatively, they may be used to evaluate surrogate markers of frailty/opportunity to measure muscle mass and osteopenia (when the studies were performed for another purpose).	Although radiologic studies can reveal a change in muscle mass, they provide no information on muscle performance needed to diagnose sarcopenia clinically.
Dual-energy x-ray absorptiometry[38]	Accepted reference values to detect sarcopenia by DXA: 7.26 kg/m^2 for men; <5.45 kg/m^2 for women.	However, DXA is not routinely performed to assess muscle mass or before surgery.
MRI[38]	Assessment of sarcopenia with MRI is being evaluated as a prognostic marker in select groups (eg, as a measure of muscle quality, assessing fat-free muscle area in patients with decompensated cirrhosis).	
Other Tests Used to Measure Frailty (Physical)		
Gait speed Timed get up and go Handgrip strength Short physical performance battery		
Other Tests Used to Measure Frailty (Functional)		
Katz Instrumental Activities of Daily Living Activities of Daily Living Eastern Cooperative Group Performance States Self-reported mobility assessment[28]		

Abbreviations: ADLs, activities of daily living; DXA, dual-energy x-ray absorptiometry; FI, Frailty Index; ICD, International Classification of Diseases; IGF-1, insulin-like growth factor 1; mFI, modified Frailty Index.

[a] This is not intended to be a complete list.

Lin HS, McBride RL, Hubbard RE. Frailty and anesthesia - risks during and post-surgery. Local Reg Anesth. 2018;11:61-73. Published 2018 Oct 5. https://doi.org/10.2147/LRA.S142996.

A high-quality frailty metric should comprise key elements of objectivity, such as the presence or absence of a comorbidity; reproducibility; and generalizability among different pathologies and surgical procedures.[21] This is reflected in the designs of mFI-11 and mFI-5, which have easy calculable scoring, and validation among various surgical specialties that enhances clinical practicality.[21] Unlike some other frailty instruments (eg, Edmonton Frailty Scale, Geriatric Consult Index), mFI-11 and mFI-5 exclude subjective components (eg, fatigue and mood) that can negatively affect external validity.

In a systematic review by Aucoin and colleagues,[30] the Fried phenotype was the most prevalent out of 35 various frailty instruments. The next most prevalent instruments included the Clinical Frailty Scale, a physical measure of frailty (gait speed, timed get up and go, handgrip strength, short physical performance battery); the FI; the Edmonton Frailty Scale; or a measure of function or disability, such as Katz Instrumental Activities of Daily Living, Activities of Daily Living, Eastern Cooperative Group Performance States, or self-reported mobility assessment. However, per Aucoin and colleagues,[30] the most common approach to assessing frailty was dichotomization of a frailty instrument (frail vs not frail). Other studies categorized frailty into three levels, and fewer studies categorized frailty into four or more levels or as a continuous measure.[30] Chan and colleagues[22] concluded that in addition to discrepancies between the frailty tools, there was heterogeneity in the methodology and research groups among studies using the same frailty index. Subsequently, results lack generalizability essential for clinical decision making. Therefore, the authors called for future research on frailty that prioritizes design precision and focused patient populations.

FUTURE DIRECTIONS

Evidence shows that frailty increases the risk for surgery while also negatively impacting acute and nonacute surgical outcomes. There is rising public health attention surrounding the development of clinical tools that will advance medical care for vulnerable, older adults.[17,18,27] Identification of superior frailty assessments with routine surveillance and electronic health record implementation will heighten clinical awareness and drive efforts to optimize the perioperative health status of older patients.[17,18,23] Frailty is also associated with higher hospital expenditure and overall health care costs thus incentivizing establishment of cost-effective interventions to treat older adults.[18] Furthermore, attaining an accurate understanding of health trajectories in older adults can help clinicians deliver patient-centered care that addresses quality of life and conveys potential high-risk surgical outcomes.[23,24] Additional research and standardization of multimodal surgical prehabilitation has fundamental potential to improve surgical outcomes and patient satisfaction, minimize postoperative complications, and reduce morbidity and mortality of older adults.[31,33,34]

SUMMARY

Precautionary measures and social isolation enforced during the COVID-19 pandemic resulted in reduced access to elective surgeries and heightened exposure to physiologically harmful conditions that caused a major decline in baseline health statuses of vulnerable populations. These disadvantaged groups, not mutually exclusive, include individuals with frail syndrome, older age, disability, and racial-ethnic minority status. Furthermore, these patient groups have known associations with higher rates of postoperative complications, hospital readmissions, longer LOS, nonhome discharges, poor patient satisfaction, and mortality. Surgical prehabilitation has potential to improve postoperative outcomes for comorbid, older populations. Frailty is a common measurement used to identify these surgically high-risk individuals. However, future research is required to help standardize frailty tools for clinical application. Optimal measurement tools will improve identification of older, frail patients, and subsequently direct designs for population-specific, multimodal prehabilitation to reduce postoperative risks and mortality.

CLINICS CARE POINTS

- Geriatric syndromes may include falls, polypharmacy, depression, cognitive impairment, and/ or delirium.
- Clinical use of comorbidity alone is an inadequate measure of health status because it excludes significant factors, such as functionality, physical endurance, and cognition, which collectively can impact medical management and surgery.
- Frailty may be a valuable predictor of poor outcomes in surgical patients.
- Clinical implementation of an effective frailty tool may be critical for risk stratification and optimal medical management and surgical decision-making.
- Multimodal prehabilitation may reduce postoperative morbidity and mortality for vulnerable, older populations including individuals with comorbidities, frail syndrome, disabilities, or racial-ethnic minority status.

AUTHOR DISCLOSURES

The authors have nothing to disclose.

SUPPLEMENTARY DATA

Supplementary data related to this article can be found online at https://doi.org/10.1016/j.pmr.2023.03.002.

REFERENCES

1. Silver JK, Santa Mina D, Bates A, et al. Physical and psychological health behavior changes during the COVID-19 pandemic that may inform surgical pre-habilitation: a narrative review. Curr Anesthesiol Rep 2022;12(1):109–24.
2. Shinall MC, Arya S, Youk A, et al. Association of preoperative patient frailty and operative stress with postoperative mortality. JAMA Surg 2020;155(1): e194620.
3. George EL, Hall DE, Youk A, et al. Association between patient frailty and post-operative mortality across multiple noncardiac surgical specialties. JAMA Surg 2021;156(1):e205152.
4. Afilalo J, Mottillo S, Eisenberg MJ, et al. Addition of frailty and disability to cardiac surgery risk scores identifies elderly patients at high risk of mortality or major morbidity. Circ: Cardiovasc Qual Outcomes 2012;5(2):222–8.
5. Kim GU, Park J, Kim HJ, et al. Definitions of unfavorable surgical outcomes and their risk factors based on disability score after spine surgery for lumbar spinal stenosis. BMC Musculoskelet Disord 2020;21(1):288.
6. Jacob KC, Patel MR, Collins AP, et al. The effect of the severity of preoperative disability on patient-reported outcomes and patient satisfaction following mini-mally invasive transforaminal lumbar interbody fusion. World Neurosurgery 2022;159:e334–46.
7. Mazzola P, Bellelli G, Broggini V, et al. Postoperative delirium and pre-fracture disability predict 6-month mortality among the oldest old hip fracture patients. Aging Clin Exp Res 2015;27(1):53–60.
8. Rudisill SS, Varady NH, Birir A, et al. Racial and ethnic disparities in total joint arthro-plasty care: a contemporary systematic review and meta-analysis. J Arthroplasty 2022. https://doi.org/10.1016/j.arth.2022.08.006. S088354032200746X.

9. Cardinal T, Bonney PA, Strickland BA, et al. Disparities in the surgical treatment of adult spine diseases: a systematic review. World Neurosurgery 2022;158: 290–304.e1.

10. Saggu RK, Barlow P, Butler J, et al. Considerations for multimodal prehabilitation in women with gynaecological cancers: a scoping review using realist principles. BMC Wom Health 2022;22(1):300.

11. Pang NQ, Tan YX, Samuel M, et al. Multimodal prehabilitation in older adults before major abdominal surgery: a systematic review and meta-analysis. Langenbeck's Arch Surg 2022;407(6):2193–204.

12. Molenaar CJ, van Rooijen SJ, Fokkenrood HJ, et al. Prehabilitation versus no prehabilitation to improve functional capacity, reduce postoperative complications and improve quality of life in colorectal cancer surgery. Cochrane Database Syst Rev 2022;5:CD013259.

13. Gillis C, Davies SJ, Carli F, et al. Current landscape of nutrition within prehabilitation oncology research: a scoping review. Front Nutr 2021;8:644723.

14. Gillis C, Buhler K, Bresee L, et al. Effects of nutritional prehabilitation, with and without exercise, on outcomes of patients who undergo colorectal surgery: a systematic review and meta-analysis. Gastroenterology 2018;155(2):391–410.e4.

15. Scheede-Bergdahl C, Minnella EM, Carli F. Multi-modal prehabilitation: addressing the why, when, what, how, who and where next? Anaesthesia 2019;74(Suppl 1):20–6.

16. Atkins D, Best D, Briss PA, et al. Grading quality of evidence and strength of recommendations. BMJ 2004;328(7454):1490.

17. Kapadia M, Obaid O, Nelson A, et al. Evaluation of frailty assessment compliance in acute care surgery: changing trends, lessons learned. J Surg Res 2022;270: 236–44.

18. Lemos JL, Welch JM, Xiao M, et al. Is frailty associated with adverse outcomes after orthopaedic surgery? A systematic review and assessment of definitions. JBJS Reviews 2021;9(12). https://doi.org/10.2106/JBJS.RVW.21.00065.

19. Panayi AC, Orkaby AR, Sakthivel D, et al. Impact of frailty on outcomes in surgical patients: a systematic review and meta-analysis. Am J Surg 2019;218(2): 393–400.

20. Arai Y, Kimura T, Takahashi Y, et al. Preoperative frailty is associated with progression of postoperative cardiac rehabilitation in patients undergoing cardiovascular surgery. Gen Thorac Cardiovasc Surg 2019;67(11):917–24.

21. Chan R, Ueno R, Afroz A, et al. Association between frailty and clinical outcomes in surgical patients admitted to intensive care units: a systematic review and meta-analysis. Br J Anaesth 2022;128(2):258–71.

22. Chan V, Wilson JRF, Ravinsky R, et al. Frailty adversely affects outcomes of patients undergoing spine surgery: a systematic review. Spine J 2021;21(6): 988–1000.

23. Lin HS, McBride RL, Hubbard RE. Frailty and anesthesia: risks during and postsurgery. Local Reg Anesth 2018;11:61–73.

24. Shaw JF, Budiansky D, Sharif F, et al. The association of frailty with outcomes after cancer surgery: a systematic review and metaanalysis. Ann Surg Oncol 2022; 29(8):4690–704.

25. Jiang X, Xu X, Ding L, et al. The association between metabolic syndrome and presence of frailty: a systematic review and meta-analysis. Eur Geriatr Med 2022. https://doi.org/10.1007/s41999-022-00688-4.

26. Subramaniam A, Shekar K, Afroz A, et al. Frailty and mortality associations in patients with COVID-19: a systematic review and meta-analysis. Intern Med J 2022; 52(5):724–39.

27. Wanhella KJ, Fernandez-Patron C. Biomarkers of ageing and frailty may predict COVID-19 severity. Ageing Res Rev 2022;73:101513.

28. Gracie TJ, Caufield-Noll C, Wang NY, et al. The association of preoperative frailty and postoperative delirium: a meta-analysis. Anesth Analg 2021. https://doi.org/10.1213/ANE.0000000000005609.

29. Tjeertes EKM, van Fessem JMK, Mattace-Raso FUS, et al. Influence of frailty on outcome in older patients undergoing non-cardiac surgery: a systematic review and meta-analysis. Aging and disease 2020;11(5):1276.

30. Aucoin SD, Hao M, Sohi R, et al. Accuracy and feasibility of clinically applied frailty instruments before surgery. Anesthesiology 2020;133(1):78–95.

31. Schuijt HJ, Morin ML, Allen E, et al. Does the frailty index predict discharge disposition and length of stay at the hospital and rehabilitation facilities? Injury 2021;52(6):1384–9.

32. Kitamura K, van Hooff M, Jacobs W, et al. Which frailty scales for patients with adult spinal deformity are feasible and adequate? A systematic review. Spine J 2022;22(7):1191–204.

33. Bai Y, Zhang XM, Sun X, et al. The association between frailty and mortality among lower limb arthroplasty patients: a systematic review and meta-analysis. BMC Geriatr 2022;22(1):702.

34. Baimas-George M, Watson M, Elhage S, et al. Prehabilitation in frail surgical patients: a systematic review. World J Surg 2020;44(11):3668–78.

35. Milder DA, Pillinger NL, Kam PCA. The role of prehabilitation in frail surgical patients: a systematic review. Acta Anaesthesiol Scand 2018;62(10):1356–66.

36. Moskven E, Charest-Morin R, Flexman AM, et al. The measurements of frailty and their possible application to spinal conditions: a systematic review. Spine J 2022; 22(9):1451–71.

37. Magnuson A, Sattar S, Nightingale G, et al. A practical guide to geriatric syndromes in older adults with cancer: a focus on falls, cognition, polypharmacy, and depression. Am Soc Clin Oncol Educ Book 2019;39:e96–109.

38. Fried LP, Tangen CM, Walston J, et al. Frailty in older adults: evidence for a phenotype. J Gerontol A Biol Sci Med Sci 2001;56(3):M146–56.

39. Kurumisawa S, Kawahito K. The psoas muscle index as a predictor of long-term survival after cardiac surgery for hemodialysis-dependent patients. J Artif Organs 2019;22(3):214–21.

40. Bentov I, Kaplan SJ, Pham TN, et al. Frailty assessment: from clinical to radiological tools. Br J Anaesth 2019;123(1):37–50.

41. Howlett SE, Rockwood MRH, Mitnitski A, et al. Standard laboratory tests to identify older adults at increased risk of death. BMC Med 2014;12:171.

42. Rockwood K, McMillan M, Mitnitski A, et al. A frailty index based on common laboratory tests in comparison with a clinical frailty index for older adults in long-term care facilities. J Am Med Dir Assoc 2015;16(10):842–7.

Neurologic and Neuromuscular Sequelae of COVID-19

Carol Li, MD[a,b,c],*, Monica Verduzco-Gutierrez, MD[a]

KEYWORDS

- Neurologic • COVID-19 • Neurorehabilitation • Encephalopathy • Stroke

KEY POINTS

- Exact pathophysiology for neurotropic features of SARS-CoV-2 is still unclear; direct neuroinvasion is becoming less probable, but more theories involving cytokine storm and activation of proinflammatory cascade leading to endothelial and blood-brain barrier disruption are more likely.
- Older patients with vascular comorbidities, such as cardiovascular disease and diabetes, are at a higher risk of cerebral microangiopathy, thromboembolism, and subsequent brain atrophy.
- Generalized muscle weakness, muscle injury, and myalgias are the most common neurologic and neuromuscular sequelae; second most common symptom is headache.
- Encephalopathy, cerebrovascular disease, Guillain Barré syndrome, and critical illness myopathy are generally associated with higher mortality and poorer prognosis; depending on severity and medical stability, early rehabilitation intervention may be key to recovery, although long-term sequelae may still be possible.
- Pharmacologic options for specific neurologic symptoms may be limited to supportive management and dependent on existing guidelines for respective diagnoses, although novel interventions and related research are underway.

INTRODUCTION

The impact of postacute sequelae of SARS-CoV-2 infection (PASC) on the central nervous system (CNS) and peripheral nervous system (PNS) is widely known and can disproportionally affect the aging patient population.[1] These complications can manifest as a result of direct neuroinvasion, autoimmunity, and possibly lead to chronic

[a] Department of Rehabilitation Medicine, Long School of Medicine at University of Texas Health Science Center at San Antonio, 7703 Floyd Curl Drive, MC 7798, San Antonio, TX 78229, USA; [b] Polytrauma Outpatient Neurorehabilitation Services, Audie L. Murphy VA Medical Center; [c] Polytrauma Rehabilitation Center, P168, 7400 Merton Minter, San Antonio, TX 78229, USA
* Corresponding author. 7703 Floyd Curl Drive, Mail Code 7798, San Antonio, TX 78229.
E-mail address: CAROL.LI@VA.GOV

Phys Med Rehabil Clin N Am 34 (2023) 539–549
https://doi.org/10.1016/j.pmr.2023.04.002

neurodegenerative processes. Additionally, particularly in patients with prolonged mechanical ventilation, there could be concurrent global muscle atrophy or intensive care unit–acquired weakness that can further cloud the clinical picture of an underlying neuromuscular condition, potentially leading to underdiagnosis. The focus of this article is to present an overview of what is currently known about the clinical presentation of these various conditions, proposed pathophysiology, and the diagnostic approaches and clinical management.

PATIENT EVALUATION OVERVIEW
Pathophysiology

Neurotropism is defined as the ability to infect the brain, and SARS-CoV-2 has neurotropic qualities. The virus has known receptors, particularly the human angiotensin-converting enzyme 2 (ACE2), which in addition to be expressed in type II pneumocytes and endothelial cells, are also expressed in neurons and glial cells. The SARS-CoV-2 virus has a high affinity for ACE2 receptors in the neurons and glial cells, which has been further confirmed with few postmortem studies where viral particles have been found in the cerebrospinal fluid, cytoplasm of hypothalamus neurons, brainstem, and lower cranial nerves.[2–4]

The pathway in which the virus enters the CNS still remains debatable. Hematogenous viral spread with disruption of blood-brain barrier to CNS has been described, but the entry point through olfactory system is the most discussed. In rat studies, it has been demonstrated that viral entry starts at the olfactory bulbs before spreading to the brain and CNS, which likely explains the neurologic cause of smell loss at the onset of the infection. Viral entry through cribriform plate is does not occur all the time; a systematic review by Chowdhary and colleagues[5] states younger age (mean age, 29) may be associated with olfactory bulb involvement and abnormal neuroimaging can still be found in patients without olfactory bulb enhancement. Despite findings of viral particles in postmortem brains, cerebrospinal fluid analysis that has been collected more acutely if clinical presentation is consistent with encephalopathy or meningitis show that although there may be evidence of pleocytosis and elevated protein with some cases of intrathecal autoimmune antibodies and cytokine markers, most of the data suggest that there is limited evidence to suggest SARS-CoV-2 directly infects the CNS.[6] Similarly, although controlled animal studies can lead to overexpression of ACE2 receptors and potentially exaggerate the presence of direct viral neurotropism, SARS-CoV-2 RNA levels in human brains are still lower than what is found in the nasal cavity.[7] These findings challenge the idea of direct neuroinvasion of SARS-CoV-2 being the primary pathophysiology.

Regardless of the exact route of viral entry, damage to the neurologic system has also been hypothesized to result from the "cytokine storm" phenomenon, where the excessive cytokine secretion from glial cells can lead to cerebral edema, increased intracranial pressures, and disruption of the blood-brain barrier.[3] This combination of neuroinvasion and viral impact on endothelial cells has particularly affected elderly patients, whom are already at an increased risk for cerebrovascular disease (ie, stroke), vasculitis, and other complications of the CNS, PNS, and musculoskeletal systems. Indirect damage to CNS and PNS through secondary mechanisms, such as hypoxia, sepsis, and multiple organ failure, can also occur. Certain autoantibodies (eg, anti–hypocretin receptor antibody) generated as a response to the infection may also be associated with neurologic sequelae.[4] Additionally, chronically in the convalescence stages, it has been suggested that these viral particles can remain dormant in the CNS and be reactivated.[2] Through this proposed mechanism, SARS-CoV-2 can continue to wreak havoc on the nervous system well after resolution of the acute infection, and these neurologic sequelae can affect patients regardless of the severity of acute illness, further raising the importance of a thorough neurologic examination and continued surveillance for changes post-COVID-19.

Symptom Presentation, Biomarkers, and Neuroimaging

Worldwide, the frequency of neuromuscular and neurologic sequelae associated with COVID-19 can range from 36.4% to 88%.[4] Anosmia, dysgeusia, "brain fog," and headache are some of the most frequently reported residual neurologic symptoms after acute COVID-19.[2] However, there are growing number of cases and observational studies documenting incidence of more severe conditions, such as Guillain-Barré syndrome (GBS), stroke, de novo status epilepticus, and encephalopathy.[8] A more complete list of neurologic conditions associated with COVID-19 is found in **Box 1**.

Serum biomarkers for signs of brain injury, axonal degradation, or blood-brain barrier integrity, such as Glial Fibrillary Acidic Protein (GFAP) and neurofilament light (Nfl), have been shown to be elevated in severe cases,[9] but can also increase with age. In addition to GFAP and Nfl, other markers, such as total Tau ubiquitin carboxyl-terminal esterase L1 (UCH-L1), have also shown to correlate with severity and higher mortality.[10] Other COVID-19-specific biomarkers, such as cytokines and chemokines, is beyond the scope of this article, and there are not enough large population studies to show consistent correlation of these markers with neurologic manifestations.

Box 1
Central and peripheral neurologic/neuromuscular disorders associated with SARS-CoV-2

Guillain-Barré syndrome and variants[a]

Myasthenia gravis

Parsonage-Turner syndrome

Mononeuritis multiplex

Rhabdomyolysis

Critical illness myopathy

Nonspecific encephalopathy[b]

Generalized myoclonus

Transverse myelitis

Cerebrovascular accidents, ischemic and hemorrhagic

Acute necrotizing encephalitis

Leukoencephalopathy

Acute encephalomyelitis

Cerebral venous thrombosis

Posterior reversible leukoencephalopathy syndrome

Demyelinating disorders

Cranial nerve palsies, visual impairments

[a]Miller Fisher syndrome. [b]Examples include acute demyelinating encephalomyelitis, acute necrotizing encephalopathy, Bickerstaff encephalitis, limbic encephalitis.

Clinical and routine use of specific serum biomarkers therefore is unclear, and largely for research purposes at best.

Advanced neuroimaging studies, such as computed tomography (CT), MRI, and PET scans, may be helpful in the early stages with common findings, such as bilateral anterior and posterior white matter hyperintensities on MRI or hypodensities on CT,[11] but it's use in chronic PASC stages is not as clearly defined and can also be limited in interpretation if there is lack of premorbid imaging data. Furthermore, correlating neuroimaging findings with PASC-related neurologic sequelae is difficult when trying to distinguish between findings directly caused by SARS-CoV-2 versus neuropathology findings exacerbated by SARS-CoV-2.[6] Dynamic brain changes, such as hypoperfusion, white matter and gray matter changes, subcortical nuclei volume differences, and cortical thickness changes have been shown even in patients without neurologic manifestations, and although some patients with mild acute infection may have shown some recovery to baseline 10 months later, many patients with severe infection and oftentimes the elderly older than 60 years did not recover to baseline.[12] In the next sections, we review some specific examples as it pertains to the CNS, PNS, and neuromuscular systems.

Central Nervous System Complications

One study showed the most common new-onset central neurologic sequelae were encephalopathies (51%), seizure (12%), stroke (14%), and hypoxic/ischemic injury (11%).[13] These complications can often be associated with poorer prognosis. For example, patients with stroke and COVID-19 have a higher mortality of 39% when compared with patients with stroke without COVID-19,[14] particularly in the acute phase of illness.

Encephalopathies with alteration of consciousness and delirium can result from systemic inflammation, sepsis, and cytokine storm. Viral encephalitis can result from direct neuronal damage and immune-mediated elevated interleukin activity because of the high binding affinity of SARS-CoV-2 to ACE2 receptors. If not acutely reversed or subacutely identified, progression into more severe irreversible damage can occur and lead to worse prognosis and lower survival rate.

For cerebrovascular disease associated with COVID-19, although microbleeds can occur from disruption of blood-brain barrier, ischemic infarcts are the most common.[15,16] Pathophysiology is still largely unknown, but it has been suggested to be related to hypercoagulability because of: (1) viral neuroinvasion that secondarily induced coagulopathy through endothelial inflammation, (2) destabilization of preexisting atheroma plaques, or (3) formation of clots from myocardial damage.[16] Elderly patients with vascular comorbidities are at highest risk, and typically results in multivessel or large territory infarcts with associated severe functional impairments often requiring intensive comprehensive neurorehabilitation.

Seizure disorders associated with COVID-19 are increasing in incidence, either as a result of lowered seizure threshold or as a complication of severe hypoxic brain injury from septic encephalopathy and respiratory failure.[2] One proposal of new-onset seizures, or de novo status epilepticus, is caused by the activation of neuroinflammatory cascade causing more neuronal depolarization and metabolic derangements that can induce status.[17] Seizures are associated with worse functional outcomes and impact rehabilitation potential, so it is paramount to take measures in preventing hypoxia and controlling electrolyte imbalance acutely, optimizing pulmonary hygiene, starting respiratory exercises and progressing to aerobic exercises to improve pulmonary function to help reduce seizure risk.

There have also been reports of multiple sclerosis and antimyelin oligodendrocyte glycoprotein antibody-associated disease associated with COVID-19, but these are rare.[18,19] Cerebellar ataxia and myoclonus have been described after resolution of respiratory symptoms post-COVID-19.[20] Patients with premorbid Parkinson disease (PD) may also experience exacerbations because of COVID-19 infection, but there have also been several case and observational studies suggesting an association with SARS-CoV-2-induced PD in younger patients without family or personal history of PD.[21,22] Viral-induced parkinsonism is not new, because it has been demonstrated with other viruses (HIV, West Nile, herpesvirus), and thought mainly from indirectly causing neurodegeneration of substantia nigra through inflammatory mediators. However, a definitive correlation between SARS-CoV-2 and PD has yet to be established and larger controlled studies are still needed.

Headache is the second most common neurologic symptom post-COVID-19. Prevalence of post-COVID headaches does not seem to vary between hospitalized and nonhospitalized patients but does decrease over time.[23] Cytokine storm and proinflammatory state is thought to contribute to post-COVID-19 headaches, with migraine and tension-type phenotypes being more common. Typical headache features include localizing to bifrontal and temporal regions, throbbing nature, and associations with photophobia and phonophobia. Further discussion of post-COVID headaches is found later in this article.

Other common symptoms, such as smell and taste disturbances, may also persist beyond acute COVID-19 infection, although recent variants (ie, delta and omicron) have been associated with decreased frequency of these symptoms as compared with the alpha strain. Pathophysiology is presumed to be related to damage to olfactory centers of the brain, olfactory receptor neurons, cytokine storm, nasal obstruction, and rhinorrhea.[24] Obtaining an MRI with focus on olfactory bulbs may show thinning and less hyperintensity; however, it can also be normal in patients with anosmia. For gustatory disturbances, there are also a high number of ACE2 receptors in salivary glands and taste buds,[25] making them easy viral targets.

Cognitive impairment post-COVID-19 is consistent with dysexecutive function and more commonly known as "brain fog." In a large retrospective cohort study on neurologic and psychiatric risk trajectories after SARS-CoV-2 infection, risk of cognitive deficits was increased at a 2-year follow-up period up to 36%.[26] Symptoms are primarily impaired short-term memory, decreased attention and concentration, word finding difficulties, and poor executive function. This can also be associated with neuropsychiatric disorders, such as depression, anxiety, posttraumatic stress disorder, and insomnia. More information on this topic is found elsewhere in this issue.

Peripheral Nervous System Complications

PNS involvement can manifest in various ways, such as peripheral neuropathy, nonspecific paresthesias, brachial plexopathies, isolated peripheral facial paralysis, sensorineuronal hearing loss, and compression neuropathies.[4]

GBS is a known, although rare, acute complication of COVID-19. In a systematic review, median onset of GBS post-COVID-19 was 10 days, and typically the demyelinating form.[27] Independent from COVID-19, the ascending paralysis and neuropathy that can occur in more severe cases of GBS can frequently involve the respiratory system. With SARS-CoV-2 being a primarily respiratory illness, concurrent development of GBS because of the proinflammatory cascade activation may further compound an already weakened pulmonary function and lead to more fatality. A subvariant, Miller Fisher syndrome, has been identified in a case study.[28] After acute infection resolution, long-term neurologic sequelae may persist and neurorehabilitation including admission to an inpatient rehabilitation unit may be indicated once pulmonary status is stabilized.

Cranial neuropathies, such as trigeminal neuropathy and abducens nerve palsy, have been reported.[8] Compression neuropathies can also occur, particularly because of supine positioning from prolonged bedrest. Order from most to least common peripheral nerve compression are ulnar, radial, sciatic, brachial plexus, and median nerves.[4] Frequent repositioning and range of motion to avoid prolonged pressure points along elbow and shoulder is important during acute phase of illness.

Implications of autonomic nervous system involvement can manifest as dysautonomia or even postural orthostatic tachycardia syndrome, which is discussed further elsewhere in this issue.

Neuromuscular Complications

Muscle injury and myalgia is a common neurologic sequelae after COVID-19, and in one systematic review, found to be the most common symptom.[29] Generalized nonspecific muscle weakness from prolonged hospital course from severe cases has been described, but there have also been cases where weakness has preceded acute infection as a prodromal symptom.[29] Muscle soreness or myalgias may result from direct injury to muscle secondary to viral inflammation, which may correlate with elevated levels of creatinine kinase. Intensive care unit–acquired weakness can result from myopathic causes, such as critical illness myopathy, critical illness polyneuropathy, or a combination of both. A high clinical suspicion and knowledge of risk factors for critical illness myopathy/critical illness polyneuropathy (meta-analysis data from Yang and colleagues[30] are summarized in **Table 1**) should prompt an electrodiagnostic work-up to better guide rehabilitation interventions.

SARS-CoV-2 can also be associated with neuromuscular junction disorders and autoimmune induced myositis. There have been several case studies describing systemic myasthenia gravis occurring 5 to 7 days after acute COVID-19.[31,32] Like other infections inducing autoimmune neurologic conditions, COVID-19 can potentially trigger this by similar mechanisms. In the case of myasthenia gravis, antibodies against SARS-CoV-2 can potentially interact with acetylcholine receptor subunits or have similarities to components of the neuromuscular junction.[31] Other autoimmune conditions reported include dermatomyositis, which may also induce myositis through activation of the antiviral cytokine type I interferon.[4]

Table 1 Risk factors for intensive care unit–acquired weakness	
Demographics	Female gender
Comorbidities	Multiple organ failure Systemic inflammatory response syndrome Sepsis
Pharmacologic	Neuromuscular blocking agents Aminoglycosides Norepinephrine use
Laboratory studies	Electrolyte disturbance Hyperglycemia Hyperosmolarity Elevated lactate
Others	Parenteral nutrition Duration of mechanical ventilation

Special Discussion: Postvaccination Neurologic Sequelae

Although rare, mRNA vaccines for SARS-CoV-2 have known neurologic adverse re-actions. Several studies have linked certain COVID-19 vaccines to vaccine-induced immune thrombocytopenia, cerebral venous thrombosis, cerebral hemorrhage, bilateral facial nerve palsy, encephalitis, opsoclonus myoclonus syndrome, and GBS.[4] Functional movement disorders have also been reported to be associated with COVID-19 vaccines, which has contributed to vaccine hesitancy and closely related to information spreading from social networking services.[33] Continuing to remain up to date on vaccine guidelines and understanding and weighing the benefits over risks can help inform health care providers to give the best recommendations regarding vaccination.

TREATMENT AND MANAGEMENT APPROACHES

Treatment of most neuromuscular and neurologic symptoms related to COVID-19 is mostly supportive. A multidisciplinary approach is recommended when approaching rehabilitation management for surviving long COVID patients with neurologic and neuromuscular complications. Patients should be considered for intensive inpatient rehabilitation early on and only after medical stability has been achieved to prevent re-lapses during rehabilitation course. Given that these patients may have potential auto-nomic dysfunction and multiorgan involvement, strict monitoring of vital signs should be initiated during dynamic exercises targeting balance, gait, and strength. It is also recommended to develop a gradual progressive exercise program,[34] but also devel-oping an individualized plan depending on patient's specific deficits. Collaboration with subspecialists in physiatry, neurology, cardiology, pulmonary medicine, psychol-ogy, neuropsychology, and psychiatry may be necessary to provide a comprehensive level of care in symptom management and long-term prognosis. General approach to management of a few selected COVID-19-related neurologic symptoms is highlighted in the next subsections.

Headache

A complete history including identifying headache phenotype, triggers, associated symptoms, and premorbid headache history is important. A comprehensive neurologic and musculoskeletal examination that encompasses cranial nerves, sensorimotor evaluation, reflexes, proprioception, and gait assessment is helpful in identifying any findings that may indicate a more focal pathology requiring imaging work-up. Premor-bid headaches can potentially be exacerbated by COVID-19 infection; however, new-onset migraine headaches with auras and positional headaches should prompt more work-up and advanced neuroimaging (CT, MRI) should be considered. Because post-COVID headaches can correlate with neuropsychiatric conditions, optimization of other factors that can worsen headaches, such as sleep disturbances, depression, anxiety, and posttraumatic stress disorder, is also important.

A consensus for pharmacologic management does not exist specifically for post-COVID headaches but given that the migraine phenotype tends to be more com-mon,[35] American Academy of Neurology guidelines for episodic migraine prevention can be followed for management. For example, there is strong Level A evidence for use of antiepileptics (sodium valproate, topiramate, divalproex sodium) and β-blockers (metoprolol, propranolol, timolol) for preventative treatment. Triptans are effective abortive agents in general; however, frovatriptan has strong Level A evidence for menstrual-associated migraines prophylaxis. Magnesium oxide and riboflavin are also effective for migraine prevention.

Smell and Taste Disturbances

Smell disturbances (parosmia) or smell loss (anosmia) can persist beyond the acute infectious period and be a common PASC symptom. There are no current standardized treatment recommendations for smell dysfunction; however, research trials are ongoing. Interventions, such as oral corticosteroids combined with nasal irrigation, palmitoylethanolamide, and luteolin, have been studied but have uncertain conclusive outcomes given small study size.[36] Many other agents, such as intranasal insulin, phosphodiesterase inhibitors, intranasal vitamin A, and zinc, have been studied, but all yielded mostly weak, moderate evidence of efficacy or no benefit or harm identified.[24] Olfactory training with four categories of scents (citrus, flower, spice, herbaceous) done at least twice daily, 10 seconds each nostril, for at least 12 weeks has been the most well-studied and effective therapeutic intervention for postviral anosmia.[37] α-Lipoic acid, often an over-the-counter antioxidant and insulin-memetic supplement, can be prescribed at 600 mg daily for smell dysfunction associated with viral infections,[38] and it is in this author's experience that it has been effective when paired with smell therapy in treating post-COVID anosmia, but it can take at least 3 months of medication administration before effect and further research is still needed to establish more definitive efficacy. However, recently some providers have noticed an increasing number of case reports evidence of neural epidermal growth factor-like 1 (NELL1) associated glomerulonephritis linked to α-lipoic acid administration,[39] with acute presentation of proteinuria and acute nephrotic syndrome that resolved with medication cessation. Although still rare and more studies are needed for formal guidelines to be established, consideration of checking for proteinuria and hypoalbuminemia may be indicated should a patient develop acute-onset edema.

Taste disturbances or dysgeusia can also occur and be challenging to treat. In a case series, stellate ganglion block has been shown to reduce PASC symptoms including dysgeusia, suggesting dysautonomia may play a role.[40] Similar to olfactory dysfunction, data about specific treatment options remain limited.

Other Symptoms

Parkinsonism associated with COVID-19 may respond to traditional dopamine agonists, whereas other cases have described using other agents, such as levodopa/benserazide, pramipexole, and biperiden, to help with motor symptoms.[22] At this time, direct causation between COVID-19 and parkinsonism is still out for debate.

SUMMARY AND FUTURE DIRECTIONS

A wide variety of neurologic and neuromuscular manifestations can occur after COVID-19, and certain complications are associated worse prognosis, lower functional outcome, and higher mortality. Early recognition and continued surveillance for emergence of new neurologic symptoms or persistence of symptoms beyond acute infection as in the case of PASC is challenging given general lack of consensus in diagnostic and therapeutic interventions. Other medical comorbidities and concurrent neuropsychiatric conditions can further confound the clinical picture, so a multidisciplinary approach would be beneficial in providing a comprehensive and individualized care plan.

More research is needed for better understanding of neuropathophysiology to possibly elucidate potential drug targets. Larger scale research studies are still needed to demonstrate efficacy for certain interventions (ie, smell and taste dysfunction). Although there may be evidence of atrophy to certain parts of the brain, changes in cerebral blood flow and cortical thickness associated with post-COVID-19 neurologic changes,[12] correlation of neurologic sequelae, and risk of neurogenerative disorders is speculation at best; however, elderly patients with premorbid vascular risk factors may be at an increased risk of more long-term cognitive impairment.

CLINICS CARE POINTS

- Exact pathophysiology for neurotropic features of SARS-CoV-2 is still unclear; direct neuroinvasion is becoming less probable, but more theories involving cytokine storm and activation of proinflammatory cascade leading to endothelial and blood-brain barrier disruption are more likely.

- Older patients with vascular comorbidities, such as cardiovascular disease and diabetes, are at a higher risk of cerebral microangiopathy, thromboembolism, and subsequent brain atrophy.

- Generalized muscle weakness, muscle injury, and myalgias are the most common neurologic and neuromuscular sequelae; second most common symptom is headache.

- Encephalopathy, cerebrovascular disease, Guillain Barré syndrome, and critical illness myopathy are generally associated with higher mortality and poorer prognosis; depending on severity and medical stability, early rehabilitation intervention may be key to recovery, although long-term sequelae may still be possible.

- Pharmacologic options for specific neurologic symptoms may be limited to supportive management and dependent on existing guidelines for respective diagnoses, although novel interventions and related research are underway.

DISCLOSURE

None.

REFERENCES

1. Jacob S, Kapadia R, Soule T, et al. Neuromuscular complications of SARS-CoV-2 and other viral infections. Front Neurol 2022;13:914411.
2. Camargo-Martínez W, Lozada-Martínez I, Escobar-Collazos A, et al. Post-COVID 19 neurological syndrome: implications for sequelae's treatment. J Clin Neurosci 2021;88:219–25.
3. Monroy-Gómez J, Torres-Fernández O. Effects of the severe acute respiratory syndrome coronavirus (SARS-CoV) and the Middle East respiratory syndrome coronavirus (MERS-CoV) on the nervous system. What can we expect from SARS -CoV-2? Biomedical 2020;40(Suppl. 2):173–9.
4. Shimohata T. Neuro-COVID-19. Clin Exp Neuroimmunol 2022;13(1):17–23.
5. Chowdhary A, Subedi R, Tandon M, et al. Relevance and clinical significance of magnetic resonance imaging of neurological manifestations in COVID-19: a systematic review of case reports and case series. Brain Sci 2020;10(12):1017.
6. Doyle MF. Central nervous system outcomes of COVID-19. Transl Res 2022;241:41–51.
7. Thakur KT, Miller EH, Glendinning MD, et al. COVID-19 neuropathology at Columbia University Irving Medical Center/New York Presbyterian Hospital. Brain 2021;144(9):2696–708.
8. Sharifian-Dorche M, Huot P, Osherov M, et al. Neurological complications of coronavirus infection; a comparative review and lessons learned during the COVID-19 pandemic. J Neurol Sci 2020;417:117085.

9. Kanberg N, Ashton NJ, Andersson LM, et al. Neurochemical evidence of astrocytic and neuronal injury commonly found in COVID-19. Neurology 2020;95: e1754.e9.

10. De Lorenzo R, Lore NI, Finardi A, et al. Blood neurofilament light chain and total tau levels at admission predict death in COVID-19 patients. J Neurol 2021; 268(12):4436–42.

11. Egbert AR, Cankurtaran S, Karpiak S. Brain abnormalities in COVID-19 acute/subacute phase: a rapid systematic review. Brain Behav Immun 2020;89:543–54.

12. Tian T, Wu J, Chen T, et al. Long-term follow-up of dynamic brain changes in patients recovered from COVID-19 without neurological manifestations. JCI Insight 2022;7(4):e155827.

13. Frontera JA, Sabadia S, Lalchan R, et al. A prospective study of neurologic disorders in hospitalized patients with COVID-19 in New York City. Neurology 2021; 96:e575–86.

14. Trejo-Gabriel-Galán JM. Stroke as a complication and prognostic factor of COVID-19. Neurology (Engl Ed) 2020;35(5):318–22.

15. Hernández-Fernández F, Sandoval Valencia H, Barbella-Aponte RA, et al. Cerebrovascular disease in patients with COVID-19: neuroimaging, histological and clinical description. Brain 2020;143(10):3089–103.

16. Fraiman P, Godeiro Junior C, Moro E, et al. COVID-19 and cerebrovascular diseases: a systematic review and perspectives for stroke management. Front Neurol 2020;11:574694.

17. Asadi-Pooya AA. Seizures associated with coronavirus infections. Seizure 2020; 79:49–52.

18. Palao M, Fernández-Díaz E, Gracia-Gil J, et al. Multiple sclerosis following SARS-CoV-2 infection. Mult Scler Relat Disord 2020;45:102377.

19. Pinto AA, Carroll LS, Nar V, et al. CNS inflammatory vasculopathy with antimyelin oligodendrocyte glycoprotein antibodies in COVID-19. Neurol Neuroimmunol Neuroinflamm 2020;7(5):e813.

20. ábano-Suárez P, Bermejo-Guerrero L, Méndez-Guerrero A, et al. Generalized myoclonus in COVID-19. Neurology 2020;95:e767–72.

21. Méndez-Guerrero A, Laespada-García MI, Gómez-Grande A, et al. Acute hypokinetic-rigid syndrome following SARS-CoV-2 infection. Neurology 2020;95: e2109–18.

22. Bouali-Benazzouz R, Benazzouz A. Covid-19 infection and parkinsonism: is there a link? Mov Disord 2021;36(8):1737–43.

23. Fernández-de-Las-Peñas C, Navarro-Santana M, Gómez-Mayordomo V, et al. Headache as an acute and post-COVID-19 symptom in COVID-19 survivors: a meta-analysis of the current literature. Eur J Neurol 2021;28(11):3820–5.

24. Khani E, Khiali S, Beheshtirouy S, et al. Potential pharmacologic treatments for COVID-19 smell and taste loss: a comprehensive review. Eur J Pharmacol 2021;912:174582.

25. Doyle ME, Appleton A, Liu QR, et al. Human type II taste cells express angiotensin-converting enzyme 2 and are infected by severe acute respiratory syndrome coronavirus 2 (SARS-CoV-2). Am J Pathol 2021;191(9):1511–9.

26. Taquet M, Sillett R, Zhu L, et al. Neurological and psychiatric risk trajectories after SARS-CoV-2 infection: an analysis of 2-year retrospective cohort studies including 1 284 437 patients. Lancet Psychiatr 2022;9(10):815–27.

27. De Sanctis P, Doneddu PE, Viganò L, et al. Guillain-Barré syndrome associated with SARS-CoV-2 infection. A systematic review. Eur J Neurol 2020;27:2361–70.

28. Gutiérrez-Ortiz C, Méndez-Guerrero A, Rodrigo-Rey S, et al. Miller Fisher syndrome and polyneuritis cranialis in COVID-19. Neurology 2020;95(5):e601–5.
29. Pinzon RT, Wijaya VO, Buana RB, et al. Neurologic characteristics in coronavirus disease 2019 (COVID-19): a systematic review and meta-analysis. Front Neurol 2020;11:565.
30. Yang T, Li Z, Jiang L, et al. Risk factors for intensive care unit-acquired weakness: a systematic review and meta-analysis. Acta Neurol Scand 2018;138(2):104–14.
31. Restivo DA, Centonze D, Alesina A, et al. Myasthenia gravis associated with SARS-CoV-2 infection. Ann Intern Med 2020;173(12):1027–8.
32. Assini A, Gandoglia I, Damato V, et al. Myasthenia gravis associated with anti-MuSK antibodies developed after SARS-CoV-2 infection. Eur J Neurol 2021; 28(10):3537–9.
33. Hull M, Parnes M. Tics and TikTok: functional tics spread through social media. Mov Disord Clin Pract 2021;8(8):1248–52.
34. Herrera JE, Niehaus WN, Whiteson J, et al. Multidisciplinary collaborative consensus guidance statement on the assessment and treatment of fatigue in postacute sequelae of SARS-CoV-2 infection (PASC) patients. Pharm Manag PM R 2021;13(9):1027–43.
35. Al-Hashel JY, Abokalawa F, Alenzi M, et al. Coronavirus disease-19 and headache; impact on pre-existing and characteristics of de novo: a cross-sectional study. J Headache Pain 2021;22(1):97.
36. O'Byrne L, Webster KE, MacKeith S, et al. Interventions for the treatment of persistent post-COVID-19 olfactory dysfunction. Cochrane Database Syst Rev 2022;9(9):CD013876.
37. Hummel T, Rissom K, Reden J, et al. Effects of olfactory training in patients with olfactory loss. Laryngoscope 2009;119(3):496–9.
38. Hummel T, Heilmann S, Hüttenbriuk KB. Lipoic acid in the treatment of smell dysfunction following viral infection of the upper respiratory tract. Laryngoscope 2002;112(11):2076–80.
39. Spain RI, Andeen NK, Gibson PC, et al. Lipoic acid supplementation associated with neural epidermal growth factor-like 1 (NELL1)-associated membranous nephropathy. Kidney Int 2021;100(6):1208–13.
40. Liu LD, Duricka DL. Stellate ganglion block reduces symptoms of long COVID: a case series. J Neuroimmunol 2022;362:577784.

Cardiovascular Complications of Coronavirus Disease-2019

Carmen M. Terzic, MD, PhD[a,b,*], Betsy J. Medina-Inojosa, MD[b]

KEYWORDS

- COVID-19 • Cardiovascular complications COVID-19
- Post-acute sequelae of SARS-CoV-2 infection • Cardiac • Myocarditis
- Dysrhythmia • Heart failure

KEY POINTS

- Cardiovascular complications are a common manifestation of acute and post-acute coronavirus disease-2019 (COVID-19) infection.
- Complications include cardiomyopathy, myocardial infarction, arrhythmias, heart failure, and deep venous thrombosis.
- Pathophysiology remains poorly defined and complex.
- No single study has proven a distinct treatment of post-COVID-19-associated cardiovascular disease; therefore, it is recommended to follow established guidelines for treating specific cardiovascular conditions.
- Cardiac rehabilitation program is advised for individuals who meet the established criteria for cardiac rehabilitation.

INTRODUCTION

In the initial 3 years of the pandemic, the severe acute respiratory syndrome coronavirus 2 (SARS-CoV-2), the etiologic agent of coronavirus disease-2019 (COVID-19), has infected more than 600 million individuals causing over 6 million deaths.[1] COVID-19 can target multiple systems in the body, including the cardiovascular (CV) system. Multisystemic involvement can be present during the acute phase of the infection and may continue or develop even long-term. This extended presentation of COVID-19 is referred to long COVID, long-haul COVID, and post-acute sequela of SARS-CoV-2 infection (PASC).[2] CV manifestations associated with COVID-19 are

[a] Department of Physical Medicine and Rehabilitation, Cardiovascular Rehabilitation, Rehabilitation Medicine Research Center, Mayo Clinic, 200 First Street Southwest, Rochester, MN 55905, USA; [b] Division of Preventive Cardiology, Department of Cardiovascular Medicine, Mayo Clinic, 200 First Street Southwest, Rochester, MN 55905, USA
* Corresponding author. Mayo Clinic, 200 First Street Southwest, Rochester, MN 55905.
E-mail address: Terzic.carmen@mayo.edu

Phys Med Rehabil Clin N Am 34 (2023) 551–561
https://doi.org/10.1016/j.pmr.2023.03.003

diverse. The spectrum includes symptoms ranging from dyspnea, impaired activity tolerance, palpitations, and chest pain, to more complex syndromes such as cardiomyopathy, myocardial infarction, arrhythmias, heart failure (HF), and deep venous thrombosis.[3] The global burden from cardiovascular disease (CVD) include nearly 18 million death.[4] Owing to the COVID-19 pandemic, this number is to growth, aggravating heart disease's incidence, prevalence, and economic load. The epidemiology of CVD in the setting of prevalent COVID-19 is an area of active investigation, with a particular focus on establishing the paradigm of disease course and its impact on CV health outcomes.

BACKGROUND AND DISCUSSION
Acute Cardiovascular Manifestations of Coronavirus Disease-2019

Acute myocardial injury, defined by an elevation of serum cardiac troponins in the absence of electrocardiographic or echocardiographic evidence of acute ischemia, has been described as the most common and early cardiac abnormality during the acute phase of COVID-19. Initial studies at the pandemic's beginning reported incidences ranging from 1%-100%.[5] More recent studies have placed the incidence of acute myocardial injury in the setting of COVID-19 at ~31%.[6] The reported differences may reflect the significant heterogeneity of the definitions used and the population studied. Despite the difference in reported incidence, all studies showed that levels of cardiac troponin in COVID-19 correlate with clinical disease severity, inflammatory and prothrombotic markers, older age, and the presence of CV risk factors. Moreover, elevated troponin levels were found to be associated with increased in-hospital mortality and arrhythmias.[5,6]

Mechanisms of cardiac injury during the acute phase of COVID-19 include direct and indirect routes. The unique affinity of SARS-CoV-2 for the host angiotensin-converting enzyme 2 (ACE2) receptor raises the possibility of direct viral infection of the vascular endothelium and myocardium.[7] SARS-CoV-2 viral particles have been identified in cardiomyocytes obtained from heart biopsies,[1] supporting the notion of virus invasion.[8] In addition, SARS-CoV-2 can invade endothelial cells and cause endotheliitis. Furthermore, the cytokine storm triggered by the immune response against SARS-CoV-2 might also cause direct cardiac injury. In this regard, a multicenter pathology study found inflammatory cardiac changes, including interstitial macrophage infiltration affecting 86% of the studied patients.[9]

Several lines of evidence also support an indirect mechanism for cardiac injury. Namely, respiratory failure may induce hypoxic injury with an acute imbalance in myocardial oxygen supply without atherothrombosis (type 2 myocardial infarction).[10] In addition, overwhelming cytokine release and excessive Angiotensin II activity may lead to endothelial activation, increased endothelial permeability, vascular inflammation, and inflammation-induced hypercoagulability with intracoronary thrombosis (type I myocardial infarction).[11] In fact, histopathologic and immunohistochemical analysis of COVID-19 cases have shown cardiac fibrin microthrombi and megakaryocytes within the cardiac microvasculature, suggesting that thrombosis may play an important role in myocardial injury during the disease.[11,12] In addition, atherosclerotic plaque instability and rupture, increased metabolic demand, and reduced cardiac reserve with myocardial dysfunction have also been described as potential mechanisms of cardiac injury[13] (**Fig. 1**).

The incidence of myocardial infarction in patients with acute COVID-19 infection remains unclear. A precise diagnosis of ST-elevation myocardial infarction (STEMI) is

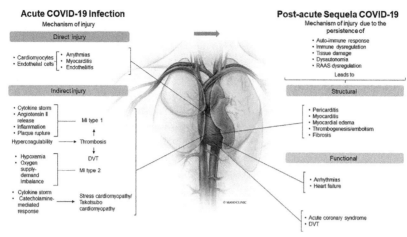

Fig. 1. Summary of potential mechanisms involved in the acute and post-acute cardiac complications of COVID-19 infections. During the acute phase of the infection, myocarditis and arrhythmias are associated with direct viral injury of the myocardium. In contrast, indirect injuries associated with exaggerated inflammatory and hypercoagulability state are postulated to be involved in ischemic events. Long-term complications are linked with persistent autoimmune and inflammatory responses leading to structural changes and functional abnormalities. DVT, deep venous thrombosis; MI, myocardial infarction; RAAS, renin–angiotensin–aldosterone system. (Central illustration Courtesy of [Mayo Foundation for Medical Education and Research, Rochester, Minnesota]; with permission.)

difficult as COVID-19 can cause myocarditis, coronary spasm, and stress cardiomyopathy, all mimicking STEMI. Moreover, during the initial stages of the pandemic, significant concerns regarding the safety of hospital personnel delayed diagnostic and treatment procedures such as percutaneous coronary interventions, limiting an accurate diagnosis of the acute ischemic coronary syndrome.[14] It has been reported that approximately 40% of COVID-19 patients with STEMI did not have obstructive coronary disease suggesting oxygen supply-demand imbalance as the pathophysiological mechanism.[14]

COVID-19 is a significant risk factor for myocarditis, with risk varying by age group. A comprehensive study using an extensive US hospital-based administrative database of health care encounters from >900 hospitals found that among patients with myocarditis ~42% had a history of COVID-19.[15] Although direct myocardial injury is the most common mechanism of viral myocarditis, the exact mechanisms in SARS-CoV-2 infection remain largely unknown.[16,17]

Cardiac arrhythmias are associated with high morbidity and mortality among patients hospitalized with COVID-19 infection, with only half of them reported surviving hospital discharge. Atrial fibrillation was the most common occurring in approximately 80% of patients with arrhythmias, followed by bradyarrhythmia (~23%) and ventricular arrhythmias (~21%).[18] Patients with a high burden of comorbidities and preexisting CVD, including congestive HF and coronary artery disease, were more predisposed to develop arrhythmias during COVID-19 infection.[18] Multiple mechanisms have been hypothesized for the development of arrhythmias, including COVID-19-associated electrolyte disturbances such as hypomagnesemia or hypokalemia. Other influencing factors involve systemic inflammation and viral-induced injury in the cardiac conduction system.[18]

HF in patients with COVID-19 may be precipitated by acute illness, acute hemodynamic stress (eg, acute cor pulmonale), or acute myocardial injury.[19] Patients with a previous history of HF or preexisting heart disease were at risk of acute decompensation, extended hospital stays, increased risk of mechanical ventilation, and mortality.[20] However, 22% of patients with a new diagnosis of HF during acute infection did not have a history or risk factors for CVD.[20]

The presence of Takotsubo cardiomyopathy, a form of nonischemic, stress-induced cardiomyopathy (also known as Gebrochenes-Herz syndrome, transient apical ballooning syndrome, apical ballooning cardiomyopathy, and broken-heart syndrome),[21] has also been demonstrated in COVID-19 patients. It is associated with higher cardiac and inflammatory biomarkers, critical illness, lower ejection fraction, and higher mortality.[22] The mechanism may involve the overwhelming stress caused by the infection with a catecholamine surge, the overactive immune response from cytokine storm, and the development of coronary vasculature dysfunction.[22]

Patients with SARS-CoV-2 infection appear to have a high risk for thromboembolic complications of up to 71%.[14] Localized clot formation rather than diffuse thrombi is also a unique feature in COVID-19 and is seen primarily in the lung vessels.[14] Multiple studies have reported widespread procoagulant/hypercoagulable states, including thrombotic microangiopathy, endothelial dysfunction, bleeding disorder, and thrombosis. The proposed mechanism involves the cytokine storm from excessive inflammation causing endothelial injury and platelet and coagulation factors activation.[23] However, we should remember the traditional Virchow's triad: stasis of flow due to immobilization, intravascular vessel wall damage, and a hypercoagulable state, all present in COVID-19 infection.[24]

Post-acute cardiovascular manifestations of coronavirus disease-2019

The post-acute sequelae or long-term CV complications of COVID-19 are defined as persistent or new symptoms 4 or more weeks after the initial infection. Symptoms and signs may include chest pain, palpitations, impaired activity intolerance, dyspnea, fatigue, and orthostatic manifestations. The seriousness of these symptoms can be variable and are present in individuals without a history of CVD (5% to 29% of patients).[25,26] Specific CV syndromes can also be present and are associated with more severe CV complications of COVID-19 and comprise pericardial effusion, cardiac injury leading to myocarditis, myocardial infarction, left or right ventricular dysfunction, arrhythmias, congestive HF, and nonspecific findings on imaging.[27–31] In fact, 60% of patients present active myocardial inflammation on cardiac magnetic resonance (CRM).[25,26]

A recent study analyzed a cohort of more than 150,000 individuals with COVID-19 using a national health care database from the US Department of Veterans Affairs.[32] Compared with 5.8 million historical and 5.6 million contemporary controls, individuals that experienced COVID-19 infection are at increased risk of ischemic and nonischemic heart disease, myocarditis, pericarditis, arrhythmias, HF, and thromboembolic events.[32] In this study, CV complications were reported in hospitalized and nonhospitalized patients, although the seriousness of the CVD was directly associated with the severity of the initial COVID-19 infection.[32] Furthermore, CV sequela of COVID-19 was present in all age groups, either sex, races, in patients without a history of CVD, and in younger patients without CVD risk factors including hypertension, obesity, hyperlipidemia, and diabetes.[32]

Table 1 summarizes CV complications and reported prevalence during the acute and post-acute infection. A significant variability in the frequency of specific

Table 1	
Cardiovascular complications secondary to coronavirus disease-2019[2,6,14,15,18,25–31,33]	
Acute	**Post-acute Sequelae**
Asymptomatic heart disease	*Symptoms*
Myocarditis 1.4% to 42%	Chest pain 5% to 20%
Pericarditis 3.2%	Palpitations 10% to 20%
Stress-induced cardiomyopathy 2% to 4%	Effort intolerance 12% to 19%
Myocardial infarction (Type I Type 2) 7% to 40%	Dyspnea 18% to 62%
Venous thromboembolism 15% to 21%	Fatigue 32% to 36%
Arrhythmia 18% to 44%	Orthostatic intolerance 10%
Atrial fibrillation/flutter 6.6% to 80%	*Cardiovascular syndromes*
Tachycardia	Pericardial effusion 1% to 30%
Bradycardia 12.8% to 22.6%	Cardiac injury
Ventricular arrhythmia 20.7%	Myocarditis 4% to 60%
Heart failure 22% to 33%	Myocardial infarction 17% to 23%
Left ventricular dysfunction 10% to 16%	Heart failure 10% to 52%
Right ventricular dysfunction 16% to 39%	Left ventricle dysfunction 3% to 18%
Myocardial injury ~31%.	Right ventricle dysfunction 10% to 14%
Cardiogenic shock	Arrhythmias
	Atrial fibrillation 18%
	Ventricular tachycardia/fibrillation 4% to 6%
	Pericarditis 14%
	Venous thromboembolism 15% to 21%
	Myocardial edema and myocardial abnormalities on cardiac magnetic resonance (up to 78%)

symptoms or cardiac syndromes across published studies is present, mainly due to differences in cohort characteristics, study design, and SARS-CoV-2 variants.[27,28,33]

Mechanisms for continuing cardiac injury post-acute infection, are likely multifactorial. Long-term functional and structural cardiac damage due to inflammation associated with viral persistence in the heart tissue, immune dysregulation, and the development of the autoimmune response to cardiac antigens, have been proposed as potential mechanisms.[34] The perseverant inflammation may cause tissue damage and myocardial fibrosis leading to decreased ventricular compliance, impaired myocardial perfusion, increased myocardial stiffness, reduced contractility, and potential arrhythmias.[30,33,34] Neurophysiological mechanisms, such as central nervous system sensitization, have also been proposed as a potential factor to explain CV symptoms such as fatigue, dyspnea, orthostatic intolerance, and impaired activity tolerance in patients with PASC.[35] In addition, it has been shown that patients with PASC had a lower peak oxygen uptake (VO_{2peak}) 30% below predicted, suggesting that abnormal ventilation, circulatory limitations, and deconditioning could be responsible for below-normal cardiorespiratory fitness and explaining some of the cardiac symptoms present in those patients.[36]

EVALUATION AND MANAGEMENT

Considering the high prevalence of CV complications in the post-acute phase of COVID-19, it is highly recommended to perform a comprehensive CV screening in individuals with either CVD risk factors or CV complications during the acute phase. A comprehensive approach for management and follow-up care of CVD associated with COVID-19 has been presented.[33] In brief, the initial evaluation of the patient should include.

- A comprehensive review of COVID-19 past medical history.
- A thorough assessment of lingering symptoms.
- Assessment of mental, physical, and cognitive health.
- Review of risk factors for CVD (obesity, hyperglycemia/diabetes mellitus, hyperlipidemia, tobacco use, sleep apnea, sedentarism, poor nutrition, and stress).
- Assessment of previous tests, cardiology evaluations, and current CV history.
- Evaluation of current medications focusing on those prescribed for CV conditions and medications with potential CV effect (beta-blockers, calcium channel blockers, ACE inhibitors, anti-arrhythmic agents, anticoagulants, antiplatelet agents, antihistaminics, and cold decongestant medications).

A complete CV system examination and laboratory and cardiac tests should be requested to diagnose, treat, and exclude serious pulmonary, thromboembolic, and cardiac complications. These include complete blood count, electrolytes, troponin level, brain natriuretic peptide, D-dimer, C-reactive protein, sedimentation rate, lipid panel, liver function tests, glucose, creatinine, electrocardiogram, echocardiogram, functional capacity testing (stress testing, echo stress test, 6-min walking test). Ambulatory cardiac monitoring (Holter, event monitor) should be requested when palpitations, orthostatic intolerance, and arrhythmias are present. Additional testing is recommended if significant abnormalities are found, including CRM and cardiac computed tomography angiography. Invasive coronary angiography may be indicated for high-risk individuals. Referral to specialist clinics, such as arrhythmia clinic and autonomic dysfunction clinic, is highly recommended. In addition, referral to appropriate services such as physical and occupational therapy, psychology, and social services will provide the necessary support to alleviate the overall burden of the disease.[2,33,34]

In the absence of a distinct proven treatment of CV complications associated with post-acute COVID-19, controlling CVD risk factors, and managing specific CV disorders using current guidelines are recommended.[34,36] Management of viral myocarditis and stress cardiomyopathy should be based on therapy for ventricular dysfunction and arrhythmic risk. Maintaining adequate heart rate control is the preferred strategy when managing atrial fibrillation.[34,36] Primary percutaneous interventions (PCIs) remained the standard of care for STEMI. Guideline-directed medical therapy for long-term care should be administrated, including β-blockers, antiplatelet agents, nitrates, statin, and heparin therapy.[37]

Exercise Interventions

Currently, no evidence-based guidelines for returning or starting an exercise program for patients with CV symptoms associated with COVID-19 have been established. In this regard, the National Institute of Health (NIH) recommendations are valuable in guiding the acute and subacute management of activities and exercises in the setting of COVID-19.[38] In brief, NIH guidelines recommend the following.

- Patients with asymptomatic or mild illness should not exercise for 10 days after symptoms onset or positive test.
- Patients with moderate disease (O_2 saturations >94% at room air) should not exercise for 10 days after the resolution of symptoms.
- Patients with severe illness (O_2 saturations <94% and respiratory rate > 30 breaths/min on room air) requiring hospitalization or supplemental oxygen should refrain from exercises for at least 14 days after resolution of the initial COVID-19 infection symptoms, with a physician or advance practitioner assessing patient symptoms before starting an exercise program.

Box 1
Suggestions for exercise prescription

1. Patients with PASC are diverse in terms of symptom severity, exercise capacity, and perceived functional decline relative to pre-illness abilities. Exercise program individualization is a must.

2. Assessment of exercise capacity with either CPX or the 6-min walk test is advised.

3. Patients with significant functional limitations benefit from physical and/or occupational therapy before beginning a formal exercise program.

4. Start with a small dose of exercise with a gradual progression of duration and intensity.

5. Stop exercise if clinically significant symptoms occur, such as chest pain, palpitations, excessive HR, severe dyspnea, lightheadedness/dizziness, pre-syncope/syncope, excessive fatigue, peripheral edema, headache, and tunnel vision.

6. Participation in supervised exercise in a cardiopulmonary rehabilitation program (center-based, home-based, or hybrid approach) is highly desirable. However, reimbursement may not be available, and some rehabilitation staff may not be adequately prepared to treat patients with PASC.

7. Aerobic exercise prescription specifics based on the acronym FITT-P (frequency, intensity, type, time, progression) are as follows:
   a. *Frequency*: daily; consider multiple brief (<10 min) daily sessions.
   b. *Intensity*: begin with lower intensity (Borg perceived exertion ratings [RPE] of 10 to 11 on the 6- to 20-point scale, HR <60% of maximum).
   c. *Type*: consider starting with non-weight-bearing modes of exercise for individuals with limited capacities and/or orthostatic symptoms: recumbent stationary cycle, recumbent stepper, rowing ergometer.
   d. *Time*: conservative duration at first: >5 to 10 min.
   e. *Progression*: Time: increase by 1 to 3 min/session, as tolerated with a goal duration of 30 to 45 min; intensity: gradually progress to moderate intensity (RPE 12 to 13, HR >80% of maximum); and further progress to moderate to higher intensity (RPE 14 to 17, HR >80% of maximum), as tolerated.

8. Resistance exercise prescription specifics based on the *FITT-P* acronym:
   a. *Frequency*: 2 to 3 sessions/wk on nonconsecutive days.
   b. *Intensity*: perform 10 to 15 slow repetitions of each exercise, RPE 11 to 13 or 40% to 60% of one repetition maximum.
   c. *Time*: one to three sets of 8 to 10 exercises for the major muscle groups; initial focus should be on the lower extremities and body core for patients with POTS-like symptoms. For these patients, gradually add other exercises for the major muscle groups.
   d. *Type*: elastic bands, hand weights, body weight, and weight training machines.
   e. *Progression*: gradual progression of repetitions and resistance, as tolerated.

Abbreviations: CPX, cardiopulmonary exercise testing; HR, heart rate; PASC, post-acute sequelae COVID-19 syndrome; POTS, postural orthostatic tachycardia syndrome.

From: [Smer A, Squires RW, Bonikowske AR, Allison TG, Mainville RN, Williams MA. Cardiac Complications of COVID-19 Infection and the Role of Physical Activity. *J Cardiopulm Rehabil Prev.* Jul 15 2022;https://doi.org/10.1097/hcr.0000000000000701] with permission.

- Patients with myocardial injury, acute coronary syndrome, and arrhythmias require cardiology clearance before exercising and referral to cardiac rehabilitation (CR).

In addition to the NIH recommendations, patients with COVID-19-related myocarditis should not start any CR or exercise program for 3 to 6 months. In this group of patients, if the left ventricular ejection fraction (LVEF) is within normal and no arrhythmias are present, a lighter exercise program can be started 3 months' post-infection.

However, if the patient displays a low LVEF, they should be reevaluated 6 months before any exercise activity decision.[36,39]

Growing clinical experience recommended that eligible individuals who meet the established criteria for CR should be referred to specialized CR programs.[40] Qualified patients include those with evidence of an acute coronary event in the setting of COVID-19 with or without coronary intervention, new myocardial dysfunction or valve disease that required surgical intervention, worsening HF due to COVID-19, and heart transplant following COVID-19.[40] The multidisciplinary and comprehensive approach to CR provided the desirable environment to support individuals with CV complications associated with COVID-19. Rehabilitation interventions for individuals with PASC appear to improve certain clinical outcomes, including quality of life, functional exercise capacity, and dyspnea.[41]

In parallel, exercise recommendations for patients with PASC have been developed based on the comprehensive perspective from multidisciplinary experts in physical medicine and rehabilitation, CR, cardiology, internal medicine, and pulmonary and critical care.[2,36,39] A complete exercise recommendations and prescription are described in **Box 1**.

SUMMARY

CV complications are a common manifestation of acute and PASC infection. They span several CV disorders, including myocardial injury, acute coronary syndromes, myocarditis, cardiomyopathy, arrhythmias, HF, and deep venous thrombosis. The risk and burden of CVD among those who survive the disease are substantial. Studies are necessary to elucidate the interaction between SARS-CoV-2 and the CV system and the biological processes that result in cardiac dysfunction. Evidence for the treatment of CV complications associated with SARS-CoV-2 is lacking and CV manifestations are currently managed following established guidelines developed prior COVID-19 pandemic. Understanding and refining diagnosis, treatment, and exercise interventions are imperative to prevent and manage CV sequela and the progression of CVD in high-risk patients in the context of a lengthy pandemic.

CLINICS CARE POINTS

- At present, no evidence-based guidelines for the management of post-acute cardiovascular complications associated with coronavirus disease-2019 are available.
- Accordingly, implementation of established guidelines for the treatment of specific cardiovascular conditions is recommended.
- Patients who meet the established criteria for cardiac rehabilitation should be referred to specialized programs. Others may benefit from an individualized and gradually progressive exercise program as recommended by a multidisciplinary panel of experts.

DISCLOSURE

All authors declare no conflict of interest.

REFERENCES

1. Bearse M, Hung YP, Krauson AJ, et al. Factors associated with myocardial SARS-CoV-2 infection, myocarditis, and cardiac inflammation in patients with COVID-19. Mod Pathol 2021;34(7):1345–57.

2. Whiteson JH, Azola A, Barry JT, et al. Multi-disciplinary collaborative consensus guidance statement on the assessment and treatment of cardiovascular complications in patients with post-acute sequelae of SARS-CoV-2 infection (PASC). P & M (Philos Med) R 2022;14(7):855.

3. Liu F, Liu F, Wang L. COVID-19 and cardiovascular diseases. J Mol Cell Biol 2021; 13(3):161–7.

4. Tsao CW, Aday AW, Almarzooq ZI, et al. Heart Disease and Stroke Statistics-2022 Update: A Report From the American Heart Association. Circulation 2022; 145(8):e153–639.

5. Sandoval Y, Januzzi JL Jr, Jaffe AS. Cardiac troponin for assessment of myocardial injury in COVID-19: JACC review topic of the week. Journal of the American college of cardiology 2020;76(10):1244–58.

6. Smilowitz NR, Jethani N, Chen J, et al. Myocardial injury in adults hospitalized with COVID-19. Circulation 2020;142(24):2393–5.

7. Jaffe AS, Cleland JG, Katus HA. Myocardial injury in severe COVID-19 infection. Eur Heart J 2020;41(22):2080–2.

8. Weckbach LT, Curta A, Bieber S, et al. Myocardial Inflammation and Dysfunction in COVID-19–Associated Myocardial Injury. Circulation: Cardiovascular Imaging 2021;14(1):e012220.

9. Basso C, Leone O, Rizzo S, et al. Pathological features of COVID-19-associated myocardial injury: a multicentre cardiovascular pathology study. Eur Heart J 2020;41(39):3827–35.

10. Babapoor-Farrokhran S, Gill D, Walker J, et al. Myocardial injury and COVID-19: Possible mechanisms. Life Sci 2020;253:117723.

11. Pellegrini D, Kawakami R, Guagliumi G, et al. Microthrombi as a Major Cause of Cardiac Injury in COVID-19: A Pathologic Study. Circulation 2021;143(10): 1031–42.

12. Bois MC, Boire NA, Layman AJ, et al. COVID-19-Associated Nonocclusive Fibrin Microthrombi in the Heart. Circulation 2021;143(3):230–43.

13. Mitrani RD, Dabas N, Goldberger JJ. COVID-19 cardiac injury: Implications for long-term surveillance and outcomes in survivors. Heart Rhythm 2020;17(11): 1984–90.

14. Giustino G, Pinney SP, Lala A, et al. Coronavirus and Cardiovascular Disease, Myocardial Injury, and Arrhythmia: JACC Focus Seminar. J Am Coll Cardiol 2020;76(17):2011–23.

15. Boehmer TK, Kompaniyets L, Lavery AM, et al. Association between COVID-19 and myocarditis using hospital-based administrative data—United States, March 2020–January 2021. MMWR (Morb Mortal Wkly Rep) 2021;70(35):1228.

16. Escher F, Pietsch H, Aleshcheva G, et al. Detection of viral SARS-CoV-2 genomes and histopathological changes in endomyocardial biopsies. ESC Heart Fail 2020; 7(5):2440–7.

17. Castiello T, Georgiopoulos G, Finocchiaro G, et al. COVID-19 and myocarditis: a systematic review and overview of current challenges. Heart Fail Rev 2022;27(1): 251–61.

18. Coromilas EJ, Kochav S, Goldenthal I, et al. Worldwide survey of COVID-19–associated arrhythmias. Circulation: Arrhythmia and Electrophysiology 2021; 14(3):e009458.

19. Bader F, Manla Y, Atallah B, et al. Heart failure and COVID-19. Heart Fail Rev 2021;26(1):1–10.

20. Alvarez-Garcia J, Jaladanki S, Rivas-Lasarte M, et al. New heart failure diagnoses among patients hospitalized for COVID-19. J Am Coll Cardiol 2021;77(17): 2260–2.

21. Templin C, Ghadri JR, Diekmann J, et al. Clinical Features and Outcomes of Ta-kotsubo (Stress) Cardiomyopathy. N Engl J Med 2015;373(10):929–38.

22. Techasatian W, Nishimura Y, Nagamine T, et al. Characteristics of Takotsubo car-diomyopathy in patients with COVID-19: Systematic scoping review. Am Heart J 2022;100092.

23. Acharya Y, Alameer A, Calpin G, et al. A comprehensive review of vascular com-plications in COVID-19. J Thromb Thrombolysis 2021;53(3):586–93.

24. Acanfora D, Acanfora C, Ciccone MM, et al. The cross-talk between thrombosis and inflammatory storm in acute and long-COVID-19: therapeutic targets and clinical cases. Viruses 2021;13(10):1904.

25. Puntmann VO, Carerj ML, Wieters I, et al. Outcomes of Cardiovascular Magnetic Resonance Imaging in Patients Recently Recovered From Coronavirus Disease 2019 (COVID-19). JAMA Cardiol 2020;5(11):1265–73.

26. Chang W-T, Toh HS, Liao C-T, et al. Cardiac involvement of COVID-19: a compre-hensive review. Am J Med Sci 2021;361(1):14–22.

27. Alkodaymi MS, Omrani OA, Fawzy NA, et al. Prevalence of post-acute COVID-19 syndrome symptoms at different follow-up periods: a systematic review and meta-analysis. Clin Microbiol Infection 2022;28(5):657–66.

28. Groff D, Sun A, Ssentongo AE, et al. Short-term and Long-term Rates of Posta-cute Sequelae of SARS-CoV-2 Infection: A Systematic Review. JAMA Netw Open 2021;4(10):e2128568.

29. Satterfield BA, Bhatt DL, Gersh BJ. Cardiac involvement in the long-term implica-tions of COVID-19. Nat Rev Cardiol 2022;19(5):332–41.

30. Lavelle MP, Desai AD, Wan EY. Arrhythmias in the COVID-19 patient. Heart Rhythm O2 2022;3(1):8–14.

31. Ghantous E, Szekely Y, Lichter Y, et al. Pericardial Involvement in Patients Hospi-talized With COVID-19: Prevalence, Associates, and Clinical Implications. J Am Heart Assoc 2022;11(7):e024363.

32. Xie Y, Xu E, Bowe B, et al. Long-term cardiovascular outcomes of COVID-19. Nat Med 2022;28(3):583–90.

33. Raman B, Bluemke DA, Lüscher TF, et al. Long COVID: post-acute sequelae of COVID-19 with a cardiovascular focus. Eur Heart J 2022;43(11):1157–72.

34. Shah W, Hillman T, Playford ED, et al. Managing the long term effects of covid-19: summary of NICE, SIGN, and RCGP rapid guideline. BMJ 2021;372:n136.

35. Goudman L, De Smedt A, Noppen M, et al. Is Central Sensitisation the Missing Link of Persisting Symptoms after COVID-19 Infection? J Clin Med 2021;10(23): 5594.

36. Smer A, Squires RW, Bonikowske AR, et al. Cardiac Complications of COVID-19 Infection and the Role of Physical Activity. J Cardiopulm Rehabil Prev 2022; 43(1):8–14.

37. Amsterdam EA, Wenger NK, Brindis RG, et al. 2014 AHA/ACC Guideline for the Management of Patients With Non–ST-Elevation Acute Coronary Syndromes. Cir-culation 2014;130(25):e344–426.

38. Panel C-TG. Coronavirus Disease 2019 (COVID-19) Treatment Guidelines. Na-tional Institutes of Health. https://www.covid19treatmentguidelines.nih.gov/. Pub-lished 2022. Accessed 28 November, 2022.

39. Vanichkachorn G, Newcomb R, Cowl CT, et al. Post-COVID-19 Syndrome (Long Haul Syndrome): Description of a Multidisciplinary Clinic at Mayo Clinic and Characteristics of the Initial Patient Cohort. Mayo Clin Proc 2021;96(7):1782–91.
40. Taylor RS, Dalal HM, McDonagh STJ. The role of cardiac rehabilitation in improving cardiovascular outcomes. Nat Rev Cardiol 2022;19(3):180–94.
41. Fugazzaro S, Contri A, Esseroukh O, et al. Rehabilitation Interventions for Post-Acute COVID-19 Syndrome: A Systematic Review. Int J Environ Res Public Health 2022;19(9):5185.

Autonomic Dysfunction Related to Postacute SARS-CoV-2 Syndrome

Justin Haloot, DO, MS[a], Ratna Bhavaraju-Sanka, MD[b,*],
Jayasree Pillarisetti, MD, MSc[c], Monica Verduzco-Gutierrez, MD[d]

KEYWORDS

- PASC • Autonomic dysfunction • COVID-19 • Brain fog • Tilt table test

KEY POINTS

- Autonomic dysfunction related to postacute SARS-CoV-2 can present with dizziness, tachycardia, sweating, headache, syncope, labile blood pressure, exercise intolerance, and "brain fog."
- Nonpharmacologic management involves increased salt and water intake, compression garments, progressive aerobic exercises, and enhanced external counterpulsation.
- Pharmacologic treatment can include β-blockers, fludrocortisone, midodrine, pyridostigmine, and ivabradine.

INTRODUCTION

The SARS-CoV-2 virus, a member of the coronavirus family, has been responsible for the coronavirus disease-2019 (COVID-19) pandemic with an acute phase causing pneumonia and pulmonary disorders, but it has been shown to result in extrapulmonary manifestations including cardiovascular and neurologic diseases. Moreover, residual symptoms have been reported to persist past the acute phase. In a cross-sectional study of SARS-CoV-2–positive patients, at 48 days postdischarge the most common persistent symptoms were fatigue, difficulty breathing, and psychological distress.[1] In a cohort study of 1733 patients with COVID-19 from Wuhan, China, patients reported persistence of fatigue, muscle weakness, sleeping difficulties,

[a] Department of Internal Medicine, University of Texas Health Science Center at San Antonio, 7703 Floyd Curl Drive, San Antonio, TX 78229-3900, USA; [b] Department of Neurology, UT Health San Antonio, Joe R. & Theresa Lozano Long School of Medicine, 7703 Floyd Curl Drive, Mail Code 7883, San Antonio, TX 78229, USA; [c] Janey & Dolph Briscoe Division of Cardiology, 7703 Floyd Curl Drive, San Antonio, TX 78229, USA; [d] Department of Rehabilitation Medicine, Joe R. & Teresa Lozano Long School of Medicine, UT Health at San Antonio Texas, 7703 Floyd Curl Drive, Room 628E, San Antonio, TX 78229, USA
* Corresponding author.
E-mail address: BhavarajuSan@uthscsa.edu

Phys Med Rehabil Clin N Am 34 (2023) 563–572
https://doi.org/10.1016/j.pmr.2023.04.003
1047-9651/23/© 2023 Elsevier Inc. All rights reserved.

palpitations, anxiety, or depression at 6 months after initial onset.[2] Numerous other studies now indicate the presence of persistent symptoms following COVID-19 infection, with more than 200 symptoms reported. This syndrome has been coined as the postacute SARS-CoV-2 (PASC) syndrome and has been defined as the persistence of symptoms or development of new symptoms after the time of infection, which can include fatigue, brain fog, palpitations, and a plethora of other manifestations.

BACKGROUND

Infection with SARS-CoV-2 in the acute phase can lead to extrapulmonary manifestations including fatigue, myalgias, gastrointestinal dysfunction, as well as cardiovascular complications.[3–6] It has also been reported that SARS-CoV-2 infection can have neurologic involvement in more than one-third of acute infections.[7] In a meta-analysis of patients with acute COVID-19 of more than 1585 records, acute SARS-CoV-2 infection can lead to autonomic dysfunction during the acute stages in terms of cardiovascular, sudomotor, and pupillometric functions.[8]

However, there have been growing reports that patients continue to remain unwell beyond 3 weeks.[9] In a systematic review of 57 studies, it was found that 250,351 survivors of acute COVID-19 had persistent symptoms after 6 months of initial diagnosis that could be divided into 4 major categories: neurologic symptoms, generalized symptoms, mental health disorders, and mobility impairment.[10] The same study reported common symptoms including headaches, difficulty concentrating, cognitive impairment, fatigue, functional impairment, and mobility decline. Therefore, postacute COVID syndrome continues to remain an ongoing issue that requires more examination.

Currently, there have been multiple names and criteria for this postacute phase COVID-19 syndrome. The Mayo Clinic uses the term "long COVID" to refer to long-term sequelae that occurred on or after the initial positive SARS-CoV-2 test.[11] Meanwhile, the United Kingdom National Institute for Health and Care Excellence (NICE) has defined various phases of COVID-19 including "post-COVID-19 syndrome" for symptoms that develop around the acute phase and persist for more than 12 weeks that are not explained by an alternative diagnosis and "long COVID" that describes symptomatic COVID-19 and post-COVID-19 syndrome based on the criteria.[12] In addition, a common term used has been postacute COVID-19 syndrome (PACS) and PASC and defined as the persistence of symptoms for more than 3 weeks after the initial onset of COVID-19.[13]

The mechanism of postacute COVID-19 autonomic dysfunction is thought to be multifactorial.[14] One major proposed mechanism is through direct viral effects with multiple hypotheses. Persistent viremia can lead to a persistent highly inflammatory state with cellular injury.[15–19] One of the proposed pathophysiology is cytokine- and hypoxia induced injury leading to neuronal apoptosis affecting the while matter fiber bundles causing impaired neurological function. Another hypothesis is that this inflammatory pathway could lead to autonomic and small fiber neuropathies, as previously seen in viral infections from herpes simplex and infectious mononucleosis.[20,21]

POSTACUTE AUTONOMIC MANIFESTATIONS OF CORONAVIRUS DISEASE-2019

In a systematic review involving 54 articles involving 154 cases of COVID-19, the most common clinical presentation was orthostatic intolerance (including orthostatic light-headedness, dizziness, tachycardia, sweating, headache, and "brain fog") and syncope (including reflex and orthostatic hypotension-related syncope) **(Fig. 1)**.[22] Orthostatic intolerance has been defined as the inability to tolerate the upright position due to symptoms caused by cerebral hypoperfusion, sympathetic activation, or

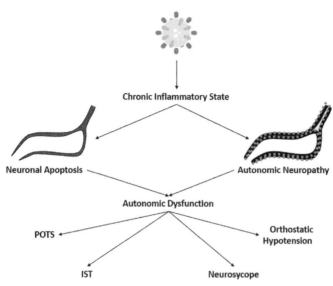

Fig. 1. Mechanism of post-acute SARS-CoV-2 autonomic dysfunction.

both and is relieved by recumbency.[23] In a prospective study of 24 patients with PASC, 23 demonstrated orthostatic intolerance based on the head-up tilt table test (HUTT).[24] In the same study, they found that these patients can present with postural orthostatic tachycardia syndrome (POTS), inappropriate sinus tachycardia, neurocardiogenic syncope (NCS), and orthostatic hypotension.

POTS, characterized by partial dysautonomia and hyperadrenergic orthostatic intolerance, typically affects young high-achieving adults, particularly Caucasian women of childbearing age who are at the beginning of their working lives.[25] POTS is heterogeneous in presentation and is associated with palpitations, dizziness, headache, fatigue, and blurry vision.[26–28] Typically, POTS is diagnosed by a tilt table test or 10-minute stand test and is characterized by an increase in heart rate of at least 30 beats per minute (bpm) from supine to standing position in the absence of orthostatic hypotension.[11,29] Before the arrival of COVID-19, approximately 50% of patients with POTS report a history of infection before symptom onset.[11,30] Most reported infections associated with POTS included mycoplasma pneumonia,[31] Epstein-Barr virus,[32,33] Trypanosoma cruzi,[34] and Borrelia burgdorferi.[35,36] Now, since the inception of the SARS-CoV-2 virus, POTS seems to be a prevalent manifestation of PASC syndrome, with this viral infection being an inciting event.

Similarly, inappropriate sinus tachycardia (IST) has been characterized by unexpected fast sinus rates (greater than 100 beats bpm) at rest and/or with minimal physical activity and can be accompanied by symptoms including palpitations, dyspnea, or dizziness.[37] Typically, IST can be diagnosed based on resting heart rate greater than 100 bpm with an average rate greater than 90 beats bpm on a 24-hour Holter monitor in symptomatic patients.[37] The underlying pathophysiology is not completely understood, although it may be related to sinus node automaticity or autonomic imbalance. It has been seen in patients with Trypanosoma cruzi antibodies that cross-react with beta receptors and stimulate tachycardia.[38,39] In a recent study of 200 patients with PASC, 20% were found to have inappropriate sinus tachycardia and can commonly affect younger women without previous comorbidities who have had a mild initial SARS-CoV-2 infection.[40] It is suggested that IST in these patients may be related to autonomic dysfunction due to decreased heart rate variability based on 24-hour electrocardiogram (ECG) monitoring.

NCS has been reported as the most common cause of syncope, with a median of 3 episodes in a lifetime and a recurrence rate of 30% within 30 months.[41] There have been case reports of NCS.[42,43] There may be some overlap between neurogenic syncope with POTS, as NCS can occur in up to 38% of patients with POTS.[35,44–46]

Orthostatic hypotension, defined as a drop of systolic blood pressure by at least 20 mm Hg or drop of diastolic blood pressure by at least 10 minutes within 3 minutes of standing from a supine position, has been accompanied by similar symptoms of dizziness and syncope. It often involves excessive pooling of blood into the splanchnic and leg circulation, leading to decreased venous return with change to standing position and resulting in decreased cardiac output.[47] Typically, the autonomic nervous system can compensate with changes in vascular tone, heart rate, and cardiac contractility. However, in neurogenic orthostatic hypotension, there may be a defective or delayed response.[47] Similarly, there have been case reports of orthostatic hypotension as a presenting symptom of autonomic dysfunction in patients with PASC.[22]

EVALUATION AND MANAGEMENT

The initial evaluation should begin with a detailed history and physical examination with particular attention to symptoms including dizziness, lightheadedness, fatigue, dyspnea, diarrhea or constipation, presyncope, anxiety, panic attacks, and brain fog.[48] Vital signs evaluation should include a review of blood pressure, heart rate, breathing rate, oxygen saturation, and pain scale. Physical examination should include a full neurologic examination (involving cranial nerve evaluation, sensory and motor function, deep tendon reflexes, and coordination), pulmonary evaluation, cardiovascular examination, musculoskeletal tone and range of motion, skin exam for rashes, and psychiatric evaluation.

The Composite Autonomic Symptom Scale (COMPASS-31) questionnaire, originally developed as an 84-question scoring instrument for autonomic symptoms,[49] has been growing in use for patients with PASC.[50] The survey has been validated in patients with autonomic dysfunction and seems to be a quick and efficient method to have patients with PASC screened.

Initial laboratory evaluation should include a complete blood cell count, renal function panel, B-type natriuretic peptide, electrolytes, thyroid stimulating hormone, morning cortisol, and resting 12-lead ECG. Based on the history, physical examination, and clinical evaluation, further laboratory testing may be warranted. There has been a high prevalence of G-protein–coupled receptor antibodies and ganglionic neuronal nicotinic acetylcholine receptor antibodies in patients with PASC and POTS.[51] POTS itself has also been reported to be associated with antinuclear, antithyroid, anti-NMDA glutamate receptor, antiphospholipid, and Sjogren antibodies and may be reasonably considered in patients with PASC with POTS if clinically appropriate.[51]

The 3-minute standing test, involving patients going from the supine position to the standing position, has been recommended by the Centers of Disease Control and Prevention and can be used as a quick and easy method for evaluating autonomic dysfunction in patients with PASC.[52] In addition to the standing test, the HUTT uses a similar concept but requires patients to be on a table with restraining belts, and the table moves into supine and upright vertical positions that can leave patients feeling uncomfortable. Despite this, the HUTT has been the most used autonomic testing mechanism in patients with PASC with concerns for cardiac autonomic dysfunction.[22]

In addition, Holter ECG monitoring and 24-hour ambulatory blood pressure monitoring can also be used in patients with PASC to evaluate for autonomic dysfunction[53]; this would particularly allow close examination for heart rate variability (HRV) in sitting and standing positions. Before COVID-19, reduced HRV has been associated with chronic fatigue syndrome and myalgic encephalomyelitis[54] and has been a tool used to evaluate autonomic nervous system functions.[8]

If further testing is needed, an examination can involve skin biopsy for intraepidermal nerve fiber density evaluating for small fiber (aδ and C fiber) neuropathy and quantitative sudomotor axon reflex test to evaluate postganglionic sympathetic cholinergic sudomotor function by evaluating sweat response time.[55] Similarly, the thermoregulatory sweat test evaluates the central and peripheral sympathetic sudomotor pathways from central nervous system to the sweat glands.[56] Electrochemical skin conductance (ESC) is a noninvasive test of sudomotor function. It is an indirect index of sympathetic nonmyelinated C-fiber activity and be estimated with ESC, due to the lack of parasympathetic innervation in the skin.[57] An abnormal ESC result can also suggest autonomic small fiber neuropathy and autonomic dysfunction in patients with PASC.

TREATMENT

With autonomic dysfunction, initial treatment can include conservative and nonpharmacological measures including increased water consumption of up to 2 to 3 L per day, increased sodium consumption of up to 10 to 12 g per day, lower limb compression stockings, and progressive aerobic exercise training programs that start in supine or sitting position for physical reconditioning. It is also important to review the existing medication and supplementation list to remove agents that can worsen the symptoms of autonomic dysfunction (anticholinergics, antihypertensives, and so forth)

Multidisciplinary care can play an essential role in the treatment and management of these patients. Primary care, neurology, physical medicine and rehabilitation, cardiology, neuropsychologists, psychiatrists, occupational therapists, physical therapists, speech therapists, and dietitians may be part of the care team to assist with the complex syndrome of PASC autonomic dysfunction.[10,58,59] Rehabilitation therapeutics include breathwork exercises, yoga/pranayama, autonomic reconditioning, symptom-titrated physical activity/movement, and functional restoration.

If symptoms persist despite the above measures, pharmacologic management may be considered. The Heart Rhythm Society recommends medical management with fludrocortisone, midodrine, pyridostigmine, β-blockers (specifically propranolol), or ivabradine.[37] However, ivabradine is still being studied for safety and efficacy in patients with a specific subtype of POTS.[60] These therapies can theoretically help with volume expansion (fludrocortisone), heart rate inhibition (propranolol, ivabradine, and pyridostigmine), and vasoconstriction (midodrine) that may help with autonomic dysfunction response (**Table 1**).

There have been case reports where enhanced external counterpulsation (EECP), a noninvasive therapy that involves retrograde aortic flow to decrease the number of inflammatory cytokines, has been added as a suitable treatment method for patients with PASC.[61,62] EECP has been approved by Food and Drug Administration and shown to improve morbidity and mortality for patients with chronic stable angina or ischemic heart failure. The benefit has been theorized to be due to vascular changes and improve endothelial function by affecting vasodilation and proinflammatory agents.[63] Therefore, EECP may improve response to PASC autonomic dysfunction.

Blitshteyn and colleagues made additional multidisciplinary recommendations for evaluating and treating PASC-related autonomic dysfunction, and their consensus

Table 1
Options for pharmacologic treatment

Drug	Mechanism of Action	Dosing	Side Effects
Propranolol	Reduces HR by beta-adrenergic blockade	10–20 mg up to 4 times a day	Bradycardia, hypotension, fatigue, bronchospasm
Fludrocortisone	Volume expansion	0.1–0.2 mg daily	Hypokalemia, edema, headache
Desmopressin (DDAVP)	Volume expansion	0.1–0.2 mg daily	Hyponatremia, edema
Midodrine	Vasoconstriction	2.5–15 mg 3 times a day	Headache, scalp tingling, hypertension
Pyridostigmine	Cholinergic, reduces HR	30–60 mg 3 times a day	Nausea, abdominal cramps, diarrhea
Ivabradine	Reduces HR	2.5–7.5 mg twice a day	Headache, palpitations, hypertension, visual disturbance

Abbreviation: HR, heart rate.

guidance was published in 2022 and is now accessible.[64] In the authors' preliminary study looking at 42 patients with PASC-related autonomic dysfunction, despite treatments, they continue to be symptomatic at 1 year since PASC onset with mild to moderate improvement of their symptoms. Long-term follow-up and studies are needed to bring the much-needed respite for these symptoms.

CLINICS CARE POINTS

- There are several subtypes of autonomic dysfunction related to postacute SARS-CoV-2 including postural orthostatic tachycardia syndrome (POTS), inappropriate sinus tachycardia, neurocardiogenic syncope (NCS), and orthostatic hypotension.

- Evaluation beyond a history and physical, should be inclusive of a Composite Autonomic Symptom Scale (COMPASS-31) questionnaire and a 3-minute standing test. The head-up tilt table test (HUTT) can be done when there is concern for cardiac autonomic dysfunction and stand test is nondiagnostic.

- Treatment for autonomic dysfunction should include both conservative and nonpharmacological management to start. It is also imperative to consider pharmacologic management to help treat symptoms.

DISCLOSURES

None related to this work.

REFERENCES

1. Halpin SJ, McIvor C, Whyatt G, et al. Postdischarge symptoms and rehabilitation needs in survivors of Covid-19 infection: A cross-sectional evaluation. J Med Virol 2020;93(2):1013–22.
2. Huang C, Huang L, Wang Y, et al. 6-Month Consequences of COVID-19 in Patients Discharged from Hospital: A Cohort Study, Lancet, 397 (10270), 2021, 220–232.
3. Zhu N, Zhang D, Wang W, et al. A novel coronavirus from patients with pneumonia in China, 2019. N Engl J Med 2020;382:727–33.
4. Chan JF, Yuan S, Kok KH, et al. A familial cluster of pneumonia associated with the 2019 novel coronavirus indicating person-to-person transmission: a study of a family cluster. Lancet 2020;395:514–23.
5. Huang C, Wang Y, Li X, et al. Clinical features of patients infected with 2019 novel coronavirus in Wuhan, China. Lancet 2020;395:497–506.
6. Kang Y, Chen T, Mui D, et al. Cardiovascular manifestations and treatment considerations in COVID-19. Heart 2020;106:1132–41.
7. Mao L, Jin H, Wang M, et al. Neurologic Manifestations of Hospitalized Patients With Coronavirus Disease 2019 in Wuhan, China. JAMA Neurol 2020;77:683–90.
8. Scala I, Rizzo PA, Bellavia S, et al. Autonomic Dysfunction during Acute SARS-CoV-2 Infection: A Systematic Review. J Clin Med 2022;11(13):3883.
9. Kings College London. COVID symptom study. how long does COVID-19 last? 2020. Available: https://covid19. joinzoe. com/post/covid- long- term? fbclid= IwAR1RxIcmmdLEFjh_al-.
10. Groff D, Sun A, Ssentongo AE, et al. Short-term and Long-term Rates of Postacute Sequelae of SARS-CoV-2 Infection: A Systematic Review. JAMA Netw Open 2021;4(10):e2128568.

11. Thieben MJ, Sandroni P, Sletten DM, et al. Postural orthostatic tachycardia syndrome: the Mayo clinic experience. Mayo Clin Proc 2007;82(3):308–13.

12. National Institute for Health and Care Excellence (NICE) (2021) COVID-19 rapid guideline: managing the long-term effects of COVID-19. https://www. nice. org. uk/guida nce/ng188. Accessed 30 Dec 2021.

13. Dixit NM, Churchill A, Nsair A, et al. Post-Acute COVID-19 Syndrome and the cardiovascular system: What is known? Am Heart J 2021;5:100025.

14. Becker RC. Autonomic dysfunction in SARS-COV-2 infection acute and long-term implications COVID-19 editor's page series. J Thromb Thrombolysis 2021;52: 692–707.

15. Oronsky B, Larson C, Hammond TC, et al. A review of persistent post-COVID syndrome (PPCS). Clin Rev Allergy Immunol. 2021;1-9.

16. Lan L, Xu D, Ye G, et al. Positive RT-PCR test results in patients recovered from COVID-19. JAMA 2020;323(15):1502–3. https://doi.org/10.1001/jama.2020.2783.

17. Ellul MA, Benjamin L, Singh B, et al. Neurological associations of COVID-19. Lancet Neurol 2020;19(9):767–83. https://doi.org/10.1016/S1474-4422(20)30221-0.

18. Colafrancesco S, Alessandri C, Conti F, et al. COVID-19 gone bad: a new character in the spectrum of the hyperferritinemic syndrome? Autoimmun Rev 2020; 19(7):102573.

19. Baig AM, Khaleeq A, Ali U, et al. Evidence of the COVID-19 virus targeting the CNS: tissue distribution, host–virus interaction, and proposed neurotropic mechanisms. ACS Chem Neurosci 2020;11(7):995–8. https://doi.org/10.1021/acschemneuro. 0c00122.

20. Neville BG, Sladen GE. Acute autonomic neuropathy following primary herpes simplex infection. J Neurol Neurosurg Psychiatry 1984;47:648–50.

21. Vassallo M, Camilleri M, Caron BL, et al. Gastrointestinal motor dysfunction in acquired selective cholinergic dysautonomia associated with infectious mononucleosis. Gastroenterology 1991;100:252–8.

22. Reis Carneiro D, Rocha I, Habek M, et al. Clinical presentation and management strategies of cardiovascular autonomic dysfunction following a COVID-19 infection - A systematic review. Eur J Neurol 2023. https://doi.org/10.1111/ene.15714. Epub ahead of print. PMID: 36694382.

23. Cutsfort-Gregory JK. Postural tachycardia syndrome and neurally mediated syncope. Continuum 2020;26:93–115.

24. Jamal SM, Landers DB, Hollenberg SM, et al. Prospective Evaluation of Autonomic Dysfunction in Post-Acute Sequela of COVID-19. J Am Coll Cardiol 2022;79(23):2325–30.

25. Shaw BH, Stiles LE, Bourne K, et al. The face of postural tachycardia syndrome - insights from a large cross-sectional online community-based survey. J Intern Med 2019;286(4):438–48. https://doi.org/10.1111/joim.12895.

26. Fedorowski A. Postural orthostatic tachycardia syndrome: clinical presentation, aetiology and management. J Intern Med 2019;285:352–66.

27. Bryarly M, Phillips LT, Fu Q, et al. Postural orthostatic tachycardia syndrome: JACC focus seminar. J Am Coll Cardiol 2019;73:1207–28.

28. Schondorf R, Low PA. Idiopathic postural orthostatic tachycardia syndrome: an attenuated form of acute pandysautonomia? Neurology 1993;43:132–7.

29. Raj SR, Guzman JC, Harvey P, et al. Canadian Cardiovascular Society position statement on postural orthostatic tachycardia syndrome (POTS) and related disorders of chronic orthostatic intolerance. Can J Cardiol 2020;36:357–72.

30. Sandroni P, Opfer-Gehrking TL, McPhee BR, et al. Postural tachycardia syndrome: clinical features and follow-up study. Mayo Clin Proc 1999;74:1106–10. https://doi.org/10.4065/74.11.1106.

31. Kasmani R, Elkambergy H, Okoli K. Postural orthostatic tachycardia syndrome associated with mycoplasma pneumoniae. Infect Dis Clin Pract 2009;17:342–3. https://doi.org/10.1097/IPC.0b013e318191781b.

32. Pohlgeers KM, Stumbo JR. Syncope in an athlete: a case of infectious mononucleosis induced postural tachycardia syndrome. Curr Sports Med Rep 2016;15: 41–5. https://doi.org/10.1249/JSR.0000000000000227.

33. Yaxley KL. Infectious mononucleosis complicated by peritonsillar abscess and postural orthostatic tachycardia syndrome: a case report. SAGE Open Med Case Rep 2020;8. https://doi.org/10.1177/2050313X20915413. 2050313X20915413.

34. Palmero HA, Caeiro TF, Josa DJ. Distinctive abnormal responses to tilting test in chronic Chagas' disease. Klin Wochenschr 1980;58:1307–11. https://doi.org/10. 1007/BF01478139.

35. Kanjwal K, Karabin B, Kanjwal Y, et al. Postural orthostatic tachycardia syndrome following Lyme disease. Cardiol J 2011;18:63–6. https://doi.org/10.1097/MJT. 0b013e3181da0763.

36. Noyes AM, Kluger J. A tale of two syndromes: lyme disease preceding postural orthostatic tachycardia syndrome. Ann Noninvasive Electrocardiol 2015;20:82–6. https://doi.org/10.1111/anec.12158.

37. Sheldon RS, Grubb BP, Olshansky B, et al. Heart rhythm society expert consensus statement on the diagnosis and treatment of postural tachycardia syndrome, inappropriate sinus tachycardia, and vasovagal syncope. Heart Rhythm 2015;12(6):e41–63.

38. Chiale PA, Garro HA, Schmidberg J, et al. Inappropriate sinus tachycardia may be related to an immunologic disorder involving cardiac β andrenergic receptors. Heart Rhythm 2006;3(10):1182–6.

39. Baruscotti M, Bianco E, Bucchi A, et al. Current understanding of the pathophysiological mechanisms responsible for inappropriate sinus tachycardia: Role of the if "funny" current. J. Interv. Card. Electrophysiol. 2016;46:19–28.

40. Aranyó J, Bazan V, Lladós G, et al. Inappropriate sinus tachycardia in post-COVID-19 syndrome. Sci Rep 2022;12(1):298.

41. Baron-Esquivias G, Morillo CA. Definitive pacing therapy in pateints with neuromediated syncope. Lessons from the SPAIN study. Rev Esp cardio 2018;71: 320–2.

42. Shouman K, Vanichkachorn G, Cheshire WP, et al. Autonomic dysfunction following COVID-19 infection: an early experience. Clin Auton Res 2021;31(3):385–94.

43. Blitshteyn S, Whitelaw S. Postural orthostatic tachycardia syndrome (POTS) and other autonomic disorders after COVID-19 infection: a case series of 20 patients. Immunol Res 2021;69(2):205–11.

44. Ojha A, McNeeley K, Heller E, et al. Orthostatic syndromes differ in syncope frequency. Am J Med 2010;123:245–9.

45. Chouksey D, Rathi P, Sodani A, et al. Postural orthostatic tachycardia syndrome in patients of orthostatic intolerance symptoms: an ambispective study. AIMS Neurosci 2020;8(1):74–85.

46. Raj SR. The Postural Tachycardia Syndrome (POTS): pathophysiology, diagnosis & management. Indian Pacing Electrophysiol J 2006;6(2):84–99.

47. Freeman R, Wieling W, Axelrod FB, et al. Consensus statement on the definition of orthostatic hypotension, neurally mediated syncope and the postural tachycardia syndrome. Clin Auton Res 2011;21:69–72.

48. Dani M, Dirksen A, Taraborrelli P, et al. Autonomic dysfunction in 'long COVID': rationale, physiology and management strategies. Clin Med 2021;21. https://doi.org/10.7861/clinmed.2020-0896. e63–e7.
49. Sletten DM, Suarez GA, Low PA, et al. COMPASS 31: a refined and abbreviated Composite Autonomic Symptom Score. Mayo Clin Proc 2012;87(12):1196–201.
50. Buoite Stella A, Furlanis G, Frezza NA, et al. Autonomic dysfunction in post-COVID patients with and witfhout neurological symptoms: A prospective multidomain observational study. J Neurol 2021. https://doi.org/10.1007/s00415-021-10735-y.
51. Fedorowski A. Postural orthostatic tachycardia syndrome: clinical presentation, aetiology and management. J Intern Med 2019;285:352–66. https://doi.org/10.1111/joim.12852.
52. Centers for Disease Control and Prevention: evaluating and caring for patients with post-COVID conditions: interim guidance. https://www.cdc.gov/coronavirus/2019-ncov/hcp/clinical-care/post-covid-index.html (2021). Accessed March 21, 2023.
53. Davido B, Seang S, Tubiana R, et al. Post-COVID-19 chronic symptoms: a post-infectious entity? Clin Microbiol Infect 2020;26:1448–9. https://doi.org/10.1016/j.cmi.2020.07.028.
54. Escorihuela RM, Capdevila L, Castro JR, et al. Reduced heart rate variability predicts fatigue severity in individuals with chronic fatigue syndrome/myalgic encephalomyelitis. J Transl Med 2020;18:4. https://doi.org/10.1186/s12967-019-02184-z.
55. Low PA, Caskey PE, Tuck RR, et al. Quantitative sudomotor axon reflex test in normal and neuropathic subjects. Ann Neurol 1983;14:573–80.
56. Fealey RD, Low PA, Thomas JE. Thermoregulatory sweating abnormalities in diabetes mellitus. Mayo Clin Proc 1989;64:617–28.
57. Bellavia S, Scala I, Luigetti M, et al. Instrumental Evaluation of COVID-19 Related Dysautonomia in Non-Critically-Ill Patients: An Observational, Cross-Sectional Study. J Clin Med 2021;10(24):5861.
58. Nasserie T, Hittle M, Goodman SN. Assessment of the frequency and variety of persistent symptoms among patients with COVID-19: a systematic review. JAMA Netw Open 2021;4(5):e2111417. https://doi.org/10.1001/jamanetworkopen.2021.11417.
59. Sivan M, Taylor S. NICE guideline on long COVID. BMJ 2020;371:m4938. https://doi.org/10.1136/bmj.m4938.
60. Taub PR, Zadourian A, Lo HC, et al. Randomized trial of ivabradine in patients with Hyperadrenergic postural orthostatic tachycardia syndrome. J Am Coll Cardiol 2021;77:861–71.
61. Dayrit JK, Verduzco-Gutierrez M, Teal A, et al. Enhanced External Counterpulsation as a Novel Treatment for Post-acute COVID-19 Sequelae. Cureus 2021;13(4):e14358.
62. Varanasi S, Sathyamoorthy M, Chamakura S, et al. Management of Long-COVID Postural Orthostatic Tachycardia Syndrome With Enhanced External Counterpulsation. Cureus 2021;13(9):e18398.
63. Raza A, Steinberg K, Tartaglia J, et al. Enhanced external counterpulsation therapy: past, present, and future. Cardiol Rev 2017;25:59–67.
64. Blitshteyn S, Whiteson JH, Abramoff B, et al. Multi-disciplinary collaborative consensus guidance statement on the assessment and treatment of autonomic dysfunction in patients with post-acute sequelae of SARS-CoV-2 infection (PASC). Pharm Manag PM R 2022;14(10):1270–91. https://doi.org/10.1002/pmrj.12894.

Pulmonary Sequelae of Coronavirus Disease 2019

Jonathan H. Whiteson, MD

KEYWORDS

- Dyspnea • Pulmonary function • Hypoxemia • Pulmonary rehabilitation
- Post-exertional symptom exacerbation • Health care disparities

KEY POINTS

- Mild respiratory symptoms including cough, mild breathing difficulty, and chest discomfort on respiration are very common in acute COVID-19 and one of the most common features of post-acute sequelae of COVID-19 (PASC).
- Following mild acute COVID-19, persistent respiratory symptoms in PASC are not typically associated with abnormalities on standard testing. However, severe acute COVID has been associated with abnormalities in pulmonary function testing, chest imaging, and cardiopulmonary stress testing.
- Although respiratory symptoms most likely indicate involvement of the pulmonary system, a comprehensive evaluation of individuals presenting with dyspnea is indicated to identify or rule out co-existing cardiac disorders and physiologic deconditioning.
- Management of respiratory symptoms in PASC should be focused on symptom mitigation and functional recovery—pulmonary rehabilitation addresses the broad medical, functional, and emotional needs of individuals with persistent symptoms and functional limitations related to PASC.
- Although respiratory symptoms and pulmonary sequelae can persist for months to years following acute COVID-19, the majority of these individuals demonstrate significant and often complete resolution of symptoms and functional limitations with rehabilitation interventions and over time.

CORONAVIRUS DISEASE 2019 AND THE RESPIRATORY SYSTEM

The primary site of entry to the human body of severe acute respiratory syndrome coronavirus 2 (SARS-CoV-2), the virus that causes coronavirus disease 2019 (COVID-19), is through the upper and lower respiratory tracts. The angiotensin-converting enzyme 2 (ACE2) receptor is the best-characterized entry receptor for SARS-CoV-2 and is highly expressed in the lung tissue. Infection of respiratory epithelial cells with SARS-CoV-2 generates a pro-inflammatory immune response including complement activation, the severity of which appears to correlate with the severity of acute COVID-19 lung disease. It is likely that variations in gene expression dictate

The author has no financial or other conflicts of interest or funding sources to disclose.
Ambulatory Care Center, 240 East 38th Street, 15th Floor, New York, NY 10016, USA
E-mail address: jonathan.whiteson@nyulangone.org

Phys Med Rehabil Clin N Am 34 (2023) 573–584
https://doi.org/10.1016/j.pmr.2023.04.005

complement hyperactivity[1] and disease severity, accounting for the significant variability in the severity of respiratory disease seen with COVID-19.

PREVALENCE

Mild respiratory symptoms including cough, mild breathing difficulty, and chest discomfort on respiration are very common in acute COVID-19 and are typically self-limiting, resolving over days to weeks. Individuals who are unvaccinated, with pre-existing lung conditions, and multiple medical comorbidities are at higher risk of more severe respiratory involvement and prolonged respiratory symptoms. Hypoxemia as evidenced by peripheral pulse oximetry of less than 92% is a marker of more severe disease. Pneumonitis, acute COVID-19 pneumonia, and superimposed bacterial infections are less common. Rarely but most concerning is the progression to acute respiratory distress syndrome (ARDS) with more severe symptoms, significant hypoxemia, and the need for hospitalization including respiratory support. Interstitial lung disease is a known long-term pulmonary sequelae of ARDS and reported in over 60%[2] of severe acute COVID-19 ARDS survivors. Recovery from post-COVID-19 interstitial lung disease may be seen over months but has also been reported to be persistent and, in a minority, progressive.

SEVERITY

Patients with acute COVID-19 present with variable clinical symptoms, ranging from a mild upper respiratory tract illness—viral bronchitis—to a severe disease with life-threatening complications exemplified by COVID-19 viral pneumonia, ARDS with acute hypoxic respiratory failure, and susceptibility to secondary bacterial pneumonia. Individuals with milder presentations may still suffer from longer-term complications including persistent pulmonary inflammation and fibrosis. Many individuals with mild acute COVID-19 have mild but persistent and significant symptoms of shortness of breath at rest, dyspnea on exertion, cough, and chest discomfort despite a negative exam and investigations. Individuals with chronic lung diseases including chronic obstructive pulmonary disease (COPD), moderate to severe asthma, bronchiectasis, interstitial lung diseases, cystic fibrosis, and pulmonary hypertension, are at increased risk for more severe acute COVID and acute respiratory consequences, as well as post-acute sequelae of COVID-19 (PASC) and persistent respiratory symptoms and disease.

DIFFERENTIAL DIAGNOSIS

Respiratory symptoms are not only due to primary pulmonary pathology and may be caused by or exacerbated by extra-pulmonary etiologies. Primary or co-existing cardiac disease which can cause or exacerbate respiratory symptoms, uncontrolled diabetes, gastro-esophageal reflux disease (GERD), musculoskeletal conditions, and emotional distress can also contribute. The evaluation and management of these non-pulmonary conditions are beyond the scope of this review.

EVALUATION
History–Symptoms

Respiratory symptoms are among the most commonly reported by individuals with acute COVID-19 and PASC. Common respiratory symptoms in acute COVID-19 include nasal congestion and rhinorrhea, cough which is predominantly dry, shortness of breath at rest and/or on exertion that may be disproportionate to the degree of physical activity, and chest discomfort described as pain, tightness, constriction, or pressure. Although typically mild in most cases of acute COVID-19, these symptoms can progress and become more distressing in severe acute COVID-19. The same symptom group can also persist as hallmarks of PASC and may fluctuate in severity over time.

Physical Examination

In acute COVID-19, the respiratory physical examination varies with severity of the disease and in mild disease can be normal. The presence of hypoxemia with oxygen saturation less than 92% on peripheral pulse oximetry is indicative of a more significant respiratory disease. In PASC, the physical exam is often normal, especially in individuals who were never hospitalized. Examination of the respiratory system starts with observation for respiratory distress including shallow, rapid breathing pattern, cough, and cyanosis. Vital signs can reveal tachypnea, tachycardia, and hypoxemia. Auscultation of the lungs in many patients is unrevealing but in those with a history of ARDS, fine 'Velcro' rales due to COVID-19-related interstitial lung disease may be heard. Rhonchi and wheezing related to secretion retention and broncho-constriction have also been reported. Findings of pre-existing pulmonary disease and co-existing cardiac disease should be noted.

Laboratory Tests/Investigations—timing of the pulmonary workup can be guided by severity of illness and degree of symptoms. In individuals with mild to moderate acute COVID-19 and PASC-related pulmonary symptoms, it is reasonable to delay testing for 2 to 3 months following presentation as many will improve over this time. In individuals with more significant presenting symptoms and signs, symptoms/signs that progress or persist, further testing can be initiated at that time.

Pulse oximetry has become readily accessible and is reliable and many individuals have access to a pulse oximeter. Despite symptoms, oxygen saturations are often normal but may identify hypoxemia. If normal at rest, activity oximetry during a standardized 6-minute walk test can reveal exercise hypoxemia that is not present at rest. If needed, persistent hypoxemia be confirmed with blood gas analysis, but this is rarely done outside of the acute care setting.

Pulmonary function testing (PFT) in those with mild to moderate acute COVID-19 typically does not change compared to prior PFTs[3] and is often normal. In those with more severe acute COVID-19, restrictive and/or obstructive patterns of lung dysfunction have been reported. Reduced diffusing capacity can be an isolated finding in the setting of otherwise normal PFTs.[4] Baseline PFTs in individuals with mild to moderate but persisting symptoms can serve as a reference for future comparison.

Radiographic evaluations are used routinely for individuals with respiratory symptoms in acute COVID-19 and in PASC. Prescription for chest x-ray (CXR) and/or computerized tomography (CT) of the lungs is not recommended in individuals with mild to moderate symptoms but can be supported in those who had moderate to severe acute COVID-19 and in individuals with persistent low oxygen saturation by pulse oximetry (SpO2), persistent cough, abnormal pulmonary exam, and/or impairment on PFT. Although in most symptomatic patients who had initial mild acute COVID-19 CXR will be normal, the most common findings on CXR and a high-resolution non-contrast CT lungs is ground glass opacities of the lower lobes. In individuals with moderate to severe acute disease, fibrotic-like changes including traction bronchiectasis, parenchymal bands, and/or honeycombing can be seen.[5] Resolution of these findings typically mirror but may lag behind clinical improvement. A contrast-enhanced CT or a nuclear medicine ventilation/perfusion lung scan is indicated if there is clinical concern for pulmonary embolism. Echocardiography and further cardiac workup (discussed elsewhere) are recommended if co-existing cardiac disease is being considered.

Standardized Symptom Testing: Standardization of respiratory symptoms is helpful to assess the impact of symptoms on function and quality of life, guide management strategies, and assess symptom evolution over time. Recommended measures include (**Table 1**).

Standardized Functional Measures

The *Six Minute Walk Test* (6MWT)[10] is a validated measure of exercise capacity for individuals with chronic lung diseases and is useful as a standardized measure of function, respiratory symptoms, and exercise hypoxemia. For individuals with persistent respiratory symptoms following COVID-19, the 6MWT has been shown to correlate with the severity of acute disease, with functional and radiological impairment in the chronic phase of COVID-19 and progressive improvement in exercise capacity.[11]

A *Cardio-Pulmonary Exercise Test* (CPET)[12] encompasses exercise stress testing on a bike ergometer or treadmill using validated and standardized progressive exercise intensity protocols and incorporating metabolic gas analysis to determine aerobic capacity. It is helpful in determining aerobic fitness levels that correlate with activity, exercise, and vocational tolerance. CPET testing can be used to evaluate symptoms in PASC and differentiate between possible mechanisms (cardiac/pulmonary/peripheral metabolic) of activity and exercise intolerance.[13]

MANAGEMENT
General

For those with respiratory symptoms but no positive findings on examination and a negative workup, management should include a general explanation regarding the current evidence-based understanding of COVID-19 and PASC. Reassurance can be given that no pulmonary abnormalities have been identified on examination and workup and that intermittent re-assessment is recommended if symptoms persist. Recognizing that individuals typically present with multiple symptoms possibly involving many organ systems, a comprehensive approach to the evaluation and management of PASC is recommended. A general discussion of diet, hydration, sleep, coping, and activity is indicated (**Table 2**). Referral to other specialties can be discussed if the etiology of symptoms may be from other organ systems.

Medications

For individuals with pre-existing lung disorders exacerbated by acute COVID-19, modification of prior medication regimens may improve control of symptoms toward baseline. Decongestants can benefit from nasal congestion. Antitussives and expectorants benefit individuals with persistent and/or productive cough. Bronchodilators

Table 1 Recommended measures	
Measure:	**Assesses:**
Multidimensional Dyspnea Profile[6]	sensation and severity of dyspnea
Modified Borg Dyspnea Scale[7]	severity of dyspnea sensation
Modified Medical Research Council Dyspnea Scale[8]	impact of dyspnea on physical activity
Duke Activity Status Index[9]	limitations in physical activity

Table 2
General management advice for individuals with post-acute sequelae of coronavirus disease 2019

	Advice	Reasoning	Also Consider....
Diet	Mediterranean 'style'	Anti-inflammatory/antioxidant-rich diet	Avoid alcohol—negative effects reported in PASC Minimize caffeine if rapid heart rate
Hydration	2–3 L water daily	Hydrates pulmonary secretions for ease of clearing Intra-vascular volume expansion if co-existing autonomic dysfunction	Maintain adequate salt and electrolyte repletion
Sleep	Address sleep patterns and hygiene	Sleep quality as important as quantity—is sleep refreshing/restorative?	Referral to Sleep Medicine for overnight sleep study and oximetry
Coping	Evaluate coping with PASC medical status, vocational and avocational tolerance, etc.	Stress, anxiety, depression, and PTSD commonly reported	Referral for supportive therapies
Activity	Understand baseline activity tolerated without post-exertional symptom exacerbation	Pushing 'hard' beyond the baseline may result in exacerbation of post-exertional symptoms resulting in a functional setback	4 Ps of Energy Conservation: Planning Pacing Prioritizing Positioning

may improve obstructive findings on PFTs. Intermittent or continuous oxygen is indicated for hypoxemia documented by pulse oximetry at rest or on exertion and symptom improvement is typically seen as oxygen saturations normalize. Oxygen during sleep is indicated for nocturnal hypoxemia identified on overnight oximetry. Criteria exist to support the prescription of oxygen in hypoxic individuals with lung disease.[14] Oxygen flow should be titrated at rest, during sleep, and with activity to maintain oxygen saturation greater than 92%. Oral glucocorticoids have been given where organizing pneumonia, pulmonary inflammation/pneumonitis, or fibrosis is suspected or identified.[15] A number of patients will either have a static form of fibrotic lung disease or a progressive type accompanied by deterioration of lung function. Use of antifibrotic medications may be helpful in the management of COVID-19-induced interstitial lung disease[16] but definitive evidence is lacking to date.

Surgery

Lung Transplantation is reserved for those with COVID-related acute respiratory lung distress who cannot be weaned from a ventilator or in those with persistent or progressive post-COVID lung fibrosis with significant functional limitations and oxygen dependency.[17]

Rehabilitation

Rehabilitation interventions for individuals with functional limitations due to pulmonary sequelae after COVID-19 must be individualized and based on a comprehensive evaluation and rehabilitation plan taking into account other organ system involvement and related physical impairments and disabilities.

For individuals *hospitalized* due to acute COVID-19 disease, the physiatrist[18] and multidisciplinary rehabilitation team play a central and vital role in managing and coordinating rehabilitative care and enhancing outcomes. Rehabilitation interventions should start immediately after the patient is admitted and considered stable for passive or active therapies. Managing sedated and ventilated[19] or awake[20] patients in the prone position is beneficial in the management of patients with COVID-19-related ARDS and acute hypoxemic respiratory failure. Safe patient turning and positioning required for proning is the purview of the rehabilitation team and can progress to early mobilization and rehabilitation in the intensive care unit (ICU) setting which has been demonstrated to improve function and overall outcomes.[21] As well, chest therapies[22] including coughing and secretion clearance techniques, breathing retraining, and patient education for oxygen use and titration are essential in the rehabilitation of individuals hospitalized with pulmonary sequelae of acute COVID-19.

For individuals with *persistent functional limitations* once medically improved, *post-acute inpatient rehabilitation* is indicated. Appropriate settings include acute inpatient rehabilitation facilities, subacute skilled nursing facilities ,and long-term acute care facilities. Criteria exist (beyond the scope of this discussion) to determine the appropriate setting. The goals of the rehabilitation program include ongoing management and improvement of medical conditions related to COVID-19 and a return toward pre-morbid function and quality of life. Inpatient rehabilitation including a comprehensive multimodal and multidisciplinary inpatient pulmonary rehabilitation program is feasible and effective in improving function, endurance, and quality of life.[23] In the continuum of rehabilitative care, most individuals who required inpatient rehabilitation therapies will benefit from post-discharge home-based, and then, outpatient rehabilitation.

The goals of *home-care therapies* include progression of function to greater independence in self-care and community mobility. Home-care therapies may be limited by duration of services (days/weeks) and time allotted for each treatment, as well as a lack of specialized rehabilitation equipment needed for optimal functional recovery. A timely and coordinated transition to outpatient services is ideal.

Outpatient rehabilitation interventions for the pulmonary sequelae of COVID-19 are essential to help individuals with persistent respiratory symptoms and functional limitations return to pre-morbid functional state, vocational and avocational roles, and quality of life.

Individuals who had a mild or moderate acute COVID-19 course without a significant hospital or ICU stay most frequently present in the outpatient setting with generalized fatigue, as well as functionally limiting pulmonary symptoms—shortness of breath, dyspnea on exertion, cough, and chest discomfort. Outpatient chest and pulmonary rehabilitation therapies are indicated. After more severe acute COVID-19 with significant hospital and/or ICU stay, individuals may present with persistent weakness, imbalance, incoordination, and postural deficits resulting in difficulties with activities of daily living and gait post-discharge. An individualized physical and occupational therapy program focusing on these deficits is indicated. Speech and swallow issues related to critical illness as well as prior intubation should be addressed and referral to Speech Language Pathology is indicated. Persisting cognitive deficits from ICU/critical illness-associated toxic/metabolic encephalopathy or from PASC-associated cognitive deficits and brain fog should be addressed by a neuropsychologist skilled in comprehensive cognitive testing and remediation. Once the general rehabilitation program is completed, referral for chest physical therapy and pulmonary rehabilitation is indicated.

Chest physical therapies encompass techniques to relieve dyspnea, optimize secretion clearance, and normalize oxygenation. Dyspnea is a sensation or 'air hunger' often associated with elevated respiratory rate and abnormal breathing patterns and mechanics typified by shallow breathing and an inspiratory to expiratory time-phase ratio approaching 1:1—the normal being 1:2, respectively. With normal physiology at rest breathing is typically 'subconscious' and the stimulus to breathing is predominantly minor fluctuations in carbon dioxide detected in the central respiratory centers. With activity, other factors contribute to stimulating the respiratory centers including a rise in body temperature, alterations in blood chemistry (ie, lactic acidosis), and mechanical factors (lung, muscle, and joint receptors). Factors contributing to dyspnea include progressive acute hypercapnia and/or hypoxemia, hypoxemia in individuals with chronic hypercapnia (ie, COPD), acidosis (ie, sepsis, uncontrolled diabetes), acute lung diseases (ie, pneumonia, pulmonary congestion, pulmonary embolus), altered chronic lung mechanics (ie, thoracic kyphosis or scoliosis), and emotional changes (ie, stress, anxiety, fear). Breathing exercises aimed at restoring normal breathing patterns, improving respiratory mechanics, and correcting hypercapnia and hypoxemia are effective in individuals with dyspnea post-COVID-19. Training in diaphragmatic breathing, pursed lips breathing, postural correction with deep breathing, and paced breathing techniques can be initiated by a Respiratory Therapist or a Physical Therapist trained in breathing techniques and continued independently.

Optimizing secretion clearance is essential for individuals with ongoing chest congestion due to COVID-19. Adequate fluid/water intake to maintain hydration of the airway and reduce the viscosity of pulmonary secretions is indicated. Mucolytics, such as guaifenesin, help 'thin' secretions making them easier to expectorate. Antitussives are not routinely recommended unless cough suppression is necessary to minimize chest wall pain experienced with coughing or when persistent coughing limits sleep. Breathing exercises, such as the active cycle of breathing technique (ACBT) which includes breathing control techniques, chest expansion exercises, and huff (forced expiration) coughing, are effective in clearing mucous from the lungs. Postural drainage utilizes gravity through positional changes to help clear sputum and involves the patient turning from side to side, prone and supine, to drain the different anatomical lung segments. Postural drainage can be used in combination with ACBT as well as 'hands-on' percussion techniques to add vibratory forces in assisting mucous clearance. Use of hand-held mucous clearing devices, including acapella, AerobiKa, lung flute and flutter valves, and/or a high-frequency chest wall oscillating vest can facilitate mucous clearance. Use of an incentive spirometer is also beneficial in providing visual feedback to optimize deep breathing techniques and minimize atelectasis. Initial instruction and supervision in these techniques and use of devices is optimally conducted with a Respiratory Therapist or a Physical Therapist trained in chest therapeutic techniques and individuals are then able to continue these techniques independently.

Hypoxemia is noted in acute COVID-19 disease in many individuals with moderate to severe acute disease and can persist. Although typically associated with dyspnea, individuals in the community setting may experience minimal or no symptoms with significant hypoxemia as evidenced by low SpO2—so-called 'silent hypoxemia'.[24] In acutely hospitalized adult patients with COVID-19 and associated hypoxemia, optimal SpO2 is 92% to 96%[25] and supplemental oxygen can be used in conjunction with other measures to achieve this target. For many individuals never hospitalized with mild/moderate acute COVID-19 but with relative hypoxemia, supplemental oxygen is not indicated if SpO2 remains greater than 90%. In the vast majority of individuals, hypoxemia resolves over time. For individuals with more persistent, severe, and prolonged hypoxemia with SpO2 less than 89%, guidelines exist supporting the prescription and use of supplemental oxygen in the community.[26] Oxygen flow should be titrated to achieve SpO2 of at least 92% and can be increased to maintain acceptable values with increasing activity. Overnight oximetry is indicated if there is concern for nocturnal hypoxemia—typically nocturnal oxygen flow rates of 1 to 2 L over daytime resting flow rates are indicated due to shallower breathing patterns normally seen during sleep. Periodic re-evaluation of the need for supplemental oxygen should be conducted as experience to date indicates that over time most individuals with hypoxemia will improve and no longer need supplemental oxygen. Prolonged oxygen need is more likely in those who had more severe acute COVID-19—those who had ARDS, were intubated, and/or have signs of pulmonary fibrosis.

Pulmonary Rehabilitation

Outpatient pulmonary rehabilitation (PR) has been shown to be effective in improving functional limitations, dyspnea, and quality of life in individuals with pulmonary sequelae of COVID-19.[27–29] Insurance coverage for outpatient PR has been expanded[30] by the Centers for Medicare and Medicaid Services (CMS) during the emergency health declaration of the COVID-19 pandemic. PR coverage now includes individuals with suspected or confirmed COVID-19 who experience persistent symptoms that include respiratory dysfunction for at least 4 weeks.

Individuals who can most benefit from PR include those with pre-existing lung disease ([COPD]; bronchiectasis; restrictive lung diseases—interstitial lung disease; kypho-scoliosis; infiltrative lung disease—sarcoidosis) whose related functional deficits are exacerbated by COVID-19 infection, as well as individuals who have new onset of COVID-19-related lung fibrosis and restrictive lung disease. However, symptomatic (shortness of breath, fatigue) individuals with no abnormalities on PFTs may still be eligible and benefit as recognized by the CMS coverage expansion. PR is well documented to benefit individuals with obstructive[31] as well as restrictive lung diseases.[32,33]

PR is a multimodal interdisciplinary rehabilitation program centered on physician-monitored exercise interventions, education, support, and nutrition to improve strength and endurance, minimize dyspnea and fatigue, and enhance functional independence and quality of life. Individuals being considered for pulmonary rehabilitation for PASC-related functional limitations require a comprehensive evaluation before participation.[34] Functional testing pre-PR participation, including a 2-minute step test, 6MWT, and CPET, helps assess current functional ability and endurance, propensity to PASC post-exertional symptoms, and assist in exercise prescription. Prescribed exercise interventions include peripheral muscle strengthening, postural training, breathing/respiratory exercises, and aerobic training. Individuals typically attend 2 to 3 times a week for up to 36 sessions. Vital signs are monitored before, during, and in recovery from exercise. Oxygen supplementation is indicated during exercise if saturations trend below 92%, with a goal saturation of greater than 94%. Integration of breathing and pacing techniques during monitored exercise helps maintain acceptable oxygen saturations. Patient education and improving self-efficacy is an essential goal of PR as long-term (life-long) compliance with all elements of PR after the monitored program has concluded is essential for ongoing improvements and long-term health, well-being, and quality of life. Functional testing is repeated after conclusion of the PR program to quantify functional and physiologic gains. Results are used to update exercise training parameters.

Challenges of PR in PASC. Some individuals with PASC experience *post-exertional symptom exacerbation* (PESE), often out of proportion to the preceding 'dose' of exercise. Symptoms are varied, may be similar to symptoms of the acute COVID-19 episode, and can include fatigue, malaise (post-exertional malaise— PEM), brain fog, sense of fever, and chest pains. PESE may last a few days to many weeks and relative rest is indicated to help resolve. Management of PESE and PEM[35] includes a significant reduction in the dose of activity and exercise to minimize recurrence and a subsequent very slow progression of activity is indicated. Significant PESE may preclude participation in or continuation of PR. Individual components, such as breathing, postural and gentle strength exercises may be tolerated in limited doses even if the aerobic component is not.

Co-existing *cardiovascular disorders* and *autonomic dysfunction* of PASC need to be considered in individuals with PASC-related pulmonary sequelae. Evaluation and management of cardiovascular[36] and autonomic disorders[37] in PASC are discussed in detail elsewhere. Similarly, *cognitive* and *neurologic dysfunction* may be present in individuals with pulmonary sequelae of PASC. Evaluation and management of cognitive[38] and neurologic disorders (pending publication) in PASC are discussed in detail elsewhere.

It is important to consider *health equity* in regard to the pulmonary sequelae of PASC. Individuals with pre-existing disabilities and chronic lung diseases, those who identify with minority groups, and older individuals are more likely to get COVID-19, severe COVID-19, and PASC with a further decline in function making access to essential health care services more challenging.[36] Health care disparities also impact access to PR services and must be addressed at the individual, health system, regional, and national levels.

Integrative health approaches have also been identified to provide benefits for individuals with breathing discomfort in PASC. Breathing retraining through singing[39] and Yogic breathing[40] may improve the emotional and quality of life components of breathlessness in PASC.

SUMMARY

Pulmonary sequelae of acute COVID-19 are common and result in functionally limiting symptoms. In most individuals who had mild to moderate acute COVID-19, no persisting abnormalities on pulse oximetry, PFTs, or radiologic evaluation of the lungs are noted. In some with more severe acute COVID-19, evidence of lung fibrosis can persist. In general, the prognosis for most individuals with pulmonary sequelae from PASC following mild to moderate acute COVID-19 is good. For those with more severe initial disease and persisting respiratory symptoms in the setting of abnormalities on testing, long-term prognosis is unclear at this time, but prior experience of post-viral infection-associated lung fibrosis indicates a potential lifelong condition. Rehabilitation interventions are an essential part of the management of pulmonary sequelae in PASC and should be individualized based on the degree of symptoms and functional limitations. PR has been shown to improve function and quality of life for even the most significantly impacted individuals. Co-management with Primary Care, Physiatry, and Pulmonary Medicine and prescription of a multidisciplinary rehabilitation program will yield optimal patient outcomes. Health care disparities must be identified and resolved to facilitate equitable access to rehabilitation services for individuals with functionally limiting pulmonary sequelae of PASC.

REFERENCES

1. Yan B, Freiwald T, Chauss D, et al. SARS-CoV-2 drivesJAK1/2-dependent local complement hyperactivation. Sci. Immunol 2021;6:eabg0833.
2. Han X, Fan Y, Alwalid O, et al. Six-month Follow-up Chest CT Findings after Severe COVID-19 Pneumonia. Radiology 2021;299(1):E177–86.
3. Lewis KL, Helgeson SA, Tatari MM, et al. COVID-19 and the effects on pulmonary function following infection: a retrospective analysis. EClinicalMedicine 2021;39: 101079.
4. Liao T, Meng D, Xiong L, et al. Long-term effects of COVID-19on health care workers 1-year post-discharge in Wuhan. Infect Dis Ther 2021;1–19.
5. Kanne JP, Little BP, Schulte JJ, et al. Long-Term Lung Abnormalities Associated with COVID-19 Pneumonia. Radiology 2022. https://doi.org/10.1148/radiol. 221806.
6. Banzett RB, O'Donnell CR, Guilfoyle TE, et al. Multidimensional dyspnea profile: an instrument for clinical and laboratory research. Eur Respir J 2015;45(6): 1681–91.
7. Mahler DA, Horowitz MB. Perception of breathlessness during exercise in patients with respiratory disease. Med Sci Sports Exerc 1994;26:1078–81.
8. Bestall JC, Paul EA, Garrod R, et al. Usefulness of the Medical Research Council (MRC) dyspnoea scale as a measure of disability in patients with chronic obstructive pulmonary disease. Thorax 1999;54:581–6.
9. Hlatky MA, Boineau RE, Higginbotham MB, et al. A brief self-administered questionnaire to determine functional capacity (the Duke activity status index). Am J Cardiol 1989;64(10):651–4.
10. ATS Statement: Guidelines for the Six-Minute Walk Test. Am J Respir Crit Care Med 2002;166:111–7.
11. Ferioli M, Prediletto I, Bensai S, et al. The role of 6MWT in Covid-19 follow up. Eur Respir J Suppl 2021;58(suppl 65):OA4046.
12. Balady GJ, Ross A, Sietsema K, et al. on behalf of the American Heart Association Exercise, Cardiac Rehabilitation, and Prevention Committee of the Council on Clinical Cardiology; Council on Epidemiology and Prevention; Council on

Peripheral Vascular Disease; Interdisciplinary Council on Quality of Care and Outcomes Research. Clinician's Guide to cardiopulmonary exercise testing in adults: a scientific statement from the. Am Heart Assoc 2010;122(2):191–225.

13. Durstenfeld MS, Sun K, Tahir P, et al. Use of Cardiopulmonary Exercise Testing to Evaluate Long COVID-19 Symptoms in Adults: A Systematic Review and Meta-analysis. JAMA Netw Open 2022;5(10):e2236057.

14. Centers for Medicare & Medicaid Services. National Coverage Determination (NCD) for Home Use of Oxygen (240.2). Publication Number100-3; Version 1; Effective Date of this Version October 27, 1993. Available at: https://www.cms.gov/medicare-coverage-database/details/ncd-details.aspx?NCDId=169.Accessed September 3, 2021.

15. Myall KJ, Mukherjee B, Castanheira AM, et al. Persistent Post-COVID-19 Interstitial Lung Disease. An Observational Study of Corticosteroid Treatment. Ann Am Thorac Soc 2021;18(5):799–806.

16. Salvi SS, Ghorpade D, Dhoori S, et al. Role of anti-fibrotic drugs in the management of post-COVID-19 interstitial lung disease: A review of literature and report from an expert working group. Lung India 2022;39(2):177–86 [published correction appears in Lung India. 2022;39(3):310].

17. King CS, Mannem H, Kukreja J, et al. Lung Transplantation for Patients With COVID-19. Chest 2022;161(1):169–78.

18. Whiteson JH, Xavier Escalón M. Susan Maltser, Monica Verduzco-Gutierrez MD Demonstrating the vital role of physiatry throughout the health care continuum: Lessons learned from the impacts of the COVID-19 pandemic on inpatient rehabilitation. PM R 2021;13:6 554–562.

19. Langer T, Brioni M, Guzzardella A, et al. Prone position in intubated, mechanically ventilated patients with COVID-19: a multi-centric study of more than 1000 patients. Crit Care 2021;25:128.

20. Ehrmann S, Li J, Ibarra-Estrada M, et al. Awake prone positioning for COVID-19 acute hypoxaemic respiratory failure: a randomised, controlled, multinational, open-label meta-trial. Lancet Respir Med 2021;9:1387–95.

21. Corcoran JR, Herbsman JM, Bushnik T, et al. Early Rehabilitation in the Medical and Surgical Intensive Care Units for Patients With and Without Mechanical Ventilation: An Interprofessional Performance Improvement Project. PM R 2017;9(2):113–9.

22. Battaglini D, Robba C, Caiffa S, et al. Chest physiotherapy: An important adjuvant in critically ill mechanically ventilated patients with COVID-19. Respir Physiol Neurobiol 2020;282:103529.

23. Gloeckl R, Leitl D, Jarosch I, et al. Benefits of pulmonary rehabilitation in COVID-19: a prospective observational cohort study. ERJ Open Res 2021;7(2):00108–2021.

24. Herrmann J, Mori V, Bates JHT, et al. Modeling lung perfusion abnormalities to explain early COVID-19 hypoxemia. Nat Commun 2020;11:4883.

25. NIH COVID-19 Treatment Guidelines. Oxygenation and Ventilation for Adults. Available at: https://www.covid19treatmentguidelines.nih.gov/management/critical-care-for-adults/oxygenation-and-ventilation-for-adults/. Accessed April 20, 2023.

26. Centers for Medicare & Medicaid Services. National Coverage Determination – Home Use of Oxygen. Available at: https://www.cms.gov/medicare-coverage-database/view/ncd.aspx?NCDId=169. Accessed September 27, 2021.

27. Nopp S, Moik F, Klok F, et al. Outpatient Pulmonary Rehabilitation in Patients with Long COVID Improves Exercise Capacity, Functional Status, Dyspnea, Fatigue, and Quality of Life. Respiration 2022;101:593–601.
28. Spielmanns M, Pekacka-Egli A-M, Schoendorf S, et al. Effects of a Comprehensive Pulmonary Rehabilitation in Severe Post-COVID-19 Patients. Int J Environ Res Publ Health 2021;18(5):2695.
29. Chen H, Shi H, Liu X, et al. Effect of Pulmonary Rehabilitation for Patients With Post-COVID-19: A Systematic Review and Meta-Analysis. Front Med 2022;9: 837420.
30. Centers for Medicare and Medicaid Services. Changes to the pulmonary rehabilitation (PR) benefit. 12/31/2021 Available at: https://www.aarc.org/wp-content/uploads/2022/06/aarc-medicare-pulmonary-rehabilitation-update-2022.pdf. Accessed December 31, 2021.
31. Casaburi R, ZuWallack R. Pulmonary Rehabilitation for Management of Chronic Obstructive Pulmonary Disease. N Engl J Med 2009;360:1329–35.
32. Huppmann P, Sczepanski B, Boensch M, et al. Effects of inpatient pulmonary rehabilitation in patients with interstitial lung disease. Eur Respir J 2013;42: 444–53.
33. Dowman L, Hill CJ, May A, et al. Pulmonary rehabilitation for interstitial lung disease. Cochrane Database Syst Rev 2021;2(2):CD006322.
34. Maley JH, Alba GA, Barry JT, et al. Multi-disciplinary collaborative consensus guidance statement on the assessment and treatment of breathing discomfort and respiratory sequelae in patients with post-acute sequelae of SARS-CoV-2 infection (PASC). PM R 2022;14(1):77–95.
35. Herrera JE, Niehaus WN, Whiteson J, et al. Multidisciplinary collaborative consensus guidance statement on the assessment and treatment of fatigue in postacute sequelae of SARS-CoV-2 infection (PASC) patients. PM R 2021; 13(9):1027–43 [Erratum in: PM R. 2022;14(1):164. PMID: 34346558; PMCID: PMC8441628].
36. Whiteson JH, Azola A, Barry JT, et al. Multi-disciplinary collaborative consensus guidance statement on the assessment and treatment of cardiovascular complications in patients with post-acute sequelae of SARS-CoV-2 infection (PASC). PM R 2022;14(7):855–78.
37. Blitshteyn S, Whiteson JH, Abramoff B, et al. Multi-disciplinary collaborative consensus guidance statement on the assessment and treatment of autonomic dysfunction in patients with post-acute sequelae of SARS-CoV-2 infection (PASC). PM R 2022;14(10):1270–91.
38. Fine JS, Ambrose AF, Didehbani N, et al. Multi-disciplinary collaborative consensus guidance statement on the assessment and treatment of cognitive symptoms in patients with post-acute sequelae of SARS-CoV-2 infection (PASC). PM R 2022;14(1):96–111.
39. Philip KEJ, Owles H, McVey S, et al. An online breathing and wellbeing programme (ENO Breathe) for people with persistent symptoms following COVID-19: a parallel-group, single-blind, randomised controlled trial. Lancet Respir Med 2022;10(9):851–62.
40. Rain M, Puri GD, Bhalla A, et al. Effect of breathing intervention in patients with COVID and healthcare workers. Front Public Health 2022;10:945988.

Postacute Sequelae of SARS-CoV-2: Musculoskeletal Conditions and Pain

Michelle Copley, MD[a], Barbara Kozminski, MD[a],
Nicole Gentile, MD, PhD[b,c], Rachel Geyer, MPH[b],
Janna Friedly, MD, MPH[a,*]

KEYWORDS

- PASC • Long COVID • COVID-related pain • Musculoskeletal conditions • Pain

INTRODUCTION

Between December 2019 and August 2022, there were over 95 million confirmed cases of COVID-19 in the United States alone, although this is likely an underestimation of the true total infections due to limited testing and underreporting of positive cases.[1,2] Although symptoms of acute COVID-19 often last 3 to 10 days, over half of people have reported experiencing prolonged symptoms[3,4] that can be disabling and impact quality of life.[5] Postacute sequelae of COVID-19 (PASC) or "long COVID" are terms to describe the ongoing or new symptoms 3 months or more after initial COVID-19 infection.[6–8] Over 200 symptoms have been attributed to PASC, including various pain-related conditions.[9–11] There is also emerging evidence that a range of musculoskeletal conditions and injuries may occur more frequently in patients with PASC compared with people without a history of COVID infection or in those who have recovered completely. Although there are a wide range of painful conditions associated with PASC, in this review the authors focus primarily on musculoskeletal and neuropathic pain as well as the potential impact of COVID on the incidence of musculoskeletal injuries and conditions.

INCIDENCE AND PREVALENCE OF MUSCULOSKELETAL PAIN CONDITIONS AFTER COVID

Pain is often not well recognized or attributed to PASC despite being reported by nearly half of patients with COVID-19.[12] Both new pain symptoms and exacerbation

[a] Department of Rehabilitation Medicine, University of Washington, 325 Ninth Avenue, Seattle, WA 98104, USA; [b] Department of Family Medicine, University of Washington, 1959 Northeast Pacific Street, Box 356390, Seattle, WA 98195-6390, USA; [c] Department of Laboratory Medicine and Pathology, University of Washington, 1959 Northeast Pacific Street Seattle, WA 98195-6390, USA
* Corresponding author.
E-mail address: Friedlyj@uw.edu

Phys Med Rehabil Clin N Am 34 (2023) 585–605
https://doi.org/10.1016/j.pmr.2023.04.008
1047-9651/23/© 2023 Elsevier Inc. All rights reserved.
pmr.theclinics.com

of chronic pain conditions have been observed in people with PASC.[13,14] Although there is no established terminology or criteria for diagnosis of post-COVID-19 pain, new-onset chronic pain after COVID-19 infection is considered one of the five most common features of PASC.[15] These symptoms negatively impact daily function, ability to work, and often lead to a higher need for health care services.[9] It is also important to recognize that many patients with PASC report multiple concurrent pain symptoms, some of which may have different etiologies and treatment strategies. For example, patients commonly report concurrent headaches, chest pain, back and neck pain, myalgias, and arthralgias.[16,17] Although the etiology of chest pain post-COVID is not well understood, chest pain is often musculoskeletal in nature as a secondary effect of coughing and respiratory symptoms rather than from cardiopulmonary or autonomic causes.

It can also be difficult to isolate musculoskeletal pain symptoms from neurologic conditions or other organ-system issues experienced by people with PASC and studies often group pain symptoms into a single category. In addition, the musculoskeletal conditions experienced by patients recovering from COVID-19 vary depending on the underlying conditions, initial severity of infection, and the treatment received for COVID-19.

In one large cohort of people infected with COVID-19 ($n = 26,000$), 43% of patients had reports of pain in their medical records 2 to 4 months after acute illness.[12] In this cohort, joint pain (21%) and headache (20%) were the most frequently reported pain conditions.[12] A recent meta-analysis (n = 2533) of hospitalized patients with COVID-19 found that 73% of patients had neurologic symptoms including headache, myalgias, and impaired consciousness.[18] Another large meta-analysis of 28,000 patients with COVID-19 found that even among nonhospitalized populations, 16.5% reported headaches in the month after their acute illness and half of those were still experiencing headaches 6 months later.[19] More than half of the patients in this meta-analysis reported some form of musculoskeletal pain 30-days after their acute illness[20] and 10% experienced musculoskeletal symptoms 1 year after initial infection.[19] Despite the high prevalence of pain and the impact of pain symptoms on daily life, these symptoms are still not well characterized in PASC literature, and there are few studies specifically addressing the trajectory of painful conditions and effective treatment strategies.[21]

The following sections explore common musculoskeletal pain conditions in PASC, including prevalence, complicating factors, and critical illness considerations.

Myalgias and Arthralgias

Both myalgias and arthralgias are commonly reported in acute COVID and in PASC. Although they are frequently experienced together; patients may report the presence of one or the other in isolation. The prevalence of myalgias in PASC varies greatly between studies, ranging from 3% to over 64% with an estimated pooled prevalence of approximately 19%.[22,23] Myalgia is a common symptom at the initial onset of COVID-19 with up to 36% documented in one meta-analysis of 10 studies ($n = 1994$).[24] However, the presence of myalgias is not significantly associated with severity of COVID-19 and should not be considered a prognostic factor.[23] Regarding arthralgias, two pain categories, "bone and joint pain" and "neck, back, and lower back pain," were among eight post-COVID-19 symptoms to actually *increase* over the first year in the ComPaRe long COVID prospective e-cohort. The prevalence of the 45 other symptoms studied either decreased or stayed stable. Specifically, "neck, back, and lower back pain" showed the highest increase in prevalence of all symptoms evaluated over this time period.[25]

Female patients are at higher risk of experiencing myalgias and arthralgias along with fatigue.[26,27] In addition, high body mass index (BMI) is correlated with higher odds of experiencing myalgias, and arthralgias have been found at 1 month postinfection.[20] In a single-center prospective cohort study ($n = 300$) of hospitalized patients, not requiring intensive care unit (ICU)-level care, myalgias were present in 63% and were more likely to be widespread (40%) than localized (23%) with the lower leg being the most commonly localized area (69% of those reporting localized myalgias). Arthralgias (reported in 59% of patients) were also more likely to be widespread (33%) with the knee being the most common localized joint (51% of 26% localized arthralgias).[20]

In a meta-analysis of PASC symptom prevalence in hospitalized and nonhospitalized COVID-19 survivors at 60 days after onset or hospitalization, chest pain (24%) and arthralgias (19%) were the most frequently reported symptoms.[28] Furthermore, approximately 10% of all patients reported myalgias and arthralgias beyond 90 days which were more prevalent in the nonhospitalized cohort (15% vs 8%).[28] At 6 months postinfection, approximately two in five patients had at least one rheumatic or musculoskeletal symptom. Fatigue (approximately one in three), arthralgia (one in five), and myalgia (one in seven) were the most frequent.[29] Of note, these symptoms were not among the most frequently reported symptoms at 30 days postinfection, which suggests that although fewer patients in total may experience these symptoms, they tend to be more persistent compared with other commonly reported symptoms, such as ageusia and anosmia.

Neuropathic Pain

Both new onset neuropathic pain and worsening of previously acquired neuropathic pain have been reported following COVID-19.[30,31] Studies have also found that even patients who did not require hospitalization initially experienced worsening of underlying neuropathic conditions for at least several weeks following initial infection, suggesting that worsening neuropathic pain is not limited to those who were critically ill.[30] New onset neuropathic pain can have a variety of causes and it is important to recognize that it can be caused by peripheral nerve injuries, polyneuropathies, myopathies, and other neurologic conditions as well as by direct damage to sensory nerve cells from the virus itself.[30,32] Acute ischemic stroke is another sequelae that can occur from SARS-CoV-2 infection and can lead to poststroke-associated neuropathic pain.[30]

Post-Exertional Malaise

Post-exertional malaise (PEM), which occurs in a large subset of patients with PASC, is one of the hallmark symptoms of myalgic encephalitis (ME) or chronic fatigue syndrome (CFS).[29] PEM often presents as worsening fatigue, myalgias, and/or arthralgias 1 to 2 days following an increase in activities involving cognitive and/or physical exertion (including exercise). Triggers are often unknown but can be identified when patients keep detailed diaries of their activities. Although the mechanism of PEM is not fully understood, it is hypothesized to relate to dysfunctional endothelial cells and leakage of blood vessels with subsequent neuroinflammation and may involve dysregulation of the hypothalamic paraventricular nucleus, which affects the function of the hypothalamus and proximal limbic system.[33]

Myositis

From a review article in July 2021, there have been at least 23 case reports of myositis attributable to coronavirus (COVID)-19 (C19 M).[34] The presentation and severity reported are varied, ranging from dermatomyositis to paraspinal associated myositis to severe rhabdomyolysis.[35] Owing to this, it is difficult to know the true incidence as differential with myalgias and modestly elevated creatine kinase (CK) include critical illness myopathy (CIM), neurogenic muscle disease, and true myositis.[35] The proposed mechanisms include the SARS-Cov-2 directly entering muscle cells via ACE2 receptor, but this has not been proven when looking at muscle biopsies and so it is favored that myositis is due to the virus triggering an autoimmune response. As such, the timing of myositis has been seen to lag by up to a few weeks and may become more prominent in the PASC period.[36] Outcomes also vary with some patients recovering within a few weeks and half within a few weeks to months. This leaves a large portion to have lingering weakness remote from their acute COVID-19 infection.[37] For these patients with prolonged C19 M, immunosuppressants such as mycophenolate mofetil, calcineurin inhibitors, and Janus kinase (JAK) inhibitors maybe considered by their rheumatologist.[34,37,38]

Dermatomyositis
While not a direct link, an observational study of a single pediatric center showed a rise of 60% compared with average admissions in the same period from 2014 to 2019 for pediatric patients with dermatomyositis in the initial period of the pandemic.[37]

Acute viral myositis
Most cases reported were males, aged 33 to 87.[34] Initial examination findings are variable from subtle weakness to profound, and patients likely to have an elevated creatine kinase, although creatine kinase levels do not directly correlate with severity or prognosis.[34]

Paraspinal myositis
Myalgia and back pain are common symptoms reported by patients and characterized as more generalized musculoskeletal symptoms that are likely multifactorial. There has been a case series of nine patients with seven of nine patients with MRI findings showing intramuscular edema and enhancement, consistent with a diagnosis of paraspinal myositis.[39] Involvement is seen in bilateral erector spinae and multifidus paraspinal muscles exclusively in the lumbar spine.[34,39] These findings were also associated with a prolonged hospital course (>25 days) and continuation of back pain in the postinfectious period. In this case series, most of these patients underwent MRI due to known "underlying degenerative spine disease and occasional neurogenic symptoms."[34] Although literature suggests this is a more rare finding, it is important to consider that many patients are not receiving advanced imaging for low back pain so prevalence is difficult to ascertain. In a patient with a protracted course of low back pain, paraspinal myositis should be considered on the differential as it may change the treatment options than typical first-line conservative measures for new onset low back pain.

Rhabdomyolysis
Rhabdomyolysis is the rapid breakdown of skeletal muscles, resulting in muscle pain, weakness, and hallmarked by dark urine and elevated serum or plasma creatine kinase levels. Patient presentation is characterized by an acute, symmetric, lower limb-dominant muscle weakness.[34] Rhabdomyolysis has been associated with multiple viral infections including influenza, Epstein–Barr, adenovirus, and parainfluenza. Numerous case reports of rhabdomyolysis in patients that tested positive for SARS-COV-2 have been reported, being described as a presenting feature and a late complication.[40] A systematic review reported incidence ranging from 0.2% to 2.2% in

hospitalized COVID-19 patients.[41] In one case series of four patients with rhabdomyolysis, all patients required intubation, suggesting that this is likely a complication associated with severe disease rather than milder initial infections or associated with PASC. Although rhabdomyolysis is likely to be a rare manifestation in critically ill patients with COVID-19, it does have life-threatening implications and can lead to severe acute kidney injury as well as prolonged pain and recovery. Mortality has been reported as high as 30% in patients with COVID-19-related rhabdomyolysis with higher rates in patients with rapidly progressing interstitia lung disease (ILD).[41]

Critical Illness Considerations

COVID-19 infections resulting in severe illness and requiring hospitalization with intensive care unit admissions have additional musculoskeletal, neuromuscular, and neurologic conditions to consider given the nature of the treatments and inherent risk of myopathy and peripheral nerve injuries that can occur in this context.[14] Patients who have survived critical illness with COVID-19 are at higher risk of developing chronic pain than those with milder infections, which is likely multifactorial, including not only factors related to their ICU stays, which is an independent risk factor of developing chronic pain, but also due to social determinants of health, the overburdened and stretched health care system, psychological impacts, and social restrictions (loneliness and perception of increased isolation).[15,42] In addition, high BMI, female sex, and myalgias at hospital admission are risk factors for development of chronic pain.[15] Many patients who were critically ill with COVID-19 were also older adults and/or with significant comorbidities, both of which place people at higher risk of developing pain.

Peripheral Nerve Injuries

Often, the treatment itself for hospitalized patients with severe COVID-19 infections puts patients at risk for peripheral nerve and musculoskeletal injuries. For example, positioning patients in the prone position for prolonged periods of time to improve respiratory function places these critically ill patients at risk for brachial plexopathy, joint subluxation, and soft tissue damage.[43] Cases of unilateral ankle dorsiflexion weakness or foot drop have been attributed to fibular head and fibular nerve compression due to prone positioning of critically ill and ventilated/sedated patients including those with COVID-19.[28] In one study of patients recovering from acute respiratory distress syndrome (ARDS) associated with COVID-19 ($n = 83$) at a stand-alone rehabilitation center, 14% developed a peripheral nerve injury with 76% occurring in the upper limb and most frequently involving the ulnar nerve (29%).[44] At least one proning session occurred in 62% of those patients.[44] In addition to proning, these patients also spent significant time in supine positions while receiving neuromuscular blocking agents, increasing their susceptibility to nerve injuries.[30,44] There were also high rates of diabetes mellitus, obesity, and older-aged patients in this cohort, which each independently places patients at higher risk for developing these types of nerve injuries.[44]

Polyneuropathy

Painful polyneuropathy has been documented in both critically ill and non-critically ill COVID-19 survivors, although is most often associated with critical illness polyneuropathy (CIP).[45] There have also been documented cases of Guillain–Barre syndrome associated with COVID-19, which is predominately the acute inflammatory demyelinating neuropathy subtype.[46] In addition, mononeuritis multiplex has also been described after COVID-19 with risk factors including preexisting diabetes, obesity, drug use, and prolonged ICU stay.[46] Drug-induced polyneuropathy due to neurotoxic drugs such as daptomycin, linezolid, lopinavir, ritonavir, hydroxychloroquine, cisatra-curium, clindamycin, and glucocorticoids has also been described as a leading cause of polyneuropathy in patients recovering from COVID-19.[46] There is little evidence to support the role of infectious neuropathy; rather polyneuropathy in patients with COVID-19 is thought to be secondary to the medications received to treat the infection and associated conditions, critical illness itself, and underlying chronic medical conditions.[45,46]

Critical Illness Polyneuropathy

CIP is characterized by a symmetric, length-dependent sensorimotor axonal poly-neuropathy. An observational ICU cohort study (n = 111) found that CIP was associ-ated with increased illness severity and was more frequent among COVID-19 patients compared with a non-COVID-19 cohort.[47] It has also been observed in the generalized ICU population, CIP often occurs concurrently with CIM.[48] Incidence is difficult to assess due to numerous circumstances including unknown premorbid status, ongoing severity of illness and inability to perform adequate physical examination, patient's un-able to vocalize symptoms, limited resources and staff availability to perform electro-diagnostics, and mortality. There is likely an underreporting of cases. It is thought that in the generalized ICU population, CIP affects between one-third and one-half of the most severely critically ill patients.[49,50]

Critical Illness Myopathy

CIM is a primary myopathy characterized by the preferential loss of myosin.[49] It is not secondary to muscle denervation.[49] CIM impacts patients with severe COVID-19 with prolonged hospitalizations and causes generalized and symmetric muscle weakness impacting limbs as well as respiratory muscles, pain, and weakness-related musculo-skeletal injuries. This is thought to be due to muscle wasting from lack of use, impaired contractility, associated neuropathies, and muscle dysfunction with dysregulated autophagy and dysfunctional mitochondrial pathways.[51,52] Needle electromyography (EMG) will demonstrate spontaneous activity in the muscles. Risk factors include sepsis and/or shock, multiple organ failure, prolonged mechanical ventilation, and metabolic disturbances such as hyperglycemia, and age, weight, comorbidities, and exposure to neurotoxic medications.[51,52] One small study of 12 patients with COVID-19 referred for CIM or polyneuropathy electrodiagnostic testing did not find any distinctive features that differentiated patients with COVID-19 patients with CIM from the general ICU-hospitalized patient population experiencing CIM.[53] The inci-dence of CIM in COVID-19 patients has been found to increase with severity of dis-ease.[47] The incidence of CIM following COVID-19 infection is not well understood but likely mirrors the general population of patients with critical illness treated in the ICU given that it does not seem to be unique to COVID-19.[53] It is thought in the ICU population, CIM affects approximately 25% of patients.[54,55]

CIP/CIM Outcomes

For outcomes, we must extrapolate from more well-studied general ICU populations. CIM and CIP are especially important to consider in PASC patients as they often cause a significant loss of function for patients that persists for months to years after critical illness resolves. CIM is thought to have a better prognosis than CIP and combined CIM/CIP cases.[45,48] For patients in an ICU cohort study, 25% with CIM demonstrated earlier markers of electrophysiological signs of recovery and lower degrees of weak-ness at discharge from the ICU (mean 19 days), compared with none in patients with CIM/CIP patients, despite CIM/CIP patients having a longer ICU length of stay (mean

35 days).[48] CIM patients, in the CRIMYNE study ($n = 92$, ICU patients, not COVID-specific) recovered within 6 months, whereas CIP patients had a slower recovery or never recovered fully.[56]

PATHOPHYSIOLOGY/PROPOSED MECHANISMS

The pathophysiology of PASC is thought to involve a prolonged immune system response to initial COVID-19 infection leading to a cascade of inflammatory and/or auto-immune processes.[57] Studies have demonstrated that laboratory abnormalities suggestive of immunologic dysfunction can be present in patients with PASC several months after acute COVID infection.[58] Although the etiology is likely multifactorial and uncertainty remains as to the exact mechanism of PASC-related pain, immune-mediated processes may play a key role in the modulation of the inflammatory response that characterizes pain associated with COVID. Examples of potential mechanisms that may contribute to PASC-related pain and musculoskeletal injuries include dysregulation of the renin angiotensin system (RAS) and the resulting impact on macrophage activation, inflammation and neural signaling, mitochondrial dysfunction, fibrin-amyloid microclots, and secondary effects of prolonged illness, including deconditioning and muscle weakness.

Renin Angiotensin System Dysregulation

SARS-CoV-2 infects cells by attaching its spike protein to the angiotensin-converting enzyme-2 (ACE2) receptor. The ACE2 receptor is found on the surface of a variety of cells, including neurons, astrocytes, endothelial, and smooth muscle cells of cerebral blood vessels, and skeletal muscle cells, which explains the uptake of SARS-CoV-2 in the peripheral and central nervous systems and the broad range of symptoms experienced by people infected with SARS-CoV-2.[59]

By attaching to the ACE2 receptor, SARS-CoV-2 prevents degradation of angiotensin II and leads to overactivation of the angiotensin II receptor type I (AT1R). This activation of the AT1R results in downregulation of the ACE2 expression and unchecked inflammation, oxidative stress, vasoconstriction, tissue fibrosis, and a wide range of neurologic complications. This imbalance of the RAS is the primary cause of the "cytokine storm" and cellular damage that causes many of the life-threatening acute complications of COVID-19 such as ARDS and multiorgan system failure. Cytokine storming is an outpouring of pro-inflammatory cytokines including interleukin (IL)-6, tumor necrosis factor (TNF)-α, IL-1β, IL-8, and IL-12, interferon (IFN)-γ inducible protein (IP10; also termed as motif chemokine ligand 10, macrophage inflammatory protein 1A, and monocyte chemoattractant protein 1.[60] Of these pro-inflammatory cytokines, IL-1β, IL-6, IP10, and TNFα are the ones with the greatest ability to induce direct tissue injury in several organs and systems, including the peripheranl nervous system (PNS) and central nervous system (CNS) (**Fig. 1**).

The RAS imbalance is also believed to contribute to many of the longer term sequelae of COVID-19 including PASC-related pain. Given that ACE2 receptors are located in muscle tissue, attachment of the spike protein to these receptors can lead directly to inflammation and cellular damage. In addition, ACE2 receptors are also located on the dorsal root ganglia (DRG) in the skin, luminal organs, and meninges and attachment of the SARS-CoV-2 to these receptors can cause an imbalance in the neuromodulation systems of nociception and result in neuropathic pain. A recent study of human tissue donors (organ donors and tissue obtained during vertebrectomy surgeries) found that 25% of the sampled DRG neurons expressed ACE2 and these free nerve endings create an entry point for the SARS-CoV-2 into the peripheral nervous system.[61]

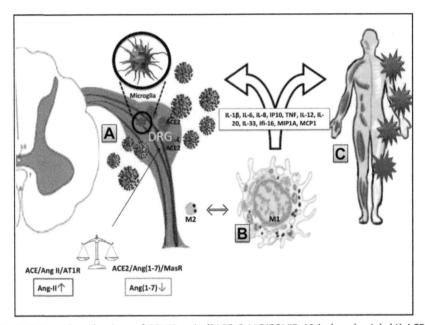

Fig. 1. Potential mechanisms of COVID-pain (SARS-CoV-2/COVID-19-induced pain). (*A*) ACE2/
RAS pathway and the direct virus-induced damage. Within the RAS, the virus/receptor
(ACE2) interaction involves unbalance of the ACE/Ang II/AT1R and the ACE2/Ang-(1–7)/
MasR axes with downregulation of ACE2 levels on cell surfaces, Ang-II accumulation, and
impairment of the anti-nociceptive Ang-(1–7) pathway. Therefore, direct damage to sensory
neurons and/or glial cells is produced. (*B*) Macrophage activation. Macrophages and other
immune cells can stimulate the production of inflammatory mediators (eg, IL-1β, TNF, and
bradykinins). These processes can facilitate the sensory cells injury and can lead to chronic
pain through sensitization/activation processes. (*C*) The exuberant immune-mediated
inflammation. It is mostly responsible for systemic damage and the triggering of long-
COVID problems (including widespread myalgia and joint pain) via peripheral and central
mechanisms. Disease-related and predisposing factors contribute to the determinism of
the damage. (*Reproduced from* Cascella M, Del Gaudio A, Vittori A, Bimonte S, Del Prete
P, Forte CA, Cuomo A, De Blasio E. COVID-Pain: Acute and Late-Onset Painful Clinical Manifestations in COVID-19 - Molecular Mechanisms and Research Perspectives. J Pain Res. 2021
Aug 10;14:2403 to 2412. https://doi.org/10.2147/JPR.S313978. PMID: 34408485; PMCID:
PMC8364364.)

Fibrin-Amyloid Microclots

Acute SARS-CoV-19 infection is associated with a variety of clotting abnormalities,
including a hypercoagulable state that can cause acute thrombosis and endotheliopa-
thies. In acute infection, markers of coagulopathies, such as the D-dimer, Von Wille-
brand factor, and fibrinogen levels, have been shown to be important markers of
prognosis. In addition, there are a number of studies that have demonstrated the presence of microclots in the lungs as well as high levels of circulating amyloid clots and
damage to platelets and erythrocytes in severe acute COVID-19 infections.[62] There
are now increasing reports of these same mechanisms being at play in many of the
PASC symptoms, including COVID-related pain. Coagulopathies are known to be
associated with a variety of autoimmune and inflammatory conditions, including
rheumatoid arthritis. However, the coagulopathies observed in patients with PASC
symptoms seem to be somewhat different in that there are high levels of circulating

amyloid-containing microclots that are more resistant to fibrinolysis.[63] In recent research, these fibrin-amyloid microclots have been observed to entrap inflammatory cells and importantly can pass through microcapillaries and cause blockages. In one study of patients with ME/CFS (which overlaps with PASC in terms of etiology and clinical manifestations), it was noted that they had levels of microclots that were 10-fold that of healthy controls. It is hypothesized that these episodic blockages of the microcapillaries with the fibrin-amyloid microclots may be one cause of some of the transient or migratory pain and neurologic symptoms that many patients with PASC experience.

Autonomic Dysregulation

Patients with PASC often experience symptoms consistent with autonomic dysregulation including instability of heart rate, blood pressure, lightheadedness when standing, chest pain, palpitations, headaches, neuropathic pain, and musculoskeletal pain. Patients may have symptoms consistent with a diagnosis of postural orthostatic tachycardia syndrome (POTS). POTS is triggered by an immunologic stress, which can include a wide range of viral infections, trauma, pregnancy, surgery, or psychosocial stressors. Although the etiology of autonomic dysregulation is not well understood, similar to other PASC symptoms, it is hypothesized to relate to an autoimmune response that involved increased sympathetic activity and potentially denervation which can cause postural central hypovolemia and reflex tachycardia.[64] It is hypothesized that autonomic dysregulation also causes exacerbation of sensory, autonomic, and small-fiber neuropathies, which may explain the worsening of neuropathic pain in people with POTS or autonomic dysregulation following COVID-19.[65]

Muscle Fatigue Due To Mitochondrial Dysfunction or Deconditioning

Another important potential mechanism for musculoskeletal injuries and pain in patients with PASC is the cumulative effect of chronic illness and inability to tolerate activity on overall strength, endurance, and flexibility. Many people with PASC symptoms have debilitating fatigue and pain that limits their ability to participate in usual activities including exercise. Given the broad range of symptoms that patients with PASC experience as well as the range of severity of organ-level consequences, there has been an increasing interest in understanding how much of what people are experiencing is related to deconditioning versus direct organ damage, mitochondrial dysfunction, or other quantifiable immune system-related processes. One potential way to evaluate this is through the use of cardiopulmonary exercise testing (CPET). In one recent cohort study of people experiencing PASC symptoms, most of the patients were not found to have any evidence of specific end organ damage (including cardiac and pulmonary damage) but had findings consistent with general deconditioning in CPET testing.[66] Another study of 71 patients with symptoms lasting up to 12 months post-COVID-19 infection found that the reduction in exercise tolerance found through CPET was most consistent with deconditioning and that patients who were initially treated in the ICU setting (more severe acute COVID-19) were much more likely to exhibit signs consistent with deconditioning.[67] However, there is emerging evidence using CPET data to suggest that at least some patients with PASC experience mitochondrial dysfunction during graded exercise that leads to reductions in fat β-oxidation and an increased buildup of blood lactate. This increase in lactic acid during exercise may play a significant role in the development of PEM.[68]

IMPACT OF POSTACUTE SEQUELAE OF COVID-19-RELATED MUSCULOSKELETAL PAIN CONDITIONS ON FUNCTION, QUALITY OF LIFE, AND RETURN TO WORK

Pain in critical illness requiring ICU level care is a known risk factor for inability to return to work and reduced quality of life for up to 5 years after hospitalization.[14,42] Given the prior research of the long-term impact of critical illness on quality of life and quality-adjusted life years, it has been proposed that ICU admission should be treated as a diagnosis that needs to be monitored and treated lifelong. Although COVID-19 is a new viral illness, research is demonstrating similar impacts of severe COVID-19 requiring ICU admission on long-term quality of life and return to work. In addition, pain seems to be one of the most disabling conditions associated with COVID-19 recovery.

In a single-center prospective study, individuals with critically ill COVID-19 were interviewed 1 month post-hospitalization. Pain was assessed using multiple scales, with 51% reporting new onset pain, 39% with clinically significant pain and those with pain were found to have worsened anxiety and depression scores. Overall, new-onset pain was associated with a lower health-related quality of life.[21]

New functional impairments are also common at 30 days after discharge among survivors of hospitalization for COVID-19, although pain is only one of the contributing factors to these impairments.[69] One prospective cohort study ($n = 92$) following individuals between 1 and 6 months after hospitalization, demonstrated that a majority (63%–67%) developed new activities of daily living (ADL) impairment, fatigue, or worsening physical function at 1 month, and of those, only 50% to 79% partially or fully recovered by 6 months.[16]

For patients with CIM, compared with their ICU counterparts without CIM, long-term complications include increased mortality, prolonged time to discharge home, and decreased physical function. Studies of ARDS patients showed that even 5 years after ICU discharge, patients still experienced varying degrees of weakness and reduced walk and exercise ability.[16,52]

Return to Work

Although not a pain or musculoskeletal issue, fatigue is a common symptom that persists for many patients who are experiencing PASC. This directly affects patient's abilities to reintegrate into their community and return to work.[28,69] In a cross-sectional study ($n = 55$), compared with pre-COVID hospitalization, 52% developed new difficulty with performing basic ADLs and 69% experienced a clinically significant worsening in their fatigue symptom severity.[69]

EVALUATION OF POSTACUTE SEQUELAE OF COVID-19-RELATED PAIN

Navigating the health care system to obtain appropriate care can be a frustrating experience for patients experiencing PASC, particularly due to the wide range of symptoms experienced and limited availability of clinicians with familiarity with PASC conditions. Many clinicians fail to recognize pain symptoms contributing to PASC and are not well trained in current guidelines related to diagnosis, treatment, or the additional hurdles of communicating with insurers or workplaces that may be necessary to help patients manage their pain.[70]

Multidisciplinary post-COVID clinics have been formed across the United States to better care for patients with PASC. In addition, multidisciplinary collaboratives such as the American Academy of Physical Medicine and Rehabilitation PASC Collaborative have been formed to help develop clinical guidance documents, develop standards of care, and advocate for additional resources to care for patients with PASC.[71] However, there are substantial gaps in the knowledge base related to optimal workups, diagnosis, and treatment of PASC symptoms, particularly PASC-related pain. Thus, PASC clinical care and research require interdisciplinary teams to address these gaps and approach PASC in a more holistic manner.[72,73] In addition, the need for this interdisciplinary approach creates an even larger care gap in rural communities that are already disproportionately impacted by COVID-19, but do not have the resources available to address patients with PASC.[74–76] Currently, post-COVID clinics and other medical practices across the country have minimal standardization in how they approach developing care teams and treating the rapidly growing numbers of patients with PASC and PASC-related pain.[71,77]

Despite the limited research available to guide diagnosis and treatment of PASC-related pain, there is a lot that can be drawn from knowledge about other related pain conditions and based on an understanding of etiology of PASC-related pain and concurrent symptoms. The following section describes some specific considerations for the evaluation of PASC-related musculoskeletal symptoms and pain.

History

In addition to a standard comprehensive musculoskeletal and pain history, providers should obtain a detailed history of COVID-19 infection, symptoms, severity, course, duration, hospitalization, and treatments received (including antivirals in both in- and outpatient settings). If patients were treated in the ICU setting, this should be noted and an attempt should be made to understand the treatments received in this setting including positioning, neuromuscular blockades, ventilatory strategies used, and other complications. Patients who were hospitalized, and especially requiring prolonged ICU care, may present with brachial plexopathy, joint subluxation, and soft tissue damage from prolonged positioning. Although pain and musculoskeletal symptoms are often widespread in PASC, it should be noted that the common location for myalgias is the lower leg and for arthralgias is the knees.[20] Patients should also be asked about frequency and timing of the most bothersome symptoms as symptoms can fluctuate over time and can be migratory. Understanding if myalgias and arthralgias are localized to specific joints or to specific times during the day can help to target treatments. Exacerbating and relieving factors should be identified whenever possible to help patients develop self-management strategies. This often requires patients to keep diaries of their symptoms and activities to try to identify factors that may be contributing to worsening symptoms. PEM, for example, is often only established after looking for patterns from patient diaries and seeing that it occurs within 1 to 2 days after heavier periods of physical or cognitive activity. As dysautonomia or POTS are common in people with PASC and are associated with pain, it is also important to ask about postural lightheadedness, tachycardia or palpitations, and heart rate and blood pressure instability.

The review of systems should include inquiry into common PASC symptoms, such as musculoskeletal symptoms including joint and muscle pain, fatigue, fever, sleep disturbance, respiratory and cardiovascular symptoms including breathlessness, cough, chest tightness, chest pain, palpitations; neurologic symptoms including "brain fog" (decreased concentration or memory), headache, paresthesias, numbness, dizziness, delirium (in older populations); gastrointestinal symptoms including abdominal pain, nausea, diarrhea, decreased appetite; psychological/psychiatric symptoms including depression and anxiety; ear, nose, and throat symptoms including tinnitus, earache, sore throat, and loss of taste and/or smell.

Examination

Physical examination can follow the standard approach to a comprehensive, history-driven physical examination of musculoskeletal and neurologic systems. In addition, evaluation of vital signs with postural changes, including the 10-minute National Aeronautics and Space Administration (NASA) lean test, can provide additional data in patients experiencing symptoms suggestive of dysautonomia or POTS.[78] Functional tests that are feasible in the clinic setting such as a 2 or 6 minute walk test with pre- and post-vital signs and timed up and go can also be helpful to measure the impact of their symptoms on endurance, cardiopulmonary function, strength, and balance. Evaluation of mood, affect, and cognitive ability are also important to assess in patients with PASC, particularly if they endorse difficulties in these areas by history.

Laboratory Testing

Laboratory tests can be useful for further evaluating the type of pain patients are experiencing (eg, inflammatory vs mechanical or other), or ruling out alternate causes of pain and related comorbidities. Some examples of laboratory tests that are recommended as part of the general PASC workup include, complete blood count with differential, c-reactive protein, erythrocyte sedimentation rate, complete metabolic panel, magnesium level, thyroid function tests, ferritin, iron panel, vitamin D level, hemoglobin A1c and when pain is present, considering uric acid, rheumatoid factor (RF), anti-cyclic citrullinated peptide (CCP) antibodies, and/or antinuclear antibody (ANA) reflexive panel with titers, among other autoantibodies depending on the patients personal and family history.

Autoantibodies as Potential Laboratory Confounders

Several studies have noted autoantibody positivity in acute COVID-19 infection and beyond.[79–86] Some examples of autoantibodies implicated include ANA, antineutrophil cytoplasmic antibodies, anti-CCP antibodies, RF, antiphospholipid antibodies, anti-interferon antibodies, anti-interleukin antibodies, anti-thyroglobulin, and among many others. ANA positivity—usually found in cases of connective tissue disease (CTD) such as systemic lupus, scleroderma, or mixed CTD—has been reported in up to one-third of acute COVID-19 cases.[79] ANA positivity has been linked to higher illness severity from COVID-19 (anti-DNA positive predictive value [PPV] 86%) and increased complications, including ICU stays.[81] Furthermore, persistent autoantibody positivity has been noted for several months after acute COVID infection. One recent study reported ANA titers greater than 1:160 in 43% of patients 12 months after onset of COVID-19 symptoms.[80] Given that PASC pain can sometimes mimic other diagnoses, such as ANA-associated CTD, ordering ANA tests has been recommended as part of the workup for PASC pain symptoms.[77] Caution should be taken, however, when contemplating ordering immunologic laboratory testing to workup PASC-related pain as the clinical relevance of autoantibody positivity post-COVID infection remains poorly understood. It is unclear if a positive test represents new onset of a rheumatologic condition, latent autoimmunity, worsening of a previously diagnosed inflammatory condition, PASC as a new autoimmune condition itself, other immunologic dysfunction, or simply an incidental finding, as benign ANA (eg, anti-dense fine speckled-70 antibodies) can be found in up to 20% of healthy individuals without autoimmune disease.[87,88] Furthermore, although autoantibody positivity may be alarming as it is classically seen in cases of CTD, transient autoantibody production may be driven by the downstream activation of autoreactive B and T cells triggered by cytokines or by the B and T cells themselves recognizing viral antigens (molecular mimicry).[86] Therefore, careful interpretation of autoantibody laboratory tests during acute viral infections and even several months after suspected recovery is advised.

Diagnostic Testing

If patients have signs of peripheral neuropathy on physical examination and/or by history, nerve conduction/EMG testing is appropriate. If small fiber neuropathy is suspected, a single fiber EMG and/or skin biopsy may be required to diagnose. In the setting of clinical suspicion for obstructive sleep apnea (OSA), sleep studies may be indicated, as untreated OSA may aggravate acute and chronic pain conditions.[89] CPET, if available, may also be particularly useful in distinguishing mitochondrial dysfunction from deconditioning or cardiopulmonary causes of exercise intolerance and PEM.

REHABILITATION/TREATMENT STRATEGIES

Much of the approach to PASC rehabilitation and therapeutics will overlap with typical pain- and musculoskeletal-related strategies. However, special consideration is needed for concurrent neurologic, autonomic, inflammatory, and cardiopulmonary symptoms and dysfunction. In addition, it is important to recognize the impact of insomnia, mental health issues and coping strategies on the experience of post-COVID pain and PASC.

Rehabilitation Strategies

Rehabilitation approaches can consider gradual return to activity as tolerated, although no validated protocols exist at this time. Physical therapy can play an integral role in structured rehabilitation addressing deconditioning, poor balance, and moving safely in pain and fatigue, as well as addressing specific pulmonary and cardiovascular considerations such as shortness of breath and POTS/dysautonomia. For patients at risk for PEM, it is important that activity-based rehabilitation be mindful of the potential impact of exertion on PEM and to not exceed the threshold of activity that triggers PEM for a given patient. Over time, this threshold can be gradually increased in many patients. In general, restorative exercises such as breathing exercises, stretching, yoga, and gentle low-intensity aerobic exercise tend to be more well tolerated than high-intensity aerobic exercise or weight training. High-intensity aerobic exercise and weight training are associated with temporary increases in inflammation and cortisol levels, which may exacerbate pain conditions and trigger PEM.[90] In addition, for patients with postural tachycardia, recumbent exercises tend to be more well tolerated.

Respiratory issues are common in PASC and may be interpreted as barriers to physical activity by patients. Home breathing exercises can help alleviate some respiratory symptoms that limit ability to engage in physical activity. This may include pursed lip breathing or incentive spirometry. Breathing and conditioning exercises can be done during the same session or separately.

Lifestyle Recommendations for Postacute Sequelae of COVID-19 Recovery and Pain Management

Given the emerging research that suggests that PASC-related pain may be mediated by an inflammatory response, reducing inflammation through diet and lifestyle may help with recovery and symptom management.[57] Anti-inflammatory lifestyle strategies include an anti-inflammatory diet,[91,92] such as the Mediterranean diet, smoking cessation, limiting alcohol intake, regular exercise/activity, good quality sleep, stress management, and weight management. As part of interdisciplinary care for PASC, nutritionists can be particularly helpful for some patients to engage in health eating and weight-loss strategies, particularly those with coexisting medical conditions or dietary restrictions.

Quality sleep may be supported by interventions such as education on sleep hygiene, evaluation for sleep apnea, and medications such as melatonin. Patients may also experience depression, anxiety, regret, trauma, re-experiencing hospitalization, and loneliness following COVID-19 infections. Evaluation and treatment for concurrent mental health issues are important to support pain management. Rehab psychology and counseling are an important component of management of chronic pain conditions, particularly when there are concurrent mental health issues that may impact recovery.

Clinician-moderated support groups that focus on behavioral strategies to manage PASC-related symptoms, including pain, are one strategy developed for PASC and currently being evaluated. These interventions may be particularly helpful in providing patients with peer support in a moderated setting in which they are guided to evidence-based strategies for self-management of symptoms and have previously been found to be effective in ICU recovery.[93]

Pain Medications in Postacute Sequelae of COVID-19-Related Pain

The approach to medication management of PASC-related pain can be similar to typical pain management strategies but with important considerations specific to PASC. For example, patients with PASC may be particularly sensitive to the sedating and cognitive impairment side effects of commonly used pain medications such as gabapentin and other anticonvulsants, sedating antidepressants, muscle relaxants, and opioids as many experience a PASC-related "brain fog." Interestingly, low-dose naltrexone (LDN) has shown promise in its use for PASC-related pain, fatigue, and mood, though data are limited to small non-randomized studies, and more rigorous evaluation is needed.[94] Side effects of LDN include diarrhea and fatigue and may limit use.[94] In addition, cost and availability of pharmacies able to compound LDN may be additional barriers to use.

Disability and Return to Work Considerations

Considering the broad constellation of symptoms of PASC and PASC-related pain conditions on daily function, patients benefit from a comprehensive approach to disability accommodations. Symptoms can fluctuate during the day or over time, which can make it challenging for employers to understand how to make reasonable accommodations. In addition, the delayed responses to overexertion seen in PEM can make it more challenging to communicate the need for accommodations to prevent these worsening symptoms of pain and/or fatigue. Return to work evaluations should consider work intensity, duration, responsibilities, and physical and mental demands. When available, vocational counseling can be particularly important to help patients navigate return to work strategies, appropriate work accommodations, and the disability system.

HEALTH EQUITY CONSIDERATIONS

It is well-documented that COVID-19 has had disparate impact on lower socioeconomic and minority communities.[56] This includes not only a higher risk of experiencing COVID-19 infection but more severe illness and higher rates of death. Although research in this area is sparse, these increased risks likely extend further into the impact on pain and musculoskeletal health issues. The social determinants of health, including access to care, insurance status, financial security, housing stability, and health literacy have a direct impact on many of the comorbidities and risk factors for worse outcomes following infection with COVID-19, such as obesity, hypertension, renal disease, and diabetes.

In addition, for some of the most pervasive and impactful symptoms, including fatigue, myalgias, and arthralgias, female patients are at higher risk than men. Fatigue is often one of the largest contributors to a delay in return to work or need for reduced work hours and can therefore cause further financial stress, particularly in women.

Furthermore, given that PASC is still an emerging public health issue, most PASC care is clustered in urban, academic settings, which disproportionately limits access to care to those living outside of those communities or without the means to travel to these clinics. The rapid expansion of telemedicine has increased the ability to provide care to patients in less accessible communities, but still requires that patients have financial and geographic access to Internet connection and technical skills to manage a telecommunication platform.

Financial considerations should also be considered when offering diagnostics and counseling to patients. Laboratory tests, advanced imaging, medications, therapies, and procedures such as electrodiagnostics are costly for an uninsured or underinsured patient or may not be covered by a patient's insurance. There is also the added financial burden if the patient or their caregiver has to take time off work to attend appointments. Furthermore, most of the supplements that we can offer patients are not covered by insurance and specialty medications, such as LDN have the added burden of needing a specialty compounding pharmacy, which can be challenging.

RESEARCH GAPS

Although there is rapidly emerging research related to the etiology, risk factors and experiences of people with PASC, there are critical gaps in our understanding of PASC-related pain. Although we are starting to better understand the pathophysiology of PASC-related pain, it is clear that more research is needed as there are many different phenotypes of pain and likely many different associated causes of PASC-related pain and different phenotypes. In addition, there is even more limited data on health disparities, particularly as they relate to the experience of pain and access to treatment for PASC-related pain conditions. There are emerging data suggesting that musculoskeletal injuries may be increased after COVID-19 particularly among athletes, but this relationship is not clear and needs further exploration.[95–97] In addition, although there are a number of evidence-based treatment strategies for many of the painful conditions experienced in PASC, there are very few ongoing clinical trials of treatments specifically for PASC-related pain.

SUMMARY

Pain is common in people who are recovering from COVID-19, and patients may experience a wide range of painful conditions including musculoskeletal-related and neuropathic pain. Patients may experience multiple different painful conditions and other concurrent symptoms that complicate their experience of pain. Although the pathophysiology of pain in PASC is still largely unproven, it likely relates to a variety of immune system changes including inflammation, the presence of auto-antibodies, autonomic dysregulation, and changes in clotting. A thorough history and diagnostic evaluation are important given the myriad symptoms, concurrent conditions, and exacerbating factors that can impact recovery from pain. Despite the limited availability of clinical trials of specific treatment strategies for PASC-related pain, there are many rehabilitation strategies that can be used to address COVID-related pain and a number of emerging and promising treatments that are under evaluation.

DISCLOSURES

None.

CLINICS CARE POINTS

- Painful musculoskeletal conditions are common in patients with post-acute sequelae of COVID-19 (PASC).
- Many patients with PASC experience multiple concomitant pain symptoms.
- Pathophysiology of pain in PASC is still unproven but a variety of immune system changes including inflammation, the presence of autoantibodies, mitochondrial dysfunction, autonomic dysregulation, and changes in clotting have been hypothesized.
- Treatment strategies should be holistic and take into consideration other concurrent PASC symptoms and a biopsychosocial treatment approach.

REFERENCES

1. Centers for Disease Control and Prevention. COVID Data Tracker. Available at: https://covid.cdc.gov/covid-data-tracker. Accessed May, 03 2022.
2. Centers for Disease Control and Prevention. COVID Data Tracker Weekly Review. Available at: https://www.cdc.gov/coronavirus/2019-ncov/covid-data/covidview/index.html. Accessed August 30, 2022.
3. Groff D, Sun A, Ssentongo AE, et al. Short-term and Long-term Rates of Postacute Sequelae of SARS-CoV-2 Infection: A Systematic Review. JAMA Netw Open 2021;4(10):e2128568.
4. Samrah SM, Al-Mistarehi AH, Kewan T, et al. Viral Clearance Course of COVID-19 Outbreaks. J Multidiscip Healthc 2021;14:555–65.
5. Malik P, Patel K, Pinto C, et al. Post-acute COVID-19 syndrome (PCS) and health-related quality of life (HRQoL)-A systematic review and meta-analysis. J Med Virol 2022;94(1):253–62.
6. Venkatesan P. NICE guideline on long COVID. Lancet Respir Med 2021;9(2):129.
7. World Health Organization. Coronavirus disease (COVID-19): Post COVID-19 condition. Available at: https://www.who.int/news-room/questions-and-answers/item/coronavirus-disease-(covid-19)-post-covid-19-condition. Accessed August 22, 2022.
8. Center for Disease Control and Prevention. Long COVID or Post-COVID Conditions. Available at: https://www.cdc.gov/coronavirus/2019-ncov/long-term-effects/index.html#print. Accessed August 22, 2022.
9. Davis HE, Assaf GS, McCorkell L, et al. Characterizing long COVID in an international cohort: 7 months of symptoms and their impact. EClinicalMedicine 2021;38:101019.
10. Hernandez-Romieu AC, Carton TW, Saydah S, et al. Prevalence of Select New Symptoms and Conditions Among Persons Aged Younger Than 20 Years and 20 Years or Older at 31 to 150 Days After Testing Positive or Negative for SARS-CoV-2. JAMA Netw Open 2022;5(2):e2147053.
11. Michelen M, Manoharan L, Elkheir N, et al. Characterising long COVID: a living systematic review. BMJ Glob Health 2021;6(9). https://doi.org/10.1136/bmjgh-2021-005427.

12. Wang L, Foer D, MacPhaul E, et al. PASCLex: A comprehensive post-acute sequelae of COVID-19 (PASC) symptom lexicon derived from electronic health record clinical notes. J Biomed Inform 2022;125:103951.
13. Alizadeh R, Aghsaeifard Z. Does COVID19 activates previous chronic pain? A case series. Ann Med Surg (Lond) 2021;61:169–71.
14. Kemp HI, Corner E, Colvin LA. Chronic pain after COVID-19: implications for rehabilitation. Br J Anaesth 2020;125(4):436–40.
15. Shanthanna H, Nelson AM, Kissoon N, et al. The COVID-19 pandemic and its consequences for chronic pain: a narrative review. Anaesthesia 2022;77(9): 1039–50.
16. Qin ES, Gold LS, Singh N, et al. Physical function and fatigue recovery at 6 months after hospitalization for COVID-19. PMR 2022. https://doi.org/10.1002/pmrj.12866.
17. Khoja O, Silva Passadouro B, Mulvey M, et al. Clinical Characteristics and Mechanisms of Musculoskeletal Pain in Long COVID. J Pain Res 2022;15:1729–48.
18. Maury A, Lyoubi A, Peiffer-Smadja N, et al. Neurological manifestations associated with SARS-CoV-2 and other coronaviruses: A narrative review for clinicians. Rev Neurol 2021;177(1–2):51–64.
19. Fernández-de-Las-Peñas C, Navarro-Santana M, Plaza-Manzano G, et al. Time course prevalence of post-COVID pain symptoms of musculoskeletal origin in patients who had survived severe acute respiratory syndrome coronavirus 2 infection: a systematic review and meta-analysis. Pain 2022;163(7):1220–31.
20. Karaarslan F, Demircioğlu Güneri F, Kardeş S. Postdischarge rheumatic and musculoskeletal symptoms following hospitalization for COVID-19: prospective follow-up by phone interviews. Rheumatol Int 2021;41(7):1263–71.
21. Ojeda A, Calvo A, Cuñat T, et al. Characteristics and influence on quality of life of new-onset pain in critical COVID-19 survivors. Eur J Pain 2022;26(3):680–94.
22. Harapan BN, Yoo HJ. Neurological symptoms, manifestations, and complications associated with severe acute respiratory syndrome coronavirus 2 (SARS-CoV-2) and coronavirus disease 19 (COVID-19). J Neurol 2021;268(9):3059–71.
23. Lippi G, Wong J, Henry BM. Myalgia may not be associated with severity of coronavirus disease 2019 (COVID-19). World J Emerg Med 2020;11(3):193–4.
24. Li LQ, Huang T, Wang YQ, et al. COVID-19 patients' clinical characteristics, discharge rate, and fatality rate of meta-analysis. J Med Virol 2020;92(6):577–83.
25. Tran VT, Porcher R, Pane I, et al. Course of post COVID-19 disease symptoms over time in the ComPaRe long COVID prospective e-cohort. Nat Commun 2022;13(1):1812.
26. Karaarslan F, Güneri FD, Kardeş S. Long COVID: rheumatologic/musculoskeletal symptoms in hospitalized COVID-19 survivors at 3 and 6 months. Clin Rheumatol 2022;41(1):289–96.
27. Tuzun S, Keles A, Okutan D, et al. Assessment of musculoskeletal pain, fatigue and grip strength in hospitalized patients with COVID-19. Eur J Phys Rehabil Med 2021;57(4):653–62.
28. Fernández-de-Las-Peñas C, Palacios-Ceña D, Gómez-Mayordomo V, et al. Prevalence of post-COVID-19 symptoms in hospitalized and non-hospitalized COVID-19 survivors: A systematic review and meta-analysis. Eur J Intern Med 2021;92: 55–70.
29. Jason LA, Islam M, Conroy K, et al. COVID-19 Symptoms Over Time: Comparing Long-Haulers to ME/CFS. Fatigue 2021;9(2):59–68.
30. Attal N, Martinez V, Bouhassira D. Potential for increased prevalence of neuropathic pain after the COVID-19 pandemic. Pain Rep 2021;6(1):e884.

31. Joshi D, Gyanpuri V, Pathak A, et al. Neuropathic Pain Associated with COVID-19: a Systematic Review of Case Reports. Curr Pain Headache Rep 2022;26(8): 595–603.

32. McFarland AJ, Yousuf MS, Shiers S, et al. Neurobiology of SARS-CoV-2 interactions with the peripheral nervous system: implications for COVID-19 and pain. Pain Rep 2021;6(1):e885.

33. Mackay A. A Paradigm for Post-Covid-19 Fatigue Syndrome Analogous to ME/CFS. Front Neurol 2021;12:701419.

34. Saud A, Naveen R, Aggarwal R, et al. COVID-19 and Myositis: What We Know So Far. Curr Rheumatol Rep 2021;23(8):63.

35. Galluzzo C, Chiapparoli I, Corrado A, et al. Rare forms of inflammatory myopathies - part I, generalized forms. Expert Rev Clin Immunol 2023;19(2):169–83.

36. Sacchi MC, Tamiazzo S, Lauritano EC, et al. Case report of COVID-19 in an elderly patient: could SARS-CoV2 trigger myositis? Eur Rev Med Pharmacol Sci 2020;24(22):11960–3.

37. Movahedi N, Ziaee V. COVID-19 and myositis; true dermatomyositis or prolonged post viral myositis? Pediatr Rheumatol Online J 2021;19(1):86.

38. Qian J, Xu H. COVID-19 Disease and Dermatomyositis: A Mini-Review. Front Immunol 2021;12:747116.

39. Mehan WA, Yoon BC, Lang M, et al. Paraspinal Myositis in Patients with COVID-19 Infection. AJNR Am J Neuroradiol 2020;41(10):1949–52.

40. Singh B, Kaur P, Mechineni A, et al. Rhabdomyolysis in COVID-19: Report of Four Cases. Cureus 2020;12(9):e10686.

41. Hannah JR, Ali SS, Nagra D, et al. Skeletal muscles and Covid-19: a systematic review of rhabdomyolysis and myositis in SARS-CoV-2 infection. Clin Exp Rheumatol 2022;40(2):329–38.

42. Cuthbertson BH, Roughton S, Jenkinson D, et al. Quality of life in the five years after intensive care: a cohort study. Crit Care 2010;14(1):R6.

43. Goettler CE, Pryor JP, Reilly PM. Brachial plexopathy after prone positioning. Crit Care 2002;6(6):540–2.

44. Malik GR, Wolfe AR, Soriano R, et al. Injury-prone: peripheral nerve injuries associated with prone positioning for COVID-19-related acute respiratory distress syndrome. Br J Anaesth 2020;125(6):e478–80.

45. Tankisi H, de Carvalho M, Z'Graggen WJ. Critical Illness Neuropathy. J Clin Neurophysiol 2020;37(3):205–7.

46. Finsterer J, Scorza FA, Scorza CA, et al. Peripheral neuropathy in COVID-19 is due to immune-mechanisms, pre-existing risk factors, anti-viral drugs, or bedding in the Intensive Care Unit. Arq Neuropsiquiatr 2021;79(10):924–8.

47. Frithiof R, Rostami E, Kumlien E, et al. Critical illness polyneuropathy, myopathy and neuronal biomarkers in COVID-19 patients: A prospective study. Clin Neurophysiol 2021;132(7):1733–40.

48. Koch S, Spuler S, Deja M, et al. Critical illness myopathy is frequent: accompanying neuropathy protracts ICU discharge. J Neurol Neurosurg Psychiatry 2011;82(3):287–93.

49. Latronico N, Bolton CF. Critical illness polyneuropathy and myopathy: a major cause of muscle weakness and paralysis. Lancet Neurol 2011;10(10):931–41.

50. Druschky A, Herkert M, Radespiel-Tröger M, et al. Critical illness polyneuropathy: clinical findings and cell culture assay of neurotoxicity assessed by a prospective study. Intensive Care Med 2001;27(4):686–93.

51. Lad H, Saumur TM, Herridge MS, et al. Intensive Care Unit-Acquired Weakness: Not just Another Muscle Atrophying Condition. Int J Mol Sci 2020;21(21). https://doi.org/10.3390/ijms21217840.
52. Vanhorebeek I, Latronico N, Van den Berghe G. ICU-acquired weakness. Intensive Care Med 2020;46(4):637–53.
53. Cabañes-Martínez L, Villadóniga M, González-Rodríguez L, et al. Neuromuscular involvement in COVID-19 critically ill patients. Clin Neurophysiol 2020;131(12): 2809–16.
54. Bednarík J, Vondracek P, Dusek L, et al. Risk factors for critical illness polyneuromyopathy. J Neurol 2005;252(3):343–51.
55. De Jonghe B, Sharshar T, Lefaucheur JP, et al. Paresis acquired in the intensive care unit: a prospective multicenter study. JAMA 2002;288(22):2859–67.
56. Guarneri B, Bertolini G, Latronico N. Long-term outcome in patients with critical illness myopathy or neuropathy: the Italian multicentre CRIMYNE study. J Neurol Neurosurg Psychiatry 2008;79(7):838–41.
57. Soares MN, Eggelbusch M, Naddaf E, et al. Skeletal muscle alterations in patients with acute Covid-19 and post-acute sequelae of Covid-19. J Cachexia Sarcopenia Muscle 2022;13(1):11–22.
58. Phetsouphanh C, Darley DR, Wilson DB, et al. Immunological dysfunction persists for 8 months following initial mild-to-moderate SARS-CoV-2 infection. Nat Immunol 2022;23(2):210–6.
59. Khazaal S, Harb J, Rima M, et al. The pathophysiology of Long COVID throughout the renin-angiotensin system. Molecules 2022;27(9). https://doi.org/10.3390/molecules27092903.
60. Cascella M, Del Gaudio A, Vittori A, et al. COVID-pain: acute and late-onset painful clinical manifestations in covid-19 - molecular mechanisms and research perspectives. J Pain Res 2021;14:2403–12.
61. Shiers S, Ray PR, Wangzhou A, et al. ACE2 and SCARF expression in human dorsal root ganglion nociceptors: implications for SARS-CoV-2 virus neurological effects. Pain 2020;161(11):2494–501.
62. Grobbelaar LM, Venter C, Vlok M, et al. SARS-CoV-2 spike protein S1 induces fibrin(ogen) resistant to fibrinolysis: implications for microclot formation in COVID-19. Biosci Rep 2021;41(8). https://doi.org/10.1042/BSR20210611.
63. Kell DB, Pretorius E. The potential role of ischaemia-reperfusion injury in chronic, relapsing diseases such as rheumatoid arthritis, Long COVID, and ME/CFS: evidence, mechanisms, and therapeutic implications. Biochem J 2022;479(16): 1653–708.
64. Fedorowski A. Postural orthostatic tachycardia syndrome: clinical presentation, aetiology and management. J Intern Med 2019;285(4):352–66.
65. Shouman K, Vanichkachorn G, Cheshire WP, et al. Autonomic dysfunction following COVID-19 infection: an early experience. Clin Auton Res 2021;31(3): 385–94.
66. Kersten J, Baumhardt M, Hartveg P, et al. Long COVID: Distinction between Organ Damage and Deconditioning. J Clin Med Res 2021;10(17). https://doi.org/10.3390/jcm10173782.
67. Kimmig LM, Rako ZA, Ziegler S, et al. Long-term comprehensive cardiopulmonary phenotyping of COVID-19. Respir Res 2022;23(1):263.
68. de Boer E, Petrache I, Goldstein NM, et al. Decreased Fatty Acid Oxidation and Altered Lactate Production during Exercise in Patients with Post-acute COVID-19 Syndrome. Am J Respir Crit Care Med 2022;205(1):126–9.

69. Qin ES, Gold LS, Hough CL, et al. Patient-reported functional outcomes 30 days after hospitalization for COVID-19. Pharm Manag PM R 2022;14(2):173–82.

70. An Analysis of the Prolonged COVID-19 Symptoms Survey by Patient-Led Research Team. Available at: https://patientresearchcovid19.com/research/report-1/#Support_by_Medical_Stafff. Accessed March 2, 2022.

71. Dundumalla S, Barshikar S, Niehaus WN, et al. A survey of dedicated PASC clinics: Characteristics, barriers and spirit of collaboration. Pharm Manag PM R 2022;14(3):348–56.

72. Gemelli Against COVID-19 Post-Acute Care Study Group. Post-COVID-19 global health strategies: the need for an interdisciplinary approach. Aging Clin Exp Res 2020;32(8):1613–20.

73. Lopez-Leon S, Wegman-Ostrosky T, Perelman C, et al. More than 50 long-term effects of COVID-19: a systematic review and meta-analysis. Sci Rep 2021; 11(1):16144.

74. Mueller JT, McConnell K, Burow PB, et al. Impacts of the COVID-19 pandemic on rural America. Proc Natl Acad Sci U S A 2021;118(1). https://doi.org/10.1073/pnas.2019378118.

75. Cheng KJG, Sun Y, Monnat SM. COVID-19 Death Rates Are Higher in Rural Counties With Larger Shares of Blacks and Hispanics. J Rural Health 2020; 36(4):602–8.

76. Hale N, Meit M, Pettyjohn S, et al. The implications of long COVID for rural communities. J Rural Health 2022. https://doi.org/10.1111/jrh.12655.

77. Sisó-Almirall A, Brito-Zerón P, Conangla Ferrín L, et al. Long Covid-19: Proposed Primary Care Clinical Guidelines for Diagnosis and Disease Management. Int J Environ Res Public Health 2021;18(8). https://doi.org/10.3390/ijerph18084350.

78. Blitshteyn S, Whiteson JH, Abramoff B, et al. Multi-disciplinary collaborative consensus guidance statement on the assessment and treatment of autonomic dysfunction in patients with post-acute sequelae of SARS-CoV-2 infection (PASC). Pharm Manag PM R 2022. https://doi.org/10.1002/pmrj.12894.

79. Pascolini S, Vannini A, Deleonardi G, et al. COVID-19 and Immunological Dysregulation: Can Autoantibodies be Useful? Clin Transl Sci 2021;14(2):502–8.

80. Seeßle J, Waterboer T, Hippchen T, et al. Persistent Symptoms in Adult Patients 1 Year After Coronavirus Disease 2019 (COVID-19): A Prospective Cohort Study. Clin Infect Dis 2022;74(7):1191–8.

81. Gomes C, Zuniga M, Crotty KA, et al. Autoimmune anti-DNA and anti-phosphatidylserine antibodies predict development of severe COVID-19. Life Sci Alliance 2021;4(11). https://doi.org/10.26508/lsa.202101180.

82. Lingel H, Meltendorf S, Billing U, et al. Unique autoantibody prevalence in long-term recovered SARS-CoV-2-infected individuals. J Autoimmun 2021;122: 102682.

83. Xu C, Fan J, Luo Y, et al. Prevalence and Characteristics of Rheumatoid-Associated Autoantibodies in Patients with COVID-19. J Inflamm Res 2021;14: 3123–8.

84. Jordhani M, Ruci D, Ruci V. Anti-phospholipid autoantibodies in COVID-19 patients. Ann Rheum Dis 2021;80(1). Available at: https://ard.bmj.com/content/80/Suppl_1/1381.1.

85. Rojas M, Rodríguez Y, Acosta-Ampudia Y, et al. Autoimmunity is a hallmark of post-COVID syndrome. J Transl Med 2022;20(1):129.

86. Taeschler P, Cervia C, Zurbuchen Y, et al. Autoantibodies in COVID-19 correlate with antiviral humoral responses and distinct immune signatures. Allergy 2022; 77(8):2415–30.

87. Mahler M, Andrade LE, Casiano CA, et al. Anti-DFS70 antibodies: an update on our current understanding and their clinical usefulness. Expert Rev Clin Immunol 2019;15(3):241–50.

88. Conrad K, Röber N, Andrade LEC, et al. The Clinical Relevance of Anti-DFS70 Autoantibodies. Clin Rev Allergy Immunol 2017;52(2):202–16.

89. Kaczmarski P, Karuga FF, Szmyd B, et al. The Role of Inflammation, Hypoxia, and Opioid Receptor Expression in Pain Modulation in Patients Suffering from Obstructive Sleep Apnea. Int J Mol Sci 2022;23(16). https://doi.org/10.3390/ijms23169080.

90. Cerqueira É, Marinho DA, Neiva HP, et al. Inflammatory Effects of High and Moderate Intensity Exercise-A Systematic Review. Front Physiol 2019;10:1550.

91. Barrea L, Grant WB, Frias-Toral E, et al. Dietary Recommendations for Post-COVID-19 Syndrome. Nutrients 2022;14(6). https://doi.org/10.3390/nu14061305.

92. Naureen Z, Dautaj A, Nodari S, et al. Proposal of a food supplement for the management of post-COVID syndrome. Eur Rev Med Pharmacol Sci 2021;25(1 Suppl):67–73.

93. Mikkelsen ME, Jackson JC, Hopkins RO, et al. Peer Support as a Novel Strategy to Mitigate Post-Intensive Care Syndrome. AACN Adv Crit Care 2016;27(2):221–9.

94. O'Kelly B, Vidal L, McHugh T, et al. Safety and efficacy of low dose naltrexone in a long covid cohort; an interventional pre-post study. Brain Behav Immun Health 2022;24:100485.

95. Grech S, Borg JN, Cuschieri S. Back pain: An aftermath of Covid-19 pandemic? A Malta perspective. Muscoskel Care 2022;20(1):145–50.

96. Annino G, Manzi V, Alashram AR, et al. COVID-19 as a Potential Cause of Muscle Injuries in Professional Italian Serie A Soccer Players: A Retrospective Observational Study. Int J Environ Res Public Health 2022;19(17). https://doi.org/10.3390/ijerph191711117.

97. Maestro A, Varillas-Delgado D, Morencos E, et al. Injury Incidence Increases after COVID-19 Infection: A Case Study with a Male Professional Football Team. Int J Environ Res Public Health 2022;19(16). https://doi.org/10.3390/ijerph191610267.

Fatigue in Post-Acute Sequelae of Coronavirus Disease 2019

Zachary Abbott, DO[1], William Summers, MD[1], William Niehaus, MD[2],*

KEYWORDS

- PASC • Long-COVID • Fatigue • ME/CFS • Post-exertional malaise • SARS-CoV-2

KEY POINTS

- According to recent data from the US Census Bureau and CDCs National Center for Health Statistics, 7.5% or one in 13 patients diagnosed with coronavirus disease 2019 (COVID-19) reported long-term symptoms.
- Because of the varied possible etiologies causing post-acute sequelae of COVID-19 (PASC) symptoms, there does not seem to be a single-laboratory evaluation, diagnostic test, or examination finding that will best identify the etiology of PASC symptoms.
- At this time, there is continued investigation into which medication, therapy program, diet, infusion, or supplement that would best improve PASC symptoms.

INTRODUCTION/HISTORY/DEFINITIONS/BACKGROUND

As of July 19, 2022, the novel severe acute respiratory syndrome coronavirus 2 (SARS-CoV-2) virus and its associated infectious disease coronavirus disease 2019 (COVID-19) have amassed over 600 million confirmed cases worldwide.[1] Multiple authors cite significant underreporting of infections with true infection rates somewhere in the range of 2 to 20 times higher than documented.[2,3] In the United States alone, these infections have led to nearly 5 million hospital admissions[4] and over 1 million deaths.[5] Hospitalization rates are widely variable with differences in virus variant, vaccination status, and age, though most estimates place the percentage of hospitalization in the single digits.[6] Despite low incidence of hospitalization, most research to date has focused on sequelae and management of acute disease in patients hospitalized with severe disease.

Department of Physical Medicine and Rehabilitation, University of Colorado School of Medicine, 12631 East 17th Avenue, Academic Office One, Mail Stop F493, Aurora, CO 80045, USA
[1] Co-First Author.
[2] Senior Author.
* Corresponding author.
E-mail address: WILLIAM.NIEHAUS@CUANSCHUTZ.EDU

Phys Med Rehabil Clin N Am 34 (2023) 607–621
https://doi.org/10.1016/j.pmr.2023.04.006
1047-9651/23/© 2023 Elsevier Inc. All rights reserved.
pmr.theclinics.com

Recently, attention has focused on long-term impacts of COVID-19. A clinical profile has emerged known as "long-COVID" to describe the prolonged impacts of infection. Commonly described sequelae include fatigue, post-exertional malaise, and cognitive dysfunction, although sufferers of long-COVID often experience a multitude of symptoms from various organ systems.[7] This constellation of symptoms has been termed "Post-Acute Sequelae of COVID" (PASC).[8] According to recent data from the US Census Bureau and centers for disease control and prevention (CDCs) National Center for Health Statistics, 7.5% or one in 13 patients diagnosed with COVID-19 reported long-term symptoms.[a] These individuals were more likely to be younger than 59 years, female, and Hispanic, comparatively. Long-COVID has been documented in less symptomatic nonhospitalized patients[7,9,10] and among more severe cases that required hospitalization and critical care.

One of the most reported symptoms of long-COVID is fatigue.[11,12] In general, fatigue is a subjective, nonspecific term that is pervasive in the outpatient setting with one in five primary care provider visits discussing the topic.[13] Fatigue is often described as akin to feeling tired (reported more often by male patients) or depression/anxiety (reported more often by female patients).[13] The etiology of fatigue can be physiologic, secondary, or chronic. Physiologic fatigue refers to day-to-day variation in energy levels and is often related to sleep patterns, exercise habits, and diet, among other factors. This form of fatigue improves with rest. Pathologic or secondary fatigue is attributable to a medical condition (eg, anemia) and often lasts greater than 1 month but less than 6 months and often improves with treatment of the underlying medical etiology. Chronic fatigue is defined as lasting greater than 6 months and not improving with rest or medical treatment. Another form of fatigue is "post-exertional malaise," which refers to worsening of fatigue following physical, cognitive, or emotional stressors that under normal circumstances would not cause symptoms.[14] Data from the International Committee on Fatigue Following Infection[15] suggest that the rates of clinically significant post-COVID infection fatigue are in the range of 10% to 35% at 6 months after controlling for medical and psychiatric causes.

This high prevalence has drawn comparisons between the PASC and post-viral fatigue syndrome/myalgic encephalomyelitis and chronic fatigue syndrome (ME/CFS). Chronic fatigue syndrome is a constellation of symptoms that accompanies severe fatigue for a period of longer than 6 months. The etiology of this condition is debated with early discussions centered on post-viral sequelae[16] and more recent criteria being updated to include considerations for a neurologic basis of disease. However, sources agree that ME/CFS encompasses a variety of organ systems with pathophysiology related to the metabolic, neurologic, and myofibrillar components.[17] ME/CFS requires a thorough medical and psychological workup to rule out other etiologies (see Evaluation section [**Box 1**]). ME/CFS is often a debilitating constellation of symptoms and has led to an estimated loss of billions of dollars of productivity in both households and the labor force.[18]

ME/CFS provides a striking example of the medical, psychological, and societal impact of post-viral and chronic fatigue conditions. Given the similarities of this condition with the new construct of PASC, it is essential to describe the pathophysiology, evaluation, and treatment of fatigue as it relates to long-COVID to better inform clinicians and patients moving forward. With this goal in mind, multiple entities have begun to provide guidance on PASC and, specifically, prolonged fatigue.[20,21] This article serves as a review of the known and hypothesized pathophysiology surrounding

---

[a] Defined as symptoms lasting 3 or more months after first contracting the virus.

> **Box 1**
> **Institute of Medicine proposed criteria for myalgic encephalomyelitis and chronic fatigue syndrome[19]**
>
> Proposed Diagnostic Criteria for ME/CFS
> - A significant reduction or impairment in the ability to engage in premorbid activities for greater than 6 months, accompanied by new and profound fatigue, not the result of excessive exertion and is not substantially improved with rest
> - Post-exertional malaise
> - Unrefreshing sleep
>
> AND ≥1 of the following:
> - Cognitive impairment
> - Orthostatic dysfunction

fatigue as a PASC and provides clinicians with guidance regarding the evaluation and treatment of this complex symptom.

Pathophysiology of Fatigue/Post-Exertional Fatigue Related to Coronavirus Disease 2019

There are currently limited data regarding the pathophysiology of fatigue as a PASC. Mackay[22] posited that SARS-CoV-2 infection, as with other triggers of ME/CFS such as vaccination, severe emotional distress, and viral infection, may act as a severe physiological stressor that could lead to fatigue by impacting hypothalamic dysfunction, spurring systemic inflammation via cytokine storm, and causing chronic damage to the pulmonary, cardiac, neurologic (including psychiatric), and myofascial systems.

Hypothalamic–pituitary axis dysfunction

Given the role of SARS-CoV-2 as a severe physiological stressor, a logical driver of COVID-related fatigue may be an altered response by the brain's stress center, the hypothalamic paraventricular nucleus (PVN). The hypothalamic PVN plays a crucial role in the body's hypothalamic–pituitary axis (HPA), a series of feedback mechanisms that regulate the release of glucocorticoids and the body's autonomic response to stimuli. Neurons within the PVN secrete the first hormone in this cascade, known as corticotrophin-releasing hormone or corticotropin-releasing hormone (CRH). These cells show significant plasticity in response to acute and chronic stress and have been suggested as a potential source of ME/CFS.[22]

The trigger of PVN dysfunction in cases of COVID-19 is not yet fully defined. In cases of ME/CFS, multiple mechanisms of damage have been described. A study by De Bellis and colleagues[23] investigated the role of an autoimmune response targeting the pituitary and hypothalamus. Their study assessed anti-pituitary antibody (APA) and anti-hypothalamic antibody (AHA) blood levels among 30 adult women diagnosed with ME/CSF using validated criteria[23] compared with 25 healthy controls. Patients diagnosed with ME/CFS had AHA and APA levels that were significantly higher (56% and 33%, respectively) than control patients. Further, important markers of appropriate stress response including adrenocorticotropic hormone (ACTH), cortisol, and insulin-like growth factor 1 (IGF-1) were lower in ME/CFS patients compared with controls. Studies have recently suggested that acute COVID-19 can be associated with similar autoimmune hypothalamic and pituitary involvement. Gonen and colleagues[24] performed a prospective, case-control study (49 COVID + patients, 28 healthy controls) which assessed prevalence of adrenal insufficiency and HPA antibodies. Their data identified AHA in 31% of patients and APA in 51% of patients.

Adrenal insufficiency was present in 4 (8.1%) of the 49 cases. We did not find any data regarding the prevalence of these antibodies and/or adrenal insufficiency in cases of PASC.

Primary adrenal insufficiency

Some authors[25] have suggested that primary adrenal gland insufficiency specifically may be underdiagnosed among PASC. COVID-19 infection may impact the adrenal glands by both direct and indirect mechanisms. From a cellular level, SARS-CoV-2 binds preferentially to angiotensin-converting enzyme 2 (ACE-2). Various studies have suggested that ACE-2 is expressed on adrenal glands and that SARS-CoV-2 may have a propensity to replicate within these cells.[25] However, there has been no direct evidence of cellular damage in these tissues. More concerning are the potential impacts of COVID-19 infection on the adrenal vasculature. Autopsy studies of patients with severe COVID-19 have found evidence of adrenal hemorrhage and infarct.[26,27] From a histopathologic level, there is evidence of coagulation sequelae such as fibrin and microthrombi in the adrenal vasculature.[27] Multiple studies have suggested the potential for these hypercoagulable sequelae to persist following initial infection even in mild cases of COVID-19.[28] With these potential impacts in mind, it is essential to consider the role of adrenal damage and insufficiency in producing common PASC including fatigue.

Cytokine storm

Beyond autoimmune dysfunction, the body's initial inflammatory response to COVID-19 may directly impact the PVNs ability to regulate stress. Acute COVID-19 infection has been shown to cause what is known as a "cytokine storm," a dramatic, systemic immune response that involves pro-inflammatory cytokines such as interleukin (IL)-1, IL-6, and tumor necrosis factor (TNF).[29] The magnitude of the body's response to infection has been correlated with the severity of this inflammatory response. For example, dramatic surges of inflammatory markers in severe COVID-19 infection have been linked with worse outcomes, including the development of acute respiratory distress syndrome and multiorgan failure.[30] In the case of COVID-related fatigue, cytokine expression patterns may play a role. Previous work has suggested that the expression of Th1 and Th17, important factors in cell mediated immunity, is downregulated in patients with ME/CFS.[25] Further, studies in populations following infection with Epstein–Barr virus and West Nile virus found that patients who experienced post-viral fatigue had higher expression of pro-inflammatory cytokines IL-2 and IL-6 compared with controls who recovered from infection without fatigue.[31,32] In patients experiencing PASC, increased levels of pro-inflammatory biomarkers such as IL-6, c-reactive protein (CRP), D-dimer have been identified.[33] Imaging studies of COVID-19 with ongoing symptoms greater than 30 days from infection found higher levels of FDG uptake in bone marrow and blood vessels, signifying increased inflammation.[34] These prolonged pro-inflammatory states have been hypothesized as a potential cause of long-COVID-related fatigue and are being targeted as potential therapeutic targets.[35]

Pulmonary dysfunction

Aside from inflammatory and endocrinologic pathways, COVID-19 has been implicated in damage to cardiac, pulmonary, myofascial, and neurologic systems. Given its tropism for pulmonary tissue, it is expected that COVID-19 would be linked to long-term pulmonary sequelae. Patients with COVID-19 have been found to have radiological lung abnormalities, including fibrosis, and impaired pulmonary function (including diffusion capacity) months after initial infection.[10] Impaired gas exchange and pulmonary function may play a role in fatigue both directly (hypoxemia or hypercarbia) and indirectly (increased respiratory effort), in addition to causing more common pulmonary symptoms such as dyspnea and cough which will be covered elsewhere in this series.

Cardiac dysfunction

Closely linked to COVID-19-related respiratory compromise is the cardiovascular system. Sars-CoV-2 has been linked to both microvascular damage and direct cardiac myocyte invasion. Autopsy studies of patients with COVID-19 have shown evidence of direct viral invasion in both cardiac myocytes and endothelial cells associated with inflammation and dysfunction.[36] A cohort study performed by Puntmann and colleagues[37] investigated a group of 100 COVID-19 recovered individuals at a median time frame of 2 to 3 months postinfection and found evidence of cardiac involvement (including fibrosis) in 78%, with evidence of ongoing myocardial inflammation in 60%, independent from preexisting cardiovascular conditions. This significantly high prevalence has been brought into question by Malek,[38] who performed a similar analysis and identified similar pathology in a twofold lower frequency. Despite this controversy, there is further evidence of cardiac inflammation, including subclinical myocarditis, in healthy, recovered COVID-19 patients.[39] A cardinal symptom of cardiac dysfunction, including heart failure and myocarditis, is fatigue. This highlights the potential for cardiac damage to drive chronic fatigue symptoms in COVID-19.

Myopathy

In conjunction with fatigue, myalgia has been a commonly reported PASC. This has led to an investigation of myopathy as a driver of physical fatigue during both acute and post-acute periods of COVID-19 infection. Agergaard and colleagues[40] investigated the presence of neuropathy and myopathy in 20 patients recovered from COVID-19 (median 216 days) who experienced persistent neuromuscular symptoms (including fatigue) using nerve conduction studies and electromyography (EMG) needle examination. Nerve conduction studies were normal in all 20 patients. However, myopathic changes were present in 55% based on EMG. In the acute phase, there is more definitive evidence of structural myopathic changes. Multiple studies[41–43] performed biopsies on patients deceased from severe COVID-19 and identified patterns consistent with inflammatory myopathy and critical illness myopathy. Case reports have corroborated the presence of critical illness myopathy[44] in cases of severe COVID-19. There have also been case reports of myositis during or after mild/moderate COVID-19 infection, though these data lack power to draw conclusions regarding causation.[45,46] According to a systemic review by Soares and colleagues,[47] there are some similarities between skeletal muscle changes in PASC and chronic fatigue syndrome. These similarities have yet to be fully investigated. In addition to structural and inflammatory muscle changes, metabolic changes may also play a role in myalgia and fatigue as PASC. For example, elevated levels of growth/differentiation factor-15 (GDF-15), an indirect marker of mitochondrial stress, have been found in a significant proportion of patients hospitalized with COVID-19.[48] Further, mitochondrial stress and skeletal muscle metabolic changes are associated with critical illness myopathy, a well-known sequela of severe COVID-19 infection. Little data exist regarding metabolic or myopathic changes in patients with mild–moderate COVID-19 infection who experience PASC.

Neuropsychiatric dysfunction

Fatigue can be a common manifestation of both central and peripheral neurologic dysfunction. The pathophysiology of PASC as it relates to the central and peripheral neurologic system will be discussed elsewhere in this series. Importantly, coronaviruses are known to invade neurologic tissues, potentially leading to alterations in cognition, behavior, mood, and function.[49] Recent data have emerged regarding the neuro-*psychiatric* sequelae of COVID-19 in driving fatigue. In a systemic review, Renaud-Charest and colleagues[50] found that depressive symptoms were present in 11% to 28% of patients greater than 12 weeks following initial infection, irrespective of initiation infection severity. Further, Ortelli and colleagues[51] performed thorough neuropsychological assessments on recovered COVID-19 patients. They found that, compared with controls, patients had higher levels of perceived exertion and fatigue. They also exhibited apathy, executive deficits, and impaired cognition compared with controls. Physiologic testing suggested that these outcomes may be related to GABA dysfunction though further testing is needed to clarify this hypothesis. Penninx[49] suggested that previously described altered inflammatory/immunologic pathways may contribute to the development of depression and anxiety in patients with PASC. Conversely, Stengel and colleagues[45] considered the potential for COVID-19 to trigger a functional disease or bodily distress disorder, akin to postinfectious irritable bowel syndrome, for which there is no clear pathophysiological basis.

Sleep disturbance

Dysfunctional sleep is a commonly reported symptom in both acute and chronic COVID-19 infection.[52–54] Estimates from Pataka and colleagues[55] suggest that 50% to 75% of all patients who suffer from COVID-19 infection experience sleep disturbance. Insomnia and fatigue often persist concurrently in patients once acute COVID-19 infection.[54] Fernández-De-Las-Peñas and colleagues[56] reported data from a multicenter cohort study including individuals previously diagnosed with COVID-19 and focused on reported symptoms of anxiety, depression, and sleep disturbance. They found that 33.2% of randomly selected patients experienced sleep disturbance at 6 to 10 months and that number decreased to 27.7% in the 11 to 15-month window. These data were modeled on trajectory curves and found to decrease at a slower rate than other major medical events such as cardiac surgery, suggesting that poor sleep quality could be longer lasting PASC, even when compared with anxiety and depression.

Gut dysregulation

Recently, literature has linked the gut microbiome to chronic fatigue syndrome.[57] Similar findings have started to emerge for PASC. Yeoh and colleagues[58] analyzed fecal microbiota from 100 patients with confirmed COVID-19 infection, including serial samples from 27 of those patients at least 30 days after virus resolution. They identified a significant difference in microbiome for patients with COVID-19 compared with controls, regardless of medication use. Further, samples greater than 30 days from infection resolution continued to exhibit lower levels of immunomodulating bacteria, potentially leading to prolonged symptoms and changes in the inflammatory cascade. Liu and colleagues[59] recently published data from a prospective cohort study suggesting the gut microbiome profile may affect both susceptibility to PASC and the symptom profile of patients experience. In their panel of 106 COVID-19 recovered patients, fatigue was the most reported PASC.

EVALUATION

The prevalence of people suffering from symptoms of PASC required professionals to develop guidelines to establish a cohesive and standardized treatment approach. Herrera and colleagues[20] provided guidance through the American Academy of Physical Medicine and Rehabilitation (AAPM&R) Multi-Disciplinary PASC Collaborative. With the help of multiple professionals and patient representatives, they created a cohesive approach to the care of people with PASC with a focus on fatigue. To improve access to interventions, this group recommends early evaluation, diagnosis, and treatment. With this goal in mind, assessment should begin if symptoms of PASC are not improving after 1 month from acute symptom onset, if symptoms are severe, or if symptoms are significantly interfering with quality of life. It is common for fluctuations in symptoms over the course of 1 to 2 months. Therefore, mild fatigue that is not functionally limiting can be closely monitored without extensive management.

Gathering a thorough history of the patient's experience with their initial illness can help guide assessments as well. The severity of illness related to COVID-19 has been associated with the risk of long-term sequelae and impairment. Approximately two-third of outpatients diagnosed with COVID-19 return to full health by the fourth week. On the other hand, patients diagnosed in an emergency room, two-third of which were eventually hospitalized, 50.9% developed chronic symptoms. Other risk factors include increased age, number of medical comorbidities, and premorbid psychological disorders. Special consideration should be given to assessment for mental health disorders. Acute mental health disorders (55%), anxiety (4.7%), depression (2%), and pos-traumatic stress disorder (PTSD) (23.5% of ward survivors, 46.9% of intensive care unit [ICU] survivors) need to be fully evaluated, all of which can contribute to a patient's activity level.[60–62] Vulnerable populations including pregnant women, minority racial and ethnic groups, and low socioeconomic status should be considered at higher risk for post-COVID-related illnesses, as outlined by the PASC Collaborative review. A broad differential for contributors to these symptoms should be considered when evaluating these patients. These include, but are not limited to, critical illness myopathy and polyneuropathy, circadian rhythm disorders, and mood disorders.

Further, Herrera and colleagues[20] provided the following recommendations when assessing patients with PASC should include.

- Detailed impacts on functional limitations throughout the day
- Impact of activity and activity intensity on fatigue
- Fatigue's impact on activities of daily living, occupational activities, and vocational activities
- Utilization of physical function tools such as timed walked tests and timed sit to stand should be used to guide targeted therapies
- A detailed history of premorbid health conditions and activity level
- Consideration of other etiologies that may exacerbate fatigue symptoms including areas of mood, sleep, nutrition, endocrine, immunology cardiopulmonary
- A review of medication adverse effects that could exacerbate fatigue. Drug classes include antihistamines, anticholinergic, pain medications, and anxiolytics.

Given the similarities between PASC and ME/CFS, as previously discussed, a similar initial assessment can be considered. The CDC and National Institute of Health and Clinical Excellence (NICE) recommend a minimal set of tests for patients presenting with fatigue. The CDC recommends initial evaluation with urinalysis; complete blood count; comprehensive metabolic panel; and measurement of phosphorus, thyroid-stimulating hormone, and C-reactive protein. NICE also recommends using immunoglobulin A endomysial antibodies to screen for celiac disease, and if indicated by the history or physical examination, urine drug screening, rheumatoid factor testing, and antinuclear antibody testing. Viral titers are not recommended unless the patient's history is suggestive of an infectious process, because they do not confirm or eliminate the diagnosis of ME/CFS. The National Collaborating Centre for

Primary care identified red flag symptoms and associated conditions. This includes Chest Pain (cardiac etiology), Focal Neurologic Deficits (central nervous system pathology), Shortness of Breath (pulmonary etiology), Inflammatory Signs or Joint Pain (autoimmune processes), and Wight Loss or Lymphadenopathy (malignancy).[16] It is important to note that PASC-related fatigue may be a unique diagnosis but can also be manifestation of ME/CFS. The diagnosis can also be multifactorial without an identifiable, singular cause.

TREATMENT

Although counseling patients with diminished activity level related to PASC, practitioners should be comfortable discussing the unknowns of PASC treatments. Most patients who present to multidisciplinary clinics report moderate to severe symptoms.[63] Overall, PASC treatment centers have noted gradual improvement in symptoms. Treatment involves a highly multidisciplinary group of specialists ranging from pulmonologists, physiatrists, neurologists, cardiologists, physical therapists, occupational therapists, psychologists, neuropsychologists, psychiatrists, speech therapists, infectious disease specialists, and nutritionists. Telemedicine can also be used to help guide treatment approaches, but the effectiveness has not been quantified. The CDC has developed guidelines for treating ME/CFS that helped guide the treatment recommendations for PASC-related fatigue. Treatment recommendations should be like the evaluation and be tailored to the patient based on their history, comorbidities, confounders for fatigue, and activity limitations.

NICE published guidelines in 2007 to help quantify fatigue severity in the context of ME/CFS.[64] The PASC Collaborative further defined fatigue severity to help guide treatment options (**Table 1**). Most patients who present to multidisciplinary clinics report moderate to severe symptoms.[63]

The PASC Collaborative has developed guidelines which have helped symptoms in patients when no identifiable, contributing cause has been determined. These include beginning an individualized return to activity program, discussing energy conservation

Table 1 American Academy of Physical Medicine and Rehabilitation post-acute sequelae of COVID-19 collaborative guidance statement recommendations[20]	
Mild fatigue	• Intact mobility • Can perform activities of daily living and do light housework (often with difficulty). • Able to continue working or going to school but may have stopped other, nonessential activities. • Often take time off, require modifications to their schedule, and use weekends to recover from their work week.
Moderate fatigue	• Decreased community mobility • Limited in their performance of instrumental activities of daily living (particularly preparing meals, shopping, doing laundry, using transportation, and performing housework). • Require frequent rest periods and naps • Generally stopped work or school.
Severe fatigue	• Mostly confined to the home • May have difficulty with activities of daily living (eating, bathing, dressing, transferring, toileting, mobility) • Leaving the home is very limited and often leads to prolonged/severe after-effects.

strategies, education and encouragement of a healthy diet and fluid intake, and treating comorbidities such as sleep hygiene, mood disorders, and pain with the assistance of other medical specialists.

Return to Activity Program

The goal of this program is to return to premorbid activity levels. This should start slowly, avoiding strenuous activities such as high-intensity workouts or heavy resistance training, as these activities can exacerbate an individual's symptoms. Patients should be counseled on perceived exertion and educated on metrics used to quantify this. Scales, such as the Borg Rating of Perceived Exertion Scale, can be used to target submaximal exertion. Recommended programs are also determined based on the severity of PASC-related fatigue and gauged using the Rate of Perceived Exertion scale (RPE scale, **Table 2**).

Those with mild fatigue, they can continue household and community activities. A slow return to higher intensity activity using a "rule of 10's" is recommended. This is defined as increasing activity duration, frequency, and intensity by 10% every 10 days. Using the RPE scale, progression from Light (10–11) to Hard (15–16) is recommended.

Those with moderate fatigue can continue household and previously tolerated community activities. Activity or aerobics should begin at Very Light-Light (RPE: 9–11) and can be slowly advanced depending on patient tolerance. If acute or delayed worsening symptoms occur, the activity should be returned to the previously tolerated level.

Those with severe fatigue can continue household activities that are tolerated without symptomatic exacerbation. Upper and lower extremity stretching with light strengthening should occur before any aerobic activity. Once tolerating these well, a light aerobic activity can be engaged at Extremely Light to Very Light (RPE: 7–9). Activity levels can be slowly advanced depending on the patient tolerance. If acute or delayed worsening symptoms occur, the activity should be returned to the previously

Table 2	
Borg's rating of perceived exertion scale[65]	
RPE	**Descriptor**
6	Most minimal exertion; sedentary
7	Extremely light exertion; conversational with ease
8	
9	Very light; comfortable
10	
11	Light; increase in breathing but able to maintain
12	
13	Somewhat hard; some breathlessness with activity
14	
15	Hard; sweating
16	
17	Very hard; able to maintain for short period
18	
19	Extremely Hard; difficulty breathing, near exhaustion
20	Maximal exertion; total exhaustion

tolerated level. A home health program can be considered for those with very limited activity tolerance. If a patient is not tolerating their return to activity program, consider a referral to a specialist familiar with post-COVID care (such as a physiatrist) to help guide the rehabilitation program.

Energy Conservation Strategies

Patient education regarding energy conservation can also aid the recovery process. Remembering the "4 Ps": Pacing, Prioritizing, Positioning, and Planning[66] can be useful for patients. Pacing refers to the concept of shorter duration activities with frequent rest to avoid prolonged recovery. Moderation of activities that increase recovery phases should be monitored. Prioritizing activities that have increased weight or importance and deferring those that can wait can help lessen overexertion and the need for extended recovery periods. Positioning is the idea of emphasizing ergonomics and focusing on energy efficiency. An example of this could include using a shower chair or bench instead of standing. Planning can help patients identify when energy expenditure is optimal or suboptimal. Periods of time during which energy is higher, coined "energy windows," are common. A personalized energy diary can help identify and plan tasks for a given day. Planning can also help schedule a gradual return to activity and work. All these tools can be used to inform employers and work with them to ensure a successful return to work. A vocational rehabilitation specialist can assist with these steps as well. A focus on quality of sleep and sleep hygiene should also be a point of emphasis to maximize recovery.

Nutritional Education

There is no diet prescription that can be universal for all patients to help combat the associated immune dysfunction related to COVID-19. Instead, nutrition guidance should be provided to account for patient preferences, allergies, and comorbidities. In general, counseling and education should be provided to encourage a well-balanced diet. Pro-inflammatory states have been linked to chronic fatigue syndromes. Clinical studies have demonstrated a well-rounded diet high in "whole grains high in fibers, polyphenol-rich vegetables, and omega-3 fatty acid-rich foods might be able to improve disease-related fatigue symptoms.[67]" There is currently no evidence to support the supplementation of B vitamins, omega-3 fatty acids, or coenzyme Q10. Muscle atrophy associated with disuse or deconditioning can also contribute to fatigue. More evidence is needed to strengthen the association of anti-inflammatory diets and fatigue improvement but is a safe addition to add as a treatment approach for PASC.

An effective treatment approach for severe cases will rely on a multidisciplinary approach. The involvement of multiple specialties including pulmonology, cardiology, physiatry, primary care, nutrition, psychiatry, infectious disease, speech therapy, occupational therapy, and physical therapy should be considered to maximize recovery and optimize function for patients with PASC symptoms. A transdisciplinary approach will allow patients to receive care across the spectrum of their PASC symptoms and ideally recovery as quickly as possible.

DISCUSSION

Given the recency of the SARS-Co-V-2 epidemic, there are clear limitations in the scientific community's ability to fully understand and manage the constellation of symptoms identified as PASC. In addition, it becomes cumbersome to provide specific treatment recommendations due to several different potential etiologies of PASC-related fatigue. The existing literature focused on ME/CFS, and other post-viral syndromes are the best analogs to guide interventions. This section of our publication has been focused on physical or mobility-related PASC fatigue symptoms, which excludes a full constellation of PASC symptoms that are related to psychologic, mental, and cognitive-based manifestations of PASC fatigue. Further research should help delineate improved evaluation strategies and treatment plans that can better target the various etiologies of PASC-related fatigue (ie, HPA, adrenal, cytokine, cardiac, pulmonary, myopathy, neuropsychiatric, sleep, and/or gut biome dysfunction).

Because of the varied possible etiologies causing PASC symptoms, there does not seem to be a single-laboratory evaluation, diagnostic test, or examination finding that will best identify the etiology of PASC symptoms. In addition, there is no consensus about a specific medication, therapy program, diet, infusion, or supplement that would best improve PASC symptoms.

Until the body of research is grown, the clinical community will need to work from the vantage point of expert opinion and the guidance from patient-led advocacy groups, PASC-focused clinical care sites, and consortiums that bring these groups together. Despite the lack of published research, it seems reasonable to model evaluation and treatment plans from existing knowledge in the ME/CFS and post-viral syndrome domains. It is reassuring that a proportion of patients with PASC symptoms are showing signs of improvements over time. Clinical care in this domain will continue to develop, and recommendations are likely to change with additional updates. This evolving landscape further complicates care for patients dealing with PASC symptoms.

SUMMARY

Fatigue from PASC is a complex constellation of symptoms that could be driven by a wide spectrum of underlying etiologies. Despite this, there seems to be hope for treatment plans that focus on addressing possible etiologies and creating a path to improving quality of life and a paced return to activity.

CLINICS CARE POINTS

- Collect a detailed fatigue history that includes information on the wide differential diagnoses that can impact post-acute sequelae of COVID-19 (PASC) symptoms including the endocrinologic (hypothalamic–pituitary axis, adrenal gland), inflammatory, cardiac, pulmonary, myofascial, neuropsychiatric (including sleep), and gastrointestinal systems.

- If not already completed, perform a general workup that includes complete blood count comprehensive metabolic panel, and measurement of phosphorus, thyroid-stimulating hormone, and C-reactive protein.

- If needed, refer to clinical sites and providers who have more experience assisting patients with PASC symptoms.

DISCLOSURE

The authors have nothing to disclose.

REFERENCES

1. COVID-19 Map - Johns Hopkins Coronavirus Resource Center. Available at: https://coronavirus.jhu.edu/map.html. Accessed July 19, 2022.

2. Phipps SJ, Grafton RQ, Kompas T. Robust estimates of the true (population) infection rate for COVID-19: a backcasting approach. R Soc Open Sci 2020; 7(11):200909.

3. Noh J, Danuser G. Estimation of the fraction of COVID-19 infected people in U.S. states and countries worldwide. PLoS One 2021;16(2):e0246772.

4. CDC COVID Data Tracker: Hospital Admissions. Available at: https://covid.cdc. gov/covid-data-tracker/#new-hospital-admissions. Accessed July 19, 2022.

5. CDC COVID Data Tracker: Daily and Total Trends. Available at: https://covid.cdc. gov/covid-data-tracker/#trends_dailydeaths. Accessed July 19, 2022.

6. Mahajan S, Caraballo C, Li SX, et al. SARS-CoV-2 Infection Hospitalization Rate and Infection Fatality Rate Among the Non-Congregate Population in Connecticut. Am J Med 2021;134(6):812. https://doi.org/10.1016/J.AMJMED.2021.01.020.

7. Davis HE, Assaf GS, Mccorkell L, et al. Characterizing Long COVID in an International Cohort: 7 Months of Symptoms and Their Impact. EClinicalMedicine 2021. https://doi.org/10.1101/2020.12.24.20248802.

8. Baratta JM, Tompary A, Siano S, et al. Postacute Sequelae of COVID-19 Infection and Development of a Physiatry-Led Recovery Clinic. Am J Phys Med Rehabil 2021;100(7):633.

9. Hernandez-Romieu AC, Leung S, Mbanya A, et al. Health Care Utilization and Clinical Characteristics of Nonhospitalized Adults in an Integrated Health Care System 28–180 Days After COVID-19 Diagnosis — Georgia, May 2020–March 2021. MMWR Morb Mortal Wkly Rep 2022;70(17):644–50.

10. Huang Y, Pinto MD, Borelli JL, et al. COVID Symptoms, Symptom Clusters, and Predictors for Becoming a Long-Hauler: Looking for Clarity in the Haze of the Pandemic. medRxiv 2021. https://doi.org/10.1101/2021.03.03.21252086.

11. Nasserie T, Hittle M, Goodman SN. Assessment of the Frequency and Variety of Persistent Symptoms Among Patients With COVID-19: A Systematic Review. JAMA Netw Open 2021;4(5). https://doi.org/10.1001/JAMANETWORKOPEN. 2021.11417.

12. Carfì A, Bernabei R, Landi F. Persistent Symptoms in Patients After Acute COVID-19. JAMA 2020;324(6):603–5.

13. Rosenthal TC, Pretorius R, Malik K. Fatigue: An Overview. 2008. Available at: http://familydoctor.org/online/famdocen/home/common/pain/disorders/031.html. Accessed July 20, 2022.

14. Stussman B, Williams A, Snow J, et al. Characterization of Post–exertional Malaise in Patients With Myalgic Encephalomyelitis/Chronic Fatigue Syndrome. Front Neurol 2020;11:1025.

15. Sandler CX, Wyller VBB, Moss-Morris R, et al. Long COVID and Post-infective Fatigue Syndrome: A Review. Open Forum Infect Dis 2021;8(10). https://doi.org/10. 1093/OFID/OFAB440.

16. Yancey JR, Thomas SM, Air Force Base F. Chronic Fatigue Syndrome: Diagnosis and Treatment. 2012;86(8). Available at: www.aafp.org/afp. Accessed July 20, 2022.

17. Maughan D, Toth M. Discerning Primary and Secondary Factors Responsible for Clinical Fatigue in Multisystem Diseases. Biology 2014;3(3):606.

18. Reynolds KJ, Vernon SD, Bouchery E, et al. The economic impact of chronic fatigue syndrome. Cost Eff Resour Alloc 2004;2(1). https://doi.org/10.1186/1478-7547-2-4.

19. Beyond Myalgic Encephalomyelitis/Chronic Fatigue Syndrome: Redefining an Illness. Mil Med 2015;180(7):721–3.

20. Herrera JE, Niehaus WN, Whiteson J, et al. Multidisciplinary collaborative consensus guidance statement on the assessment and treatment of fatigue in postacute sequelae of SARS-CoV-2 infection (PASC) patients. PM&R 2021; 13(9):1027–43.

21. Munblit D, O'Hara ME, Akrami A, et al. Long COVID: aiming for a consensus. Lancet Respir Med 2022;10(7):632–4.

22. Mackay A. A Paradigm for Post-Covid-19 Fatigue Syndrome Analogous to ME/CFS. Front Neurol 2021;12. https://doi.org/10.3389/FNEUR.2021.701419.

23. De Bellis A, Bellastella G, Pernice V, et al. Hypothalamic-Pituitary Autoimmunity and Related Impairment of Hormone Secretions in Chronic Fatigue Syndrome. J Clin Endocrinol Metab 2021;106(12):e5147–55.

24. Gonen MS, De Bellis A, Durcan E, et al. Assessment of Neuroendocrine Changes and Hypothalamo-Pituitary Autoimmunity in Patients with COVID-19. Horm Metab Res 2021;54(3):153–61.

25. Kanczkowski W, Gaba WH, Krone N, et al. Adrenal Gland Function and Dysfunction during COVID-19. Horm Metab Res 2022;54(8):532–9.

26. Santana MF, Borba MGS, Baía-Da-Silva DC, et al. Case Report: Adrenal Pathology Findings in Severe COVID-19: An Autopsy Study. Am J Trop Med Hyg 2020; 103(4):1604.

27. Iuga AC, Marboe CC, Yilmaz MM, et al. Adrenal Vascular Changes in COVID-19 Autopsies. Arch Pathol Lab Med 2020;144(10):1159–60.

28. Fan BE, Wong SW, Sum CLL, et al. Hypercoagulability, endotheliopathy, and inflammation approximating 1 year after recovery: Assessing the long-term outcomes in COVID-19 patients. Am J Hematol 2022;97(7):915–23.

29. Hu B, Huang S, Yin L. The cytokine storm and COVID-19. J Med Virol 2021;93(1): 250–6.

30. Wang J, Yang X, Li Y, et al. Specific cytokines in the inflammatory cytokine storm of patients with COVID-19-associated acute respiratory distress syndrome and extrapulmonary multiple-organ dysfunction. Virol J 2021;18(1):1–12.

31. Garcia MN, Hause AM, Walker CM, et al. Evaluation of prolonged fatigue post-West Nile virus infection and association of fatigue with elevated antiviral and proinflammatory cytokines. Viral Immunol 2014;27(7):327–33.

32. Broderick G, Fuite J, Kreitz A, et al. A formal analysis of cytokine networks in chronic fatigue syndrome. Brain Behav Immun 2010;24(7):1209–17.

33. Evans RA, Leavy OC, Richardson M, et al. Clinical characteristics with inflammation profiling of long COVID and association with 1-year recovery following hospitalisation in the UK: a prospective observational study. Lancet Respir Med 2022;10(8):761–75.

34. Sollini M, Morbelli S, Ciccarelli M, et al. Long COVID hallmarks on [18F]FDG-PET/CT: a case-control study. Eur J Nucl Med Mol Imaging 2021;48(10):3187–97.

35. Jarrott B, Head R, Pringle KG, et al. LONG COVID"—A hypothesis for understanding the biological basis and pharmacological treatment strategy. Pharmacol Res Perspect 2022;10(1):e00911.

36. Castanares-Zapatero D, Chalon P, Kohn L, et al. Pathophysiology and mechanism of long COVID: a comprehensive review. Ann Med 2022;54(1):1473.

37. Puntmann VO, Carerj ML, Wieters I, et al. Outcomes of Cardiovascular Magnetic Resonance Imaging in Patients Recently Recovered From Coronavirus Disease 2019 (COVID-19). JAMA Cardiol 2020;5(11):1265–73.

38. Małek ŁA, Marczak M, Miłosz-Wieczorek B, et al. Cardiac involvement in consecutive elite athletes recovered from Covid-19: A magnetic resonance study. J Magn Reson Imaging 2021;53(6):1723.

39. Daniels CJ, Rajpal S, Greenshields JT, et al. Prevalence of Clinical and Subclinical Myocarditis in Competitive Athletes With Recent SARS-CoV-2 Infection: Results From the Big Ten COVID-19 Cardiac Registry. JAMA Cardiol 2021;6(9): 1078–87.

40. Agergaard J, Leth S, Pedersen TH, et al. Myopathic changes in patients with long-term fatigue after COVID-19. Clin Neurophysiol 2021;132(8):1974–81.

41. Suh J, Mukerji SS, Collens SI, et al. Skeletal Muscle and Peripheral Nerve Histopathology in COVID-19. Neurology 2021;97(8):e849–58.

42. Duarte-Neto AN, Monteiro RAA, da Silva LFF, et al. Pulmonary and systemic involvement in COVID-19 patients assessed with ultrasound-guided minimally invasive autopsy. Histopathology 2020;77(2):186–97.

43. Manzano GS, Woods JK, Amato AA. Covid-19-Associated Myopathy Caused by Type I Interferonopathy. N Engl J Med 2020;383(24):2389–90.

44. Tankisi H, Tankisi A, Harbo T, et al. Critical illness myopathy as a consequence of Covid-19 infection. Clin Neurophysiol 2020;131(8):1931.

45. Stengel A, Malek N, Zipfel S, et al. Long Haulers—What Is the Evidence for Post-COVID Fatigue? Front Psychiatry 2021;12:657.

46. Aschman T, Stenzel W. COVID-19 associated myopathy. Curr Opin Neurol 2022; 35(5). https://doi.org/10.1097/WCO.0000000000001101.

47. Soares MN, Eggelbusch M, Naddaf E, et al. Skeletal muscle alterations in patients with acute Covid-19 and post-acute sequelae of Covid-19. J Cachexia Sarcopenia Muscle 2022;13(1):11–22.

48. Ahmed DS, Isnard S, Berini C, et al. Coping With Stress: The Mitokine GDF-15 as a Biomarker of COVID-19 Severity. Front Immunol 2022;13. https://doi.org/10. 3389/FIMMU.2022.820350.

49. Penninx BWJH. Psychiatric symptoms and cognitive impairment in "Long COVID": the relevance of immunopsychiatry. World Psychiatr 2021;20(3):357.

50. Renaud-Charest O, Lui LMW, Eskander S, et al. Onset and frequency of depression in post-COVID-19 syndrome: A systematic review. J Psychiatr Res 2021;144: 129–37.

51. Ortelli P, Ferrazzoli D, Sebastianelli L, et al. Neuropsychological and neurophysiological correlates of fatigue in post-acute patients with neurological manifestations of COVID-19: Insights into a challenging symptom. J Neurol Sci 2021;420: 117271.

52. Mandal S, Barnett J, Brill S, Brown J, Thorax ED-, 2021 undefined. "Long-COVID": a cross-sectional study of persisting symptoms, biomarker and imaging abnormalities following hospitalisation for COVID-19. thorax.bmj.com. Available at: https://thorax.bmj.com/content/76/4/396.abstract. Accessed September 12, 2022.

53. Jahrami H, BaHammam AS, Bragazzi NL, et al. Sleep problems during the COVID-19 pandemic by population: A systematic review and meta-analysis. J Clin Sleep Med 2021;17(2):299–313.

54. Becker SP, Dvorsky MR, Breaux R, et al. Prospective examination of adolescent sleep patterns and behaviors before and during COVID-19. Sleep 2021;44(8). https://doi.org/10.1093/SLEEP/ZSAB054.

55. Pataka A, Kotoulas S, Sakka E, et al. Sleep Dysfunction in COVID-19 Patients: Prevalence, Risk Factors, Mechanisms, and Management. J Pers Med 2021; 11(11):1203.

56. Fernández-De-Las-Peñas C, Martín-Guerrero JD, Cancela-Cilleruelo I, et al. Trajectory curves of post-COVID anxiety/depressive symptoms and sleep quality in

previously hospitalized COVID-19 survivors: the LONG-COVID-EXP-CM multi-center study. Psychol Med 2022;1–2. https://doi.org/10.1017/S003329172200006X.

57. Lupo GFD, Rocchetti G, Lucini L, et al. Potential role of microbiome in Chronic Fatigue Syndrome/Myalgic Encephalomyelits (CFS/ME). Sci Rep 2021;11(1). https://doi.org/10.1038/S41598-021-86425-6.

58. Yeoh YK, Zuo T, Lui GCY, et al. Gut microbiota composition reflects disease severity and dysfunctional immune responses in patients with COVID-19. Gut 2021;70(4):698–706.

59. Liu Q, Mak JWY, Su Q, et al. Gut microbiota dynamics in a prospective cohort of patients with post-acute COVID-19 syndrome. Gut 2022;71(3):544–52.

60. Halpin SJ, McIvor C, Whyatt G, et al. Postdischarge symptoms and rehabilitation needs in survivors of COVID-19 infection: A cross-sectional evaluation. J Med Virol 2021;93(2):1013–22.

61. Mazza MG, De Lorenzo R, Conte C, et al. Anxiety and depression in COVID-19 survivors: Role of inflammatory and clinical predictors. Brain Behav Immun 2020;89:594–600.

62. Taquet M, Luciano S, Geddes JR, et al. Bidirectional associations between COVID-19 and psychiatric disorder: retrospective cohort studies of 62 354 COVID-19 cases in the USA. Lancet Psychiatr 2021;8(2):130–40.

63. Whitehead L. The measurement of fatigue in chronic illness: a systematic review of unidimensional and multidimensional fatigue measures. J Pain Symptom Manage 2009;37(1):107–28.

64. National Institute for Health and Care Excellence (NICE). Clinical guideline: Chronic fatigue syndrome/myalgic encephalomyelitis (or encephalopathy): diagnosis and management; 2017. Available at: www.nice.org.uk/guidance/cg53. Accessed April 3, 2023.

65. Perceived Exertion (Borg Rating of Perceived Exertion Scale) | Physical Activity | CDC. Available at: https://www.cdc.gov/physicalactivity/basics/measuring/exertion.htm. Accessed April 3, 2023.

66. Homerton University Hospital: NHS Foundation Trust. Post COVID-19 Patient information pack: Helping you to recover and manage your symptoms following COVID-19. Available at: https://www.hackneycitizen.co.uk/wp-content/uploads/Post-COVID-19-%0Ainformation-pack-5.pdf. Accessed April 3, 2023.

67. Haß U, Herpich C, Norman K. Anti-Inflammatory Diets and Fatigue. Nutrients 2019;11(10). https://doi.org/10.3390/NU11102315.

Immunologic and Autoimmune-Related Sequelae of Severe Acute Respiratory Syndrome Coronavirus 2 Infection

Clinical Symptoms and Mechanisms of Disease

Akshara Ramasamy[a,1], Chumeng Wang, BS[a,1],
W. Michael Brode, MD[b], Monica Verduzco-Gutierrez, MD[c],
Esther Melamed, MD PhD[a,*]

KEYWORDS

- COVID-19 • PASC • Clinical symptoms • Disease mechanism
- Comorbid conditions • Autoimmunity

INTRODUCTION

The coronavirus disease 2019 (COVID-19) pandemic has presented a serious public health threat, resulting in more than 600 million infections worldwide and 6 million fatalities.[1] The clinical spectrum of acute SARS-CoV-2 infection varies, with patients experiencing asymptomatic, mild, moderate, severe, or critical illness with symptoms ranging from upper and/or lower respiratory infection to gastrointestinal (GI), cardiac, and neurologic manifestations. On average, the acute COVID-19 infection lasts between one and four weeks.[2] However, at least 10% to 30% of patients with COVID-19 experience lingering symptoms for months following infection, leading to postacute sequelae of SARS-CoV-2 infection (PASC), also known as long-COVID.[3] Similar to the acute COVID-19 disease stage, the diverse symptoms reported by PASC patients include multiorgan symptoms.

Presently, there is no standardized definition for PASC. The World Health Organization defines PASC as post-COVID-19 conditions "usually 3 months from the onset of

^a Department of Neurology, Dell Medical School, University of Texas at Austin, Health Discovery Building, 1601 Trinity Street, Austin, TX 78712, USA; ^b Department of Internal Medicine, Dell Medical School, University of Texas at Austin, 1601 Trinity Street, Austin, TX 78712, USA; ^c Department of Physical Medicine and Rehabilitation, University of Texas at San Antonio, 7703 Floyd Curl Drive, Mail Code 7798, San Antonio, TX 78229, USA
¹ Akshara Ramasamy and Chumeng Wang contributed equally to this work as co-first authors.
* Corresponding author. Health Discovery Building, Health Transformation Building, 1601 Trinity Street, Austin, TX 78712.
E-mail address: Esther.melamed@austin.utexas.edu

Phys Med Rehabil Clin N Am 34 (2023) 623–642
https://doi.org/10.1016/j.pmr.2023.04.004
1047-9651/23/© 2023 Elsevier Inc. All rights reserved.

COVID-19 with symptoms that last for at least 2 months."[4] The Centers for Disease Control and Prevention classifies PASC as "a wide range of new, returning, or ongoing health problems" experienced after infection with SARS-CoV-2.[5] Because of the absence of a widely recognized definition for the syndrome, proper diagnosis and treatment remain challenging.

Given the current prevalence of PASC of 10% to 30%, it is estimated that more than 10 to 30 million of people in the United States and more than 60 to 180 million people worldwide may develop PASC, which represents one of the largest mass disabling illnesses in modern history.[3,6,7] Thus, there is a pressing need to understand and treat acute COVID-19 infection and identify therapies for prevention and treatment of PASC.

Given the important evolving similarities and differences between the acute and chronic aspects of the COVID-19 infection, the goal of this review is to compare the clinical symptoms, pathophysiology, and comorbid disease risk factors for acute SARS-CoV-2 infection and PASC related to the immune system.

MULTIORGAN CLINICAL MANIFESTATIONS IN ACUTE COVID-19 AND POSTACUTE SEQUELAE OF SARS-CoV-2 INFECTION

Although initially COVID-19 was thought to be a respiratory disease, it has become clear that there are multiorgan manifestations of acute and postacute SARS-CoV-2 infection. Acute infection with SARS-CoV-2 commonly starts as an upper and/or lower respiratory disease with rhinorrhea, sore throat, cough, fatigue, and dyspnea.[8] However, patients can also experience neurologic symptoms, such as headache, neuropathic pain, and loss of sense and smell, as well as GI symptoms, such as nausea and diarrhea, and cardiac or endocrine dysregulation.[9,10]

Acute infection can be asymptomatic for up to 17.9% of adults.[11] Approximately 20% of patients infected with initial Wuhan and delta SARS-CoV-2 variants experienced severe disease requiring hospitalization or critical disease leading to mortality, in about 2% of cases.[12,13] With the advent of vaccinations and newer omicron variants, fewer people have required hospitalizations.[14]

CLINICAL SYMPTOMS IN POSTACUTE SEQUELAE OF SARS-CoV-2 INFECTION
Neuropsychiatric Sequelae

Neurologic sequelae are among the most frequently reported PASC symptoms. In a survey conducted by Davis and colleagues of 3762 patients, sensorimotor deficits (91.4%), cognitive dysfunction (85.4%), sleep disturbances (78.5%), headache (76.7%), memory impairment (72.8%), and smell/taste dysfunction (57.6%) were the most commonly reported neuropsychiatric symptoms in the first 6 months post-acute disease.[15] Notably, 85.1% of respondents experienced "brain fog" and cognitive impairment, including impaired attention, executive functioning, problem solving, and decision-making. Importantly, a total of 2454 (65.2%) PASC patients experienced neurologic and systemic symptoms such as fatigue, postexertional malaise, cognitive dysfunction, sensory symptoms, headaches, and memory difficulties after 6 months. Autonomic dysfunction has also emerged as a common PASC manifestation, with one study reporting 67% of patients with moderate to severe dysautonomia.[16]

Similarly, 165 PASC patients in an observational study exhibited heterogeneous symptoms at 6-month follow-up, with fatigue (34%), memory/attention (31%), and sleep difficulties (30%) as most common symptoms.[17] Interestingly, 40% of patients had neurologic abnormalities such as hyposmia (18.0%), cognitive impairments

(17.5%), postural tremor (13.8%), and modest motor/sensory deficiencies on neurologic examination (7.6%).

PASC is also characterized by psychiatric manifestations, with 23.98% of PASC patients having a mood, anxiety, or psychotic disorder in a cohort study by Taquet and colleagues and 88.2% of PASC patients experiencing emotional/mood disorders in the survey by Davis and colleagues.[15,18]

Gastrointestinal Sequelae

In a study by Weng and colleagues, 52 (44%) of 117 patients reported GI symptoms posthospital discharge, with 51 patients continuing to experience GI symptoms at 90 days post-discharge.[19] Loss of appetite (24%), nausea (18%), acid reflux (18%), and diarrhea (15%) were the most common GI sequelae in 117 patients; less common GI sequelae included abdominal distension (14%), belching (10%), vomiting (9%), abdominal pain (7%), and bloody stools (2%).

Within the first week following diagnosis, 49.2% of individuals had fecal SARS-CoV-2 RNA identified in the study by Natarajan and colleagues.[20] Although there was no continuous oropharyngeal SARS-CoV-2 RNA shedding in patients 4 months after diagnosis, 12.7% of participants had fecal RNA shedding and 3.8% at 7 months. Most interestingly, GI symptoms (abdominal pain, nausea, and vomiting) were associated with fecal SARS-CoV-2 RNA shedding. Therefore, the persistence of viral RNA in feces after resolution of initial infection suggests that SARS-CoV-2 infects the GI tract, contributing to the persistent GI symptoms found in PASC patients. It has been suggested that GI symptoms in PASC patients may be due to autoimmunity as part of autoimmune gastrointestinal dysmotility syndrome or result from postinfectious irritable bowel syndrome.[21,22]

Cardiovascular Sequelae

Comelli and colleagues conducted a long-term follow-up on patients with COVID-19 to study PASC sequelae.[23] At 12-month post-COVID, 91.7% of individuals reported at least one symptom/sequelae, with the most common symptoms as exertional dyspnea (71.7%), fatigue (54.6%), and GI problems (32.8%). In their study, Carfi and colleagues discovered that 43.4% of the patients with COVID-19 reported dyspnea and 21.7% experienced chest pain after 2 months.[24] These findings are consistent with those of Wong and colleagues, in which half of the patients reported dyspnea and 23% experienced persistent cough 3 months following discharge.[25]

Cardiovascular MRI demonstrated cardiac involvement in 78 individuals and persistent myocardial inflammation in 60 patients in a cohort study of 100 patients who had recovered from COVID-19.[26] Cardiovascular dysautonomia has also been widely reported. In a case series consisting of 20 COVID-19 patients, there were 15 cases of postural orthostatic tachycardia syndrome, 3 cases of neurocardiogenic syncope, and 2 cases of orthostatic hypotension after resolution of acute infection.[27] Stahlberg and colleagues report between 25% and 50% of patients in a tertiary post-COVID multidisciplinary clinic experience tachycardia or palpitations that last for 12 weeks or more.[28] Palpitations are reported by 9% of patients with postacute COVID-19 syndrome after 6 months, according to a systematic review by Huang and colleagues.[29] Cardiovascular sequelae are further discussed in another article in this special issue.

Other Sequelae

Tinnitus and vertigo are also common presentations of PASC, with 37.6% of 5163 COVID-19 survivors complaining of persistent dizziness and 16.7% reporting tinnitus in a survey administered by Lambert and colleagues.[30] Approximately 22% of PASC patients may also experience hair loss, up to 6 months postinfection.[29] Dermatologic PASC sequelae may include chilblains, papulosquamous, urticarial, and morbilliform eruptions.[31] Renal complications are also common, with COVID-19 survivors having a higher risk of acute kidney infection, glomerular filtration rate decrease, end-stage kidney disease, and major adverse kidney events after the first 30 days of infection.[32] Anosmia, ejaculation difficulties, decreased libido, hair loss, and sneezing are also commonly reported among PASC patients.[33]

PATHOPHYSIOLOGY OF SARS-CoV-2 IN ACUTE INFECTION AND POSTACUTE SEQUELAE OF SARS-CoV-2 INFECTION
Mechanism of Acute SARS-CoV-2 Infection

SARS-CoV-2 belongs to the Nidovirales order in the Coronaviridae family and is enveloped with a nonsegmented positive-sense single-stranded RNA genome.[34] SARS-CoV-2 gains cellular entry through the CoV Spike (S) glycoprotein, which interacts with human angiotensin-converting enzyme 2 (ACE-2) receptor.[35] ACE-2 is found ubiquitously on epithelial cells throughout the body and is widely expressed in the brain.[36–38] Interestingly, ACE-2, an X-linked gene, is found at a location on the X chromosome known to elude X chromosome inactivation, suggesting that women express a higher dose of the ACE-2 protein.[39] Intriguingly, a genetic variant that reduces ACE-2 expression by 37% also reduces the risk of SARS-CoV-2 infection by 40%.[40]

In early SARS-CoV-2 infection, immune activation leads to an organized cascade of events toward viral destruction. For example, proinflammatory cytokines such as interleukin-6 (IL-6) and tumor necrosis factor (TNF) are quickly released by surveilling immune cells to activate T cells, which direct viral clearance, and B cells, which in turn produce antibodies to neutralize viral particles.[41] These proinflammatory responses are typically tightly regulated to avoid host tissue destruction. However, in some cases, host responses may become severely dysregulated. Notably, in more than 1500 of COVID-19–positive patients tested on their first day of hospitalization, IL-6, IL-9, and TNF were extensively elevated and higher concentrations correlated with more severe disease outcomes.[13] Indeed, "cytokine storm," a massive cytokine activation syndrome, can result in multiorgan failure and possible death.[42]

Interestingly, Spike-ACE-2 signaling may affect the body's immune response. For example, spike protein can directly downregulate messenger RNA expression of type I interferons (IFN-1), especially IFN-α4.[35] IFN-1 typically is responsible for antiviral responses, such as inhibiting viral replication, bolstering antigen presentation, and triggering adaptive immune responses through direct and indirect actions on T and B cells.[43] Thus, persistent spike-IFN interactions may potentially endanger the body's ability to clear SARS-CoV-2.

Mechanism of Postacute Sequelae of SARS-CoV-2 Infection

Following the acute infection stage, which in symptomatic individuals can last anywhere from a few days up to a month, approximately 10% to 30% of patients go on to experience protracted symptoms of PASC. However, in some individuals, initial COVID-19 symptoms may completely resolve, and they may start to experience PASC symptoms after a month or several months after initial acute SARS-CoV-2 infection. Notably, PASC can affect patients who experienced severe or mild acute COVID-19 symptoms.[44,45]

Direct viral invasion
Although the exact mechanism of PASC is currently unknown, several hypotheses have been proposed. One hypothesis is that SARS-CoV-2 may cause direct organ damage, which persists after the virus is cleared from the body. For example, given

the highly prevalent PASC neurologic symptoms, such as memory, attention, and concentration difficulty (referred to by patients as "brain fog"); fatigue; dysgeusia; anosmia; and dysautonomia, it has been proposed that SARS-CoV-2 may be directly damaging the nervous system. Evidence for this hypothesis comes from studies demonstrating that the olfactory gyrus may be the first area of the central nervous system (CNS) to be invaded by SARS-CoV-2.[46] Furthermore, diffusion tensor imaging of recovered patients show disruption to structural and functional brain integrity in olfactory brain regions and hippocampus.[46] Damage to the brainstem's cardiorespiratory center, cerebrum, and cerebellum has also been noted.[47,48] In a systematic review of 36 articles, it was found that any cranial nerve could be affected by SARS-CoV-2, although cranial nerves III, VI, and VII were most frequently damaged.[49] A meta-analysis of 97 papers also documented evidence of SARS-CoV-2 or SARS-CoV-2 antibodies in the cerebrospinal fluid in 7.9% of 468 patients.[50] A number of studies have also documented the presence of SARS-CoV-2 and antibodies to SARS-CoV-2 viral proteins in the brain.[51–54] Thus, persistent PASC neurologic symptoms may be at least in part due to long-lasting neuronal damage from initial SARS-CoV-2 infection.[55,56]

However, the neurotropic nature of SARS-CoV-2 remains controversial. In a cohort of 85 patients with postmortem COVID-19, it was the sustentacular cells, the major olfactory cell type infected by SARS-CoV-2.[57] Sustentacular cells are support cells for sensory neurons, and their infection alone could account for the olfactory symptoms independent of direct infection of olfactory neurons. In addition, microvasculopathy in endothelial olfactory tissues may be another pathogenic mechanism independent of olfactory neuron damage.[58] In addition, other autopsy studies failed to identify viral presence in the CNS.[52] Thus, further research is necessary to fully evaluate the hypothesis of whether SARS-CoV-2 is directly neurotropic.

Persistent inflammation and rise of autoimmunity

Another proposed pathologic mechanism in PASC is persistent inflammation post-acute SARS-CoV-2 infection and rise of autoimmunity.[55] For example, in a cohort study of 31 PASC patients, levels of type I (IFN-β) and type III (IFN-λ1) cytokines were found to be persistently elevated 8 months post-acute SARS-CoV-2 infection.[59] Further, Ehrenfeld and colleagues reported a higher deposition of CD8+ T cells in the lungs and other organs of deceased patients with COVID-19, whereas Phetsouphanh and colleagues identified depletion of 3 clusters of naive B and T cell subsets in PASC patients at 8 months compared with matched controls.[60,61] The depletion of naive lymphocytes also suggests possible persistent conversion of naive cells to activated lymphocytes.[60,62] Other studies have also implicated presence of higher number of exhausted T cells in PASC patients.[61] These studies suggest that T cell dysregulation in PASC may be similar to known autoimmune diseases.

In addition, the humoral immune system has been noted to be dysregulated in PASC with findings of multiple autoantibodies, such as antinuclear, antimyelin oligodendrocyte glycoprotein, antiphospholipid, antiinterferon, and antiganglioside antibody antibodies.[2,63–65]

Lastly, the innate immune system may also be affected in PASC, given findings of persistently elevated activated monocytes, mast cells, and eosinophils.[66,67] Indeed, mast cell activation syndrome has been proposed as one of the therapeutic targets in PASC, with some patients benefiting from an antihistamine diet.[68–70]

SARS-CoV-2 persistence

Another possible cause proposed for continuation of PASC symptoms is persistent SARS-CoV-2 infection.[71] Viral particle shedding may continue from the upper airway for approximately 17 days, the lower respiratory tract for approximately 15 days, feces approximately for 13 days, and blood approximately for 17 days.[72] In a study of 113 individuals, Natarajan and colleagues found fecal SARS-CoV-2 RNA shedding in 12.7% of patients at 4 months and in 3.8% at 7 months.[20] In addition, studies have detected viral RNA for 59 days in the lower respiratory tract, 60 days in the blood, 83 days in the upper airway, and 126 days in the feces.[73]

Even if the virus does not fully reconstitute, the persistence of viral RNA could continue to be immunogenic and contribute to chronic inflammation. If this hypothesis is validated, therapeutics could be targeted at decreasing the SARS-CoV-2 viral load in PASC patients with treatments such as Paxlovid and other antivirals.

Comorbid Conditions

Several preexisting medical conditions have been associated with acute COVID-19 disease and PASC severity (**Table 1**), such as cardiovascular risk factors, pulmonary dysfunction, psychiatric conditions, immune dysregulation due to hypogammaglobu-linemia or common variable immunodeficiency (CVID), autoimmunity and genetic HLA haplotype, and cancer. **Fig. 1** summarizes known evidence for the links between pre-existing conditions in acute and chronic COVID-19 and the following section ex-pounds on the evidence related to immune dysregulation.

Autoimmunity

Association of pre-COVID autoimmunity with acute SARS-CoV-2 infection and postacute sequelae of SARS-CoV-2 infection. The apparent similarity between clinical symptoms in individuals with classifiable autoimmune illnesses and PASC patients has encouraged investigations into the role of autoimmunity in PASC. The questions that have yet to be effectively answered are surrounding the causal direction of SARS-CoV-2 infection and autoimmunity: does preexisting autoimmunity serve as an independent risk factor for PASC or does SARS-CoV-2 infection cause postviral autoimmunity?

In an analysis of 62 observational studies evaluating a total of 319,025 patients with autoimmune disease, the risk of severe COVID-19 was significantly higher compared with patients without autoimmune diseases diagnosed pre-COVID.[74] Moreover, using an autoantibody panel including autoantibodies commonly associ-ated with systemic lupus erythematosus, Su and colleagues75 determined that pa-tients with preexisting autoantibodies developed less anti-SARS-CoV-2 antibodies, suggesting that prior autoimmunity may interfere with humoral response to SARS-CoV-2.[75]

In addition, patients with autoimmune diseases are often treated with immunosup-pressive medications that may dampen humoral and cellular immune responses and thus result in lower ability to respond to acute SARS-CoV-2 infection, potentially pre-disposing patients to more severe viral complications.[76] For example, Dreyer and col-leagues found that autoimmune individuals with PASC were susceptible to symptoms such as persistent dyspnea and fatigue compared with nonautoimmune individuals.[77] Likewise, in patients with multiple sclerosis (MS) on B-cell–depleting therapies, there is a dampened production of SARS-CoV-2 antibodies.[78] Recent studies have also deter-mined that greater than 30% of patients with MS on disease-modifying therapies developed PASC symptoms.[79]

Further, Bastard and colleagues revealed that autoantibodies to neutralizing type I IFNs were associated with 20% of severe COVID-19 cases and were present before SARS-CoV-2 infection, suggesting an association with prior autoimmunity.[80] In line with these findings, Su and colleagues found that PASC patients with autoantibodies

Table 1
Comorbid conditions in acute COVID-19 and postacute sequelae of SARS-CoV-2 infection

Comorbidity	Study Design	Total Participants	Author	Major Findings
Asthma	Cohort	215	Cervia et al,[87] 2022	94% of patients with COVID-19 with asthma had persisting symptoms beyond 4 wk, and 71% developed symptoms lasting for more than 12 wk.
	Survey	4500	Philip et al,[95] 2022	PASC patients were more likely to report exacerbated breathing problems, increased inhaler use, and worse asthma management than those without PASC.
	Longitudinal	15,227	Holt et al,[96] 2021	Individuals with atopic disease (asthma, allergic rhinitis, eczema, and/or hay fever) had decreased odds of developing COVID-19 than those without.
	Cohort	365	Jackson et al,[97] 2020	Those with allergic sensitivity and asthma had reduced ACE2 expression. Nonatopic asthma was not associated with a decrease in ACE2 expression.
Oncological conditions	Cohort	423	Robilotti et al,[89] 2020	Among the 432 patients with cancer with COVID-19, 40% were hospitalized, 20% had severe respiratory issues, and 12% passed away within 30 d.
	Cohort	218	Mehta et al,[98] 2020	Of the 61 patients with cancer who died of COVID-19, the case fatality rate for hematologic cancers was higher than solid tumors. Six of eleven patients with lung cancer died of COVID-19.
	Cohort	1700	Sharafeldin et al,[93] 2022	PASC patients with cancer were older, more likely to have comorbidities, and be hospitalized for COVID-19 than noncancer controls.
	Cohort	2665	Meng et al,[99] 2020	Patients with hematological malignancies had exacerbated COVID-19 outcomes, with a mortality rate double that of those with solid tumors.
	Longitudinal	312	Dagher et al,[92] 2021	Of the 312 patients with cancer with COVID-19, 188 had

(continued on next page)

Table 1
(continued)

Comorbidity	Study Design	Total Participants	Author	Major Findings
				symptoms lasting for 7–14 mo. Fatigue, sleep problems, myalgias, and gastrointestinal symptoms were commonly reported.
Psychiatric disorders	Cohort	22	Apple et al,[100] 2022	Cognitive PASC participants exhibited more aberrant CSF results (77% vs 0%) and more preexisting cognitive risk factors such as anxiety, depression, ADHD, and learning disabilities.
	Case-control	473,958	Wang et al,[102] 2021	Those with preexisting mental disorders are at a higher risk of developing COVID-19 and exacerbated outcomes.
	Case-control	61,783,950	Wang et al,[103] 2021	Individuals with schizophrenia and depression had a 7-fold risk for COVID-19 compared with controls. Patients with psychiatric conditions also had higher mortality rates.
Cardiovascular disease risk factors	Longitudinal multi-omic	666	Su et al,[75] 2022	Significant correlations between type 2 diabetes and respiratory-viral symptoms such as fatigue, cough, shortness of breath, fever/chills, muscle aches, and nausea were identified.
	Case-control	108	Mittal et al,[104] 2021	Patients with COVID-19 with type 2 diabetes had a significantly higher prevalence of PASC fatigue, weight loss, and reduced exercise capacity.
	Retrospective Analysis	2839	Aminian et al,[105] 2021	The risk of hospitalization was 28% greater in individuals with moderate obesity and 30% higher in those with severe obesity.
	Cohort	5307	Kong et al,[106] 2021	Patient with these 4 cardiovascular risk factors (age≥ 60 y, male sex, hypertension, and diabetes mellitus) had a risk of severe COVID-19 that was more than 100 times higher than those without.

(continued on next page)

Table 1
(continued)

Comorbidity	Study Design	Total Participants	Author	Major Findings
	Meta-analysis	1527	Li et al,[107] 2021	In ICU patients, the rates of hypertension, cerebracardiovascular disease, and diabetes were approximately 2-fold, 3-fold, and 2-fold higher, respectively, than in non-ICU/severe cases.
	Systematic review/Meta-analysis	48,317	Bae et al,[108] 2020	Fatal outcomes in COVID-19 for patients of all ages were strongly associated with CVD and its risk factors (hypertension and diabetes).
	Longitudinal	1038	Yoo et al,[109] 2022	Higher BMI, diabetes, and hospitalization for COVID-19 were all characterized as risk factors associated with development of PASC.
Lung disease	Cohort Observational	8070	Lee et al,[110] 2021	Of 8070 patients with COVID-19, 67 individuals had ILD. Those with preexisting ILD required higher rates of oxygen therapy, intensive care unit admissions/mechanical ventilation, and mortality.
		18	Konopka et al,[111] 2021	Among 18 PASC patients, half had usual interstitial pneumonia (UIP). Only a minority of individuals without UIP exhibited histologic indications of persistent acute lung injury attributed to SARS-CoV-2.

Abbreviations: ADHD, attention-deficit/hyperactivity disorder; BMI, body mass index; CSF, cerebrospinal fluid; ICU, intensive care unit; ILD, interstitial lung disease.

at 2 to 3 months after infection already had mature (class-switched) immunoglobulin G (IgG) autoantibodies at diagnosis.[75]

Thus, patients with prior autoimmune conditions could be at higher risk for PASC due to immune dysregulation and/or immunosuppression and lower ability to clear a persistent SARS-CoV-2 infection. Further research will be necessary to determine other potential mechanisms of how underlying autoimmunity may serve as an independent risk factor for PASC.

New-onset autoimmunity postacute SARS-CoV-2 infection. It has now been demonstrated that SARS-CoV-2 infection induces an overactive immune system, resulting in autoantibodies in some patients. In a cohort study led by Chang and colleagues, autoantibodies were identified in approximately 50% of patients with COVID-19 but in less than 15% of healthy controls.[81] In this study, 25% of hospitalized patients with COVID-19 developed antinuclear antibodies. Chang and colleagues also detected anticytokine antibodies in 80% of 51 hospitalized patients with COVID-19 but not in

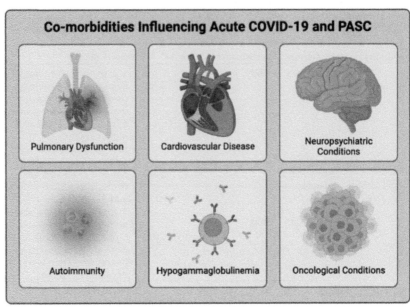

Fig. 1. Comorbidities in acute and postacute SARS-CoV-2 infection. Acute COVID-19 disease and PASC severity may be affected by preexisting medical conditions, such as pulmonary dysfunction, cardiovascular disease, neuropsychiatric conditions, autoimmunity, hypogammaglobulinemia, and cancer.

patients with mild COVID-19 or healthy controls. Moreover, Arthur and colleagues revealed the presence of ACE2 autoantibodies in patients with COVID-19.[82] Lower plasma levels of soluble ACE2 were found in patients with ACE2 antibodies.[82] Interestingly, alopecia areata, an autoimmune condition characterized by hair loss, has been reported to a be a dermatologic manifestation of acute COVID-19 infection and could be the result of the inflammation induced by SARS-CoV-2.[83–85]

Liu and colleagues found presence of sex-specific autoantibodies up to 6 months post-SARS-CoV-2 infection, further confirming prolonged autoantibody responses in PASC patients.[86] While confirming circulating autoantibodies to ACE2 as in other studies, they found autoantibodies to 59 antigens in men and another set of autoantibodies to 38 antigens in women. The autoantibodies found in men were associated with a higher frequency of symptoms compared with women. This study underlines the need to explore sex-specific outcomes of acquired autoimmunity post-COVID. As Liu and colleagues did not address the association of the discovered autoantibodies to PASC disease severity, future studies in PASC autoimmunity need to be done in larger cohorts of men and women to better understand whether specific autoantibody markers may have different sex-specific outcomes.

Overall, emerging evidence currently suggests a bidirectional relationship between autoimmunity and COVID-19 infection, with some studies showing that prior autoimmunity may predispose patients to worse COVID-19 outcomes, whereas other studies indicate new onset autoimmunity post-COVID.

Hypogammaglobulinemia

In a multicenter cohort study of 215 individuals, Cervia and colleagues found that immunoglobulin signature could predict PASC development risk.[87] These results were further validated in a cohort of 395 individuals with confirmed COVID-19 infection, in which patients with mild or severe acute COVID-19 disease who developed PASC had lower concentrations of IgG3 compared with patients with the same acute disease severity who did not develop PASC. Also, patients with high IgM titers were less likely to develop PASC. Interestingly, patients who went on to develop PASC had lower starting IgM titers before SARS-CoV-2 infection, and these concentrations remained low throughout the study. Notably, low IgG3 has been associated with chronic fatigue syndrome, which has many shared symptoms with both PASC and other autoimmune disorders. Mechanistically, low IgG3 switching is indicative of impaired immunity, as B cells are unable to properly class switch and could leave patients vulnerable to complications of COVID-19. The failure to induce Ig isotype switching to IgG3 may indicate preexisting immune cell dysfunction, which could predispose patients to PASC.

Lastly, Greenmyer and Joshi assessed the progression of SARS-CoV-2 infection in patients with CVID caused by failure in B-cell differentiation that puts patients at higher risk of infection.[88] Two patients in the cohort reported persistent symptoms consistent with PASC, and serology testing on one of the patients showed a lack of seroconversion following infection. Thus, low antibody levels resulting in hypogammaglobulinemia seem to be a significant risk factor for PASC.

Oncological Conditions

Immunocompromised individuals, such as patients with cancer, face a greater susceptibility to COVID-19. In a study by Robilotti and colleagues, 40% of 432 patients were admitted to the hospital for COVID-19, 20% had severe respiratory disease (with 9% who needed ventilatory support), and 12% died within 30 days.[89] In line with these findings, Mehta and colleagues found COVID-19 individuals with cancer to have a significantly higher mortality rate.[90] In their study, 28% of patients with cancer died of COVID-19, with COVID-19 illness resulting in the deaths of 6 out of 11 (55%) patients with lung cancer. The case fatality rate for hematologic malignancies was higher compared with solid tumors (37% vs 25%). In line with these findings, patients with hematological malignancies had fared worse in a study by Meng and colleagues, with a mortality rate double that of those with solid tumors (50% vs 26.1%).[91] There are limited data on the relationship between PASC and cancer. Notably, 60% of the patients with existing oncological conditions had persistent PASC symptoms up to 14 months postacute infection.[92] Cancer may also play a role in syndrome severity, as PASC patients with cancer were more likely to be hospitalized.[93]

SUMMARY AND FUTURE DIRECTIONS

The evidence from multiple studies suggests that both acute COVID-19 and PASC are heterogeneous conditions that affect patients differentially. Although respiratory issues are common in both conditions, patients may also experience multiorgan symptoms, including neuropsychiatric, gastrointestinal, cardiovascular, dermatologic, renal, and endocrine complications. Preexisting conditions such as autoimmunity, hypogammaglobulinemia, cancer, cardio-pulmonary and neuropsychiatric conditionsmay influence the presentation of both diseases.

With the estimated global prevalence of acute COVID-19 at greater than 600 million people and of PASC at 10% to 30% of the population, there is an urgent need to continue research to understand the underlying pathophysiology, epidemiologic factors, and immune and autoimmune implications of the SARS-CoV-2 viral infection and its sequelae.[94] With insights gained from pathophysiology of these diseases, it is also critical to develop tailored therapies that are specific to patients' clinical presentation.

To accomplish these goals, federal funding is needed both for research as well as to establish and continue to support comprehensive, specialized clinics across different states, where a cross-disciplinary approach to treatment can occur, including access to rehabilitation programs, welfare assistance, organized peer support groups, and equitable provision of services for those who face socioeconomic and geographic barriers. Most importantly, providers must continue to actively acknowledge and validate the symptoms of their patients.

CLINICS CARE POINTS

- COVID-19 has resulted in a significant number of people experiencing long-term clinical sequelae, known as long-COVID or PASC.

- PASC can involve multiorgan dysfunction and may be influenced by comorbid conditions such as autoimmunity, hypogammaglobulinemia, cancer, cardio-pulmonary and neuropsychiatric conditions.

- The mechanisms behind PASC are not fully understood but may involve persistent inflammation, the development of autoimmunity, and the potential for the virus to persist or for immunogenicity to occur from residual SARS-CoV-2 RNA.

AUTHOR'S CONTRIBUTION

A. Ramasamy: drafting/revision of the manuscript, generation of tables, study concept, and design. C. Wang: drafting/revision of the manuscript, generation of figure, study concept, and design. W.M. Brode: study concept/design, revision of the manuscript. M. Verduzco-Gutierrez: study concept/design, revision of the manuscript. E. Melamed: study concept/design, drafting/revision of the manuscript for content, generation of figures, preparation of manuscript for journal submission, funding for the study.

STUDY FUNDING

This work was supported by NIAAA, United States K08 T26-1616-11 (E. Melamed) and Institutional Dell Medical School Startup funding (E. Melamed).

DISCLOSURE

A. Ramasamy: nothing to disclose; C. Wang: nothing to disclose; M. Verduzco-Gutierrez: has received honoraria for PASC presentations and has served as a consultant for Merz, Ipsen, and AbbVie. W.M. Brode: nothing to disclose. E. Melamed: has received NIH, United States funding for COVID-19 research, honorarium from Multiple Sclerosis Association of America and National Center for Health Research, and has served on advisory boards of Genentech, Horizon, Teva, and Viela Bio.

ACKNOWLEDGMENTS

The authors are grateful to Dr Adron Harris and Diane Harris for thoughtful comments and review of the manuscript; Dr William Schwartz for helpful discussions; Jennifer Ramey, RN for helpful discussions and PASC patient advocacy; and Diana Zuckerman and Emma Roy at the National Center for Health Research for PASC advocacy and including the authors in the autoimmune PASC group that led to ideas for this manuscript. The authors also appreciate Dell Medical School Neurology Department's administrative support, by Bethaney Watson, Tran de la Torre, and Karen Rascon.

REFERENCES

1. Dong E, Du H, Gardner L. An interactive web-based dashboard to track COVID-19 in real time. Lancet Infect Dis 2020;20(5):533–4. Available at: https://www.thelancet.com/journals/laninf/article/PIIS1473-3099(20)30120-1/fulltext.
2. Proal AD, VanElzakker MB. Long COVID or Post-acute Sequelae of COVID-19 (PASC): An Overview of Biological Factors That May Contribute to Persistent Symptoms. Front Microbiol 2021;12:698169. Available at: https://www.ncbi.nlm.nih.gov/pmc/articles/PMC8260991/.
3. Logue JK, Franko NM, McCulloch DJ, et al. Sequelae in Adults at 6 Months After COVID-19 Infection. JAMA Netw Open 2021 Feb 19;4(2):e210830.
4. A clinical case definition of post COVID-19 condition by a Delphi consensus, 6 October 2021 [Internet]. [cited 2022 Jul 13]. Available at: https://www.who.int/publications-detail-redirect/WHO-2019-nCoV-Post_COVID-19_condition-Clinical_case_definition-2021.1.
5. CDC. Post-COVID Conditions [Internet]. Centers for Disease Control and Prevention. 2022 [cited 2022 Aug 4]. Available at: https://www.cdc.gov/coronavirus/2019-ncov/long-term-effects/index.html.
6. CDC. COVID Data Tracker [Internet]. Centers for Disease Control and Prevention. 2020 [cited 2022 Aug 10]. Available at:https://covid.cdc.gov/covid-data-tracker.
7. PASC Dashboard [Internet]. [cited 2022 Aug 4]. Available at: https://pascdashboard.aapmr.org/.
8. Alimohamadi Y, Sepandi M, Taghdir M, et al. Determine the most common clinical symptoms in COVID-19 patients: a systematic review and meta-analysis. J Prev Med Hyg 2020 Oct 6;61(3):E304–12. Available at: https://www.ncbi.nlm.nih.gov/pmc/articles/PMC7595075/.
9. Wang HY, Li XL, Yan ZR, et al. Potential neurological symptoms of COVID-19. Ther Adv Neurol Disord 2020;13. https://doi.org/10.1177/1756286420917830. 1756286420917830.
10. JCM | Free Full-Text | Multi-Organ Involvement in COVID-19: Beyond Pulmonary Manifestations [Internet]. [cited 2022 Oct 17]. Available at: https://www.mdpi.com/2077-0383/10/3/446.
11. Mizumoto K, Kagaya K, Zarebski A, Chowell G. Estimating the asymptomatic proportion of coronavirus disease 2019 (COVID-19) cases on board the Diamond Princess cruise ship, Yokohama, Japan, 2020. Eurosurveillance [Internet]. 2020 Mar 12 [cited 2022 Oct 17];25(10):2000180. Available at: https://www.eurosurveillance.org/content/10.2807/1560-7917.ES.2020.25.10.2000180.
12. Seyed Hosseini E, Riahi Kashani N, Nikzad H, et al. The novel coronavirus Disease-2019 (COVID-19): Mechanism of action, detection and recent therapeutic strategies. Virology 2020 Dec;551:1–9. Available at: https://www.ncbi.nlm.nih.gov/pmc/articles/PMC7513802/.
13. Buszko M, Park JH, Verthelyi D, et al. The dynamic changes in cytokine responses in COVID-19: a snapshot of the current state of knowledge. Nat Immunol 2020 Oct;21(10):1146–51. Available at: https://www.nature.com/articles/s41590-020-0779-1.
14. Signals of Significantly Increased Vaccine Breakthrough, Decreased Hospitalization Rates, and Less Severe Disease in Patients with Coronavirus Disease

2019 Caused by the Omicron Variant of Severe Acute Respiratory Syndrome Coronavirus 2 in Houston, Texas - American Journal of Pathology [Internet]. [cited 2022 Oct 17]. Available at: https://ajp.amjpathol.org/article/S0002-9440(22)00044-X/fulltext.

15. Davis HE, Assaf GS, McCorkell L, et al. Characterizing long COVID in an international cohort: 7 months of symptoms and their impact. EClinicalMedicine 2021 Aug 1;38:101019. Available at: https://www.sciencedirect.com/science/article/pii/S2589537021002996.

16. Larsen NW, Stiles LE, Shaik R, et al. Characterization of Autonomic Symptom Burden in Long COVID: A Global Survey of 2,314 Adults. medRxiv 2022; 2022(04.25):22274300. Available at: https://www.medrxiv.org/content/10.1101/2022.04.25.22274300v1.

17. Pilotto A, Cristillo V, Cotti Piccinelli S, et al. Long-term neurological manifestations of COVID-19: prevalence and predictive factors. Neurol Sci 2021 Dec 1; 42(12):4903–7.

18. Taquet M, Geddes JR, Husain M, et al. 6-month neurological and psychiatric outcomes in 236 379 survivors of COVID-19: a retrospective cohort study using electronic health records. Lancet Psychiatr 2021 May 1;8(5):416–27. Available at: https://www.thelancet.com/journals/lanpsy/article/PIIS2215-0366(21)00084-5/fulltext#seccestitle170.

19. Weng J, Li Y, Li J, et al. Gastrointestinal sequelae 90 days after discharge for COVID-19. Lancet Gastroenterol Hepatol 2021 May 1;6(5):344–6. Available at: https://www.thelancet.com/journals/langas/article/PIIS2468-1253(21)00076-5/fulltext.

20. Natarajan A, Zlitni S, Brooks EF, et al. Gastrointestinal symptoms and fecal shedding of SARS-CoV-2 RNA suggest prolonged gastrointestinal infection. Med 2022 Jun 10;3(6):371–87, e9. Available at: https://www.cell.com/med/abstract/S2666-6340(22)00167-2.

21. Montalvo M, Nallapaneni P, Hassan S, et al. Autoimmune gastrointestinal dysmotility following SARS-CoV-2 infection successfully treated with intravenous immunoglobulin. Neuro Gastroenterol Motil 2022;34(7):e14314. Available at: https://onlinelibrary.wiley.com/doi/abs/10.1111/nmo.14314.

22. Pathophysiology of irritable bowel syndrome - UpToDate [Internet]. [cited 2022 Sep 3]. Available at: https://www.uptodate.com/contents/pathophysiology-of-irritable-bowel-syndrome.

23. Comelli A, Viero G, Bettini G, et al. Patient-Reported Symptoms and Sequelae 12 Months After COVID-19 in Hospitalized Adults: A Multicenter Long-Term Follow-Up Study. Front Med 2022;9. Available at: https://www.frontiersin.org/articles/10.3389/fmed.2022.834354.

24. Carfì A, Bernabei R, Landi F. for the Gemelli Against COVID-19 Post-Acute Care Study Group. Persistent Symptoms in Patients After Acute COVID-19. JAMA 2020;324(6):603–5.

25. Wong AW, Shah AS, Johnston JC, et al. Patient-reported outcome measures after COVID-19: a prospective cohort study. Eur Respir J 2020 Nov 1;56(5). Available at: https://erj.ersjournals.com/content/56/5/2003276.

26. Puntmann VO, Carerj ML, Wieters I, et al. Outcomes of Cardiovascular Magnetic Resonance Imaging in Patients Recently Recovered From Coronavirus Disease 2019 (COVID-19). JAMA Cardiol 2020;5(11):1265–73.

27. Chadda KR, Blakey EE, Huang CLH, et al. Long COVID-19 and Postural Orthostatic Tachycardia Syndrome- Is Dysautonomia to Be Blamed? Front Cardiovasc

Med 2022. 9. Available from: https://www.frontiersin.org/articles/10.3389/fcvm. 2022.860198.

28. Ståhlberg M, Reistam U, Fedorowski A, et al. Post-COVID-19 Tachycardia Syndrome: A Distinct Phenotype of Post-Acute COVID-19 Syndrome. Am J Med 2021;134(12):1451–6. Available from: https://www.ncbi.nlm.nih.gov/pmc/articles/PMC8356730/.

29. Huang C, Huang L, Wang Y, et al. 6-month consequences of COVID-19 in patients discharged from hospital: a cohort study. Lancet 2021;397(10270): 220–32. Available from: https://www.thelancet.com/journals/lancet/article/PIIS0140-6736(20)32656-8/fulltext.

30. Lambert N, Corps S, El-Azab SA, et al. COVID-19 Survivors' Reports of the Timing, Duration, and Health Impacts of Post-Acute Sequelae of SARS-CoV-2 (PASC) Infection. medRxiv 2021;2021(03.22):21254026. Available at: https://www.medrxiv.org/content/10.1101/2021.03.22.21254026v2.

31. McMahon DE, Gallman AE, Hruza GJ, et al. Long COVID in the skin: a registry analysis of COVID-19 dermatological duration. Lancet Infect Dis 2021 Mar;21(3): 313–4. Available at: https://www.ncbi.nlm.nih.gov/pmc/articles/PMC7836995/.

32. Bowe B, Xie Y, Xu E, et al. Kidney Outcomes in Long COVID. J Am Soc Nephrol 2021 Nov 1;32(11):2851–62. Available at: https://jasn.asnjournals.org/content/32/11/2851.

33. Subramanian A, Nirantharakumar K, Hughes S, et al. Symptoms and risk factors for long COVID in non-hospitalized adults. Nat Med 2022 Jul 25;1–9. Available at: https://www.nature.com/articles/s41591-022-01909-w.

34. Insights into SARS-CoV-2 genome, structure, evolution, pathogenesis and therapies: Structural genomics approach - PMC [Internet]. [cited 2022 Aug 4]. Available at: https://www.ncbi.nlm.nih.gov/pmc/articles/PMC7293463/.

35. Sui Y, Li J, Venzon DJ, et al. SARS-CoV-2 Spike Protein Suppresses ACE2 and Type I Interferon Expression in Primary Cells From Macaque Lung Bronchoalveolar Lavage. Front Immunol 2021;12. Available at: https://www.frontiersin.org/articles/10.3389/fimmu.2021.658428.

36. Salamanna F, Maglio M, Landini MP, et al. Body Localization of ACE-2: On the Trail of the Keyhole of SARS-CoV-2. Front Med 2020;7. Available at: https://www.frontiersin.org/articles/10.3389/fmed.2020.594495.

37. Ding Y, He L, Zhang Q, et al. Organ distribution of severe acute respiratory syndrome (SARS) associated coronavirus (SARS-CoV) in SARS patients: implications for pathogenesis and virus transmission pathways. J Pathol 2004;203(2): 622–30. Available at: https://onlinelibrary.wiley.com/doi/abs/10.1002/path.1560.

38. Gu J, Gong E, Zhang B, et al. Multiple organ infection and the pathogenesis of SARS. J Exp Med 2005 Jul 25;202(3):415–24.

39. Gagliardi MC, Tieri P, Ortona E, et al. ACE2 expression and sex disparity in COVID-19. Cell Death Discov 2020;6:37. Available at: https://www.ncbi.nlm.nih.gov/pmc/articles/PMC7248455/.

40. Genome-wide analysis provides genetic evidence that ACE2 influences COVID-19 risk and yields risk scores associated with severe disease | Nat Genet [Internet]. [cited 2022 Aug 8]. Available at: https://www.nature.com/articles/s41588-021-01006-7.

41. Zhou X, Ye Q. Cellular Immune Response to COVID-19 and Potential Immune Modulators. Front Immunol 2021;12. Available at: https://www.frontiersin.org/articles/10.3389/fimmu.2021.646333.

42. Ragab D, Salah Eldin H, Taeimah M, et al. The COVID-19 Cytokine Storm; What We Know So Far. Front Immunol 2020;11. Available from: https://www.frontiersin.org/articles/10.3389/fimmu.2020.01446.

43. Murira A, Lamarre A. Type-I Interferon Responses: From Friend to Foe in the Battle against Chronic Viral Infection. Front Immunol 2016 [cited 2022 Aug 5];7. Available from: https://www.frontiersin.org/articles/10.3389/fimmu.2016.00609.

44. Blomberg B, Mohn KGI, Brokstad KA, et al. Long COVID in a prospective cohort of home-isolated patients. Nat Med 2021 Sep;27(9):1607–13. Available from: https://www.nature.com/articles/s41591-021-01433-3.

45. Respiratory and Psychophysical Sequelae Among Patients With COVID-19 Four Months After Hospital Discharge | Infectious Diseases | JAMA Network Open | JAMA Network [Internet]. [cited 2022 Oct 17]. Available at: https://jamanetwork.com/journals/jamanetworkopen/fullarticle/2775643.

46. Lu Y, Li X, Geng D, et al. Cerebral Micro-Structural Changes in COVID-19 Patients – An MRI-based 3-month Follow-up Study. EClinicalMedicine 2020 Aug; 25:100484. Available at: https://www.ncbi.nlm.nih.gov/pmc/articles/PMC7396952/.

47. Al-Dalahmah O, Thakur KT, Nordvig AS, et al. Neuronophagia and microglial nodules in a SARS-CoV-2 patient with cerebellar hemorrhage. Acta Neuropathol Commun 2020 Aug 26;8(1):147.

48. Fabbri VP, Foschini MP, Lazzarotto T, et al. Brain ischemic injury in COVID-19-infected patients: a series of 10 post-mortem cases. Brain Pathol Zurich Switz 2021 Jan;31(1):205–10.

49. Finsterer J, Scorza FA, Scorza C, et al. COVID-19 associated cranial nerve neuropathy: A systematic review. Bosn J Basic Med Sci 2022 Feb 1;22(1):39–45. Available from: https://www.bjbms.org/ojs/index.php/bjbms/article/view/6341.

50. What can cerebrospinal fluid testing and brain autopsies tell us about viral neuroinvasion of SARS-CoV-2 - Li - 2021 - Journal of Medical Virology - Wiley Online Library [Internet]. [cited 2022 Oct 17]. Available from: https://onlinelibrary.wiley.com/doi/10.1002/jmv.26943.

51. Neuropathology of patients with COVID-19 in Germany: a post-mortem case series - The Lancet Neurology [Internet]. [cited 2022 Oct 17]. Available from: https://www.thelancet.com/article/S1474-4422(20)30308-2/fulltext.

52. Neuropathologic features of four autopsied COVID-19 patients - PubMed [Internet]. [cited 2022 Oct 17]. Available from: https://pubmed.ncbi.nlm.nih.gov/32762083/.

53. Meinhardt J, Radke J, Dittmayer C, et al. Olfactory transmucosal SARS-CoV-2 invasion as port of Central Nervous System entry in COVID-19 patients. bioRxiv 2020;2020(06.04):135012. Available at: https://www.biorxiv.org/content/10.1101/2020.06.04.135012v1.

54. Duarte-Neto AN, Monteiro RAA, da Silva LFF, et al. Pulmonary and systemic involvement in COVID-19 patients assessed with ultrasound-guided minimally invasive autopsy. Histopathology 2020 Aug;77(2):186–97.

55. Yong SJ. Long COVID or post-COVID-19 syndrome: putative pathophysiology, risk factors, and treatments. Infect Dis Lond Engl 2022;1–18. Available at: https://www.ncbi.nlm.nih.gov/pmc/articles/PMC8146298/.

56. Crunfli F, Carregari VC, Veras FP, et al. Morphological, cellular, and molecular basis of brain infection in COVID-19 patients. Proc Natl Acad Sci 2022 Aug 30;119(35). e2200960119. Available at: https://www.pnas.org/doi/full/10.1073/pnas.2200960119.

57. Khan M, Yoo SJ, Clijsters M, et al. Visualizing in deceased COVID-19 patients how SARS-CoV-2 attacks the respiratory and olfactory mucosae but spares the olfactory bulb. Cell 2021 Nov 24;184(24):5932–49, e15. Available at: https://www.sciencedirect.com/science/article/pii/S0092867421012824.

58. Ho CY, Salimian M, Hegert J, et al. Postmortem Assessment of Olfactory Tissue Degeneration and Microvasculopathy in Patients With COVID-19. JAMA Neurol 2022;79(6):544–53.

59. Mehandru S, Merad M. Pathological sequelae of long-haul COVID. Nat Immunol 2022;23(2):194–202. Available at: https://www.nature.com/articles/s41590-021-01104-y.

60. Ehrenfeld M, Tincani A, Andreoli L, et al. Covid-19 and autoimmunity. Autoimmun Rev 2020 Aug;19(8):102597. Available at: https://www.ncbi.nlm.nih.gov/pmc/articles/PMC7289100/.

61. Phetsouphanh C, Darley DR, Wilson DB, et al. Immunological dysfunction persists for 8 months following initial mild-to-moderate SARS-CoV-2 infection. Nat Immunol 2022 Feb;23(2):210–6. Available at: https://www.nature.com/articles/s41590-021-01113-x.

62. Liblau RS, Wong FS, Mars LT, et al. Autoreactive CD8 T Cells in Organ-Specific Autoimmunity: Emerging Targets for Therapeutic Intervention. Immunity 2002 Jul 1;17(1):1–6. Available at: https://www.cell.com/immunity/abstract/S1074-7613(02)00338-2.

63. Seeßle J, Waterboer T, Hippchen T, et al. Persistent Symptoms in Adult Patients 1 Year After Coronavirus Disease 2019 (COVID-19): A Prospective Cohort Study. Clin Infect Dis 2021;ciab611. Available at: https://www.ncbi.nlm.nih.gov/pmc/articles/PMC8394862/.

64. Yang E, Husein A, Martinez-Perez J, et al. Post-COVID-19 Longitudinally Extensive Transverse Myelitis with Myelin Oligodendrocyte Glycoprotein Antibodies. Case Rep Neurol Med 2022;2022:1068227. Available at: https://www.ncbi.nlm.nih.gov/pmc/articles/PMC8984739/.

65. Benjamin LA, Paterson RW, Moll R, et al. Antiphospholipid antibodies and neurological manifestations in acute COVID-19: A single-centre cross-sectional study. eClinicalMedicine 2021;39. Available at: https://www.thelancet.com/journals/eclinm/article/PIIS2589-5370(21)00350-3/fulltext.

66. Patterson BK, Francisco EB, Yogendra R, et al. Persistence of SARS CoV-2 S1 Protein in CD16+ Monocytes in Post-Acute Sequelae of COVID-19 (PASC) up to 15 Months Post-Infection. Front Immunol 2022;12. Available at: https://www.frontiersin.org/articles/10.3389/fimmu.2021.746021.

67. Gebremeskel S, Schanin J, Coyle KM, et al. Mast Cell and Eosinophil Activation Are Associated With COVID-19 and TLR-Mediated Viral Inflammation: Implications for an Anti-Siglec-8 Antibody. Front Immunol 2021;12:650331. Available at: https://www.ncbi.nlm.nih.gov/pmc/articles/PMC7988091/.

68. Matito A, Escribese MM, Longo N, et al. Clinical Approach to Mast Cell Activation Syndrome: A Practical Overview. J Investig Allergol Clin Immunol 2021 Dec 21;31(6):461–70.

69. Evaluating and supporting patients presenting with fatigue following COVID-19 [Internet]. [cited 2022 Oct 17]. Available from: https://stacks.cdc.gov/view/cdc/117036.

70. Jill Schofield. Persistent Antiphospholipid Antibodies, Mast Cell Activation Syndrome, Postural Orthostatic Tachycardia Syndrome and Post-COVID Syndrome: 1 Year On. Eur J Case Rep Intern Med [Internet]. 2021 Mar 22 [cited 2022 Aug

9];(LATEST ONLINE). Available from: https://www.ejcrim.com/index.php/EJCRIM/article/view/2378.

71. Desimmie BA, Raru YY, Awadh HM, et al. Insights into SARS-CoV-2 Persistence and Its Relevance. Viruses 2021 May 29;13(6):1025.

72. Cevik M, Tate M, Lloyd O, et al. SARS-CoV-2, SARS-CoV, and MERS-CoV viral load dynamics, duration of viral shedding, and infectiousness: a systematic review and meta-analysis. Lancet Microbe 2021 Jan;2(1):e13–22.

73. Li N, Wang X, Lv T. Prolonged SARS-CoV-2 RNA shedding: Not a rare phenomenon. J Med Virol 2020 Nov;92(11):2286–7.

74. Prevalence and clinical outcomes of COVID-19 in patients with autoimmune diseases: a systematic review and meta-analysis | Annals of the Rheumatic Diseases [Internet]. [cited 2022 Aug 8]. Available from: https://ard.bmj.com/content/80/3/384.

75. Multiple early factors anticipate post-acute COVID-19 sequelae: Cell [Internet]. [cited 2022 Aug 8]. Available from: https://www.cell.com/cell/fulltext/S0092-8674(22)00072-1#secsectitle0020.

76. Jones JM, Faruqi AJ, Sullivan JK, et al. COVID-19 Outcomes in Patients Undergoing B Cell Depletion Therapy and Those with Humoral Immunodeficiency States: A Scoping Review. Pathog Immun 2021 May 14;6(1):76–103. Available at: https://www.ncbi.nlm.nih.gov/pmc/articles/PMC8150936/.

77. Dreyer N, Petruski-Ivleva N, Albert L, et al. Identification of a Vulnerable Group for Post-Acute Sequelae of SARS-CoV-2 (PASC): People with Autoimmune Diseases Recover More Slowly from COVID-19. Int J Gen Med 2021;14:3941–9. Available at: https://www.ncbi.nlm.nih.gov/pmc/articles/PMC8323859/.

78. Holroyd KB, Healy BC, Conway S, et al. Humoral response to COVID-19 vaccination in MS patients on disease modifying therapy: Immune profiles and clinical outcomes. Mult Scler Relat Disord 2022 Jul 28;67:104079.

79. Conway SE, Healy BC, Zurawski J, et al. COVID-19 severity is associated with worsened neurological outcomes in multiple sclerosis and related disorders. Mult Scler Relat Disord 2022 Jul 1;63:103946. Available at: https://www.sciencedirect.com/science/article/pii/S2211034822004576.

80. Autoantibodies neutralizing type I IFNs are present in ~ 4% of uninfected individuals over 70 years old and account for ~ 20% of COVID-19 deaths - PubMed [Internet]. [cited 2022 Aug 8]. Available at: https://pubmed.ncbi.nlm.nih.gov/34413139/.

81. Chang SE, Feng A, Meng W, et al. New-onset IgG autoantibodies in hospitalized patients with COVID-19. Nat Commun 2021 Sep 14;12(1):5417. Available at: https://www.nature.com/articles/s41467-021-25509-3.

82. Development of ACE2 autoantibodies after SARS-CoV-2 infection | PLOS ONE [Internet]. [cited 2022 Aug 8]. Available at: https://journals.plos.org/plosone/article?id=10.1371/journal.pone.0257016.

83. Androgenetic alopecia present in the majority of patients hospitalized with COVID-19: The "Gabrin sign" - Journal of the American Academy of Dermatology [Internet]. [cited 2022 Aug 28]. Available at: https://www.jaad.org/article/S0190-9622(20)30948-8/fulltext.

84. Capalbo A, Giordano D, Gagliostro N, et al. Alopecia areata in a COVID-19 patient: A case report. Dermatol Ther 2021;34(2):e14685. Available at: https://www.ncbi.nlm.nih.gov/pmc/articles/PMC7883233/.

85. Christensen RE, Jafferany M. Association between alopecia areata and COVID-19: A systematic review. JAAD Int 2022;7:57–61. Available at: https://www.ncbi.nlm.nih.gov/pmc/articles/PMC8828419/.

86. Liu Y, Ebinger JE, Mostafa R, et al. Paradoxical sex-specific patterns of autoantibody response to SARS-CoV-2 infection. J Transl Med 2021;19(1):524.
87. Cervia C, Zurbuchen Y, Taeschler P, et al. Immunoglobulin signature predicts risk of post-acute COVID-19 syndrome. Nat Commun 2022;13:446. Available at: https://www.ncbi.nlm.nih.gov/pmc/articles/PMC8789854/.
88. Greenmyer JR, Joshi AY. COVID-19 in CVID: a Case Series of 17 Patients. J Clin Immunol 2022;42(1):29–31.
89. Robilotti EV, Babady NE, Mead PA, et al. Determinants of COVID-19 disease severity in patients with cancer. Nat Med 2020;26(8):1218–23. Available at: https://www.nature.com/articles/s41591-020-0979-0.
90. Case Fatality Rate of Cancer Patients with COVID-19 in a New York Hospital System | Cancer Discovery | American Association for Cancer Research [Internet]. [cited 2022 Aug 8]. Available at: https://aacrjournals.org/cancerdiscovery/article/10/7/935/2509/Case-Fatality-Rate-of-Cancer-Patients-with-COVID.
91. Cancer history is an independent risk factor for mortality in hospitalized COVID-19 patients: a propensity score-matched analysis | Journal of Hematology & Oncology | Full Text [Internet]. [cited 2022 Aug 8]. Available at: https://jhoonline.biomedcentral.com/articles/10.1186/s13045-020-00907-0.
92. Dagher H, Malek A, Chaftari AM, et al. Long COVID in Cancer Patients: Preponderance of Symptoms in Majority of Patients Over Long Time Period. Open Forum Infect Dis 2021;8(Supplement_1):S256–7.
93. Sharafeldin N, Madhira V, Song Q, et al. Long COVID-19 in patients with cancer: Report from the National COVID Cohort Collaborative (N3C). J Clin Oncol 2022;40(16_suppl):1540. Available at: https://ascopubs.org/doi/abs/10.1200/JCO.2022.40.16_suppl.1540.
94. Global Prevalence of Post-Coronavirus Disease 2019 (COVID-19) Condition or Long COVID: A Meta-Analysis and Systematic Review | The Journal of Infectious Diseases | Oxford Academic [Internet]. [cited 2022 Aug 4]. Available at: https://academic.oup.com/jid/advance-article/doi/10.1093/infdis/jiac136/6569364#356013096.
95. Impact of COVID-19 on people with asthma: a mixed methods analysis from a UK wide survey, BMJ Open Respiratory Research [Internet]. [cited 2022 Aug 8]. Available at: https://bmjopenrespres.bmj.com/content/9/1/e001056.
96. Risk factors for developing COVID-19: a population-based longitudinal study (COVIDENCE UK), Thorax [Internet]. [cited 2022 Aug 8]. Available at: https://thorax.bmj.com/content/early/2021/11/02/thoraxjnl-2021-217487#DC1.
97. Jackson DJ, Busse WW, Bacharier LB, et al. Association of respiratory allergy, asthma, and expression of the SARS-CoV-2 receptor ACE2. J Allergy Clin Immunol [Internet] 2020;146(1):203–6.e3.
98. Case Fatality Rate of Cancer Patients with COVID-19 in a New York Hospital System | Cancer Discovery | American Association for Cancer Research [Internet]. [cited 2022 Aug 8]. Available at: https://aacrjournals.org/cancerdiscovery/article/10/7/935/2509/Case-Fatality-Rate-of-Cancer-Patients-with-COVID.
99. Cancer history is an independent risk factor for mortality in hospitalized COVID-19 patients: a propensity score-matched analysis | Journal of Hematology & Oncology | Full Text [Internet]. [cited 2022 Aug 8]. Available at: https://jhoonline.biomedcentral.com/articles/10.1186/s13045-020-00907-0.
100. Risk factors and abnormal cerebrospinal fluid associate with cognitive symptoms after mild COVID-19 - Apple - 2022 - Annals of Clinical and Translational

Neurology - Wiley Online Library [Internet]. [cited 2022 Aug 8]. Available at: https://onlinelibrary.wiley.com/doi/10.1002/acn3.51498.

102. Wang Y., Yang Y., Ren L., et al., Preexisting Mental Disorders Increase the Risk of COVID-19 Infection and Associated Mortality. Front Public Health [Internet]. 2021 [cited 2022 Aug 28];9. Available at: https://www.frontiersin.org/articles/10.3389/fpubh.2021.684112.

103. Wang Q., Xu R., Volkow N.D., Increased risk of COVID-19 infection and mortality in people with mental disorders: analysis from electronic health records in the United States. World Psychiatry [Internet]. 2021 [cited 2022 Aug 28];20(1):124–130. Available at: https://onlinelibrary.wiley.com/doi/abs/10.1002/wps.20806.

104. Mittal J., Ghosh A., Bhatt S.P., et al., High prevalence of post COVID-19 fatigue in patients with type 2 diabetes: A case-control study. Diabetes Metab Syndr Clin Res Rev [Internet]. 2021 [cited 2022 Aug 8];15(6):102302. Available at: https://www.sciencedirect.com/science/article/pii/S1871402121003222.

105. Association of obesity with postacute sequelae of COVID-19 - Aminian - 2021 - Diabetes, Obesity and Metabolism - Wiley Online Library [Internet]. [cited 2022 Aug 8]. Available at: https://dom-pubs.onlinelibrary.wiley.com/doi/10.1111/dom.14454.

106. Kong K.A., Jung S., Yu M., et al., Association Between Cardiovascular Risk Factors and the Severity of Coronavirus Disease 2019: Nationwide Epidemiological Study in Korea. Front Cardiovasc Med [Internet]. 2021 [cited 2022 Aug 8];8. Available at: https://www.frontiersin.org/articles/10.3389/fcvm.2021.732518.

107. Prevalence and impact of cardiovascular metabolic diseases on COVID-19 in China | SpringerLink [Internet]. [cited 2022 Aug 8]. Available at: https://link.springer.com/article/10.1007/s00392-020-01626-9.

108. Impact of cardiovascular disease and risk factors on fatal outcomes in patients with COVID-19 according to age: a systematic review and meta-analysis | Heart [Internet]. [cited 2022 Aug 8]. Available at: https://heart.bmj.com/content/107/5/373.

109. Yoo S.M., Liu T.C., Motwani Y., et al., Factors Associated with Post-Acute Sequelae of SARS-CoV-2 (PASC) After Diagnosis of Symptomatic COVID-19 in the Inpatient and Outpatient Setting in a Diverse Cohort. J Gen Intern Med [Internet]. 2022 [cited 2022 Aug 8];37(8):1988–1995. Available at: https://doi.org/10.1007/s11606-022-07523-3.

110. Interstitial lung disease increases susceptibility to and severity of COVID-19 | European Respiratory Society [Internet]. [cited 2022 Aug 8]. Available at: https://erj.ersjournals.com/content/58/6/2004125.

111. Usual Interstitial Pneumonia is the Most Common Finding in Surgical Lung Biopsies from Patients with Persistent Interstitial Lung Disease Following Infection with SARS-CoV-2 - eClinicalMedicine [Internet]. [cited 2022 Aug 8]. Available at: https://www.thelancet.com/journals/eclinm/article/PIIS2589-5370(21)00490-9/fulltext#seccesectitle0019.

Considerations in Children and Adolescents Related to Coronavirus Disease 2019 (COVID-19)

Erin Y. Chen, BS[a], Justin M. Burton, MD[b], Alicia Johnston, MD[c],
Amanda K. Morrow, MD[d,e], Alexandra B. Yonts, MD[f],
Laura A. Malone, MD, PhD[d,e,g],*

KEYWORDS

- Post-acute sequelae of SARS-CoV-2 • Long COVID • Multidisciplinary care
- SARS-CoV-2 • Pediatrics • Rehabilitation • Fatigue • Quality of life

KEY POINTS

- Primary care providers should screen for post-acute sequelae of SARS-CoV-2 (PASC) in children with a history of SARS-CoV-2 infection.
- PASC is a complex multisystemic disease that benefits from a multifaceted treatment approach.
- Lifestyle interventions, physical rehabilitation, and mental health management are important in improving pediatric PASC patients' quality of life.

INTRODUCTION

Since the start of the Coronavirus Disease 2019 (COVID-19) pandemic, over 14.6 million pediatric COVID-19 cases have been reported in the United States—about 18.4% of all total cases.[1] Owing to the Omicron variant surge, severe acute respiratory syndrome coronavirus 2 (SARS-CoV-2) in children has become increasingly prevalent, as 6.7 million of these cases have occurred in 2022.[1] Fortunately, only 0.1% to 1.5% of

[a] Johns Hopkins School Medicine, 733 North Broadway, Baltimore, MD 21205, USA; [b] Division of Pediatric Rehabilitation Medicine, Children's National Health System, 111 Michigan Avenue Northwest, Washington, DC 20010, USA; [c] Division of Infectious Disease, Boston Children's Hospital, 300 Longwood Avenue, Boston, MA 02115, USA; [d] Kennedy Krieger Institute, 707 North Broadway, Baltimore, MD 21205, USA; [e] Department of Physical Medicine and Rehabilitation, Johns Hopkins School of Medicine, 600 North Wolfe Street, Baltimore, MD 21287, USA; [f] Division of Infectious Diseases, Children's National Health System, 111 Michigan Avenue Northwest, Washington, DC 20010, USA; [g] Department of Neurology, Johns Hopkins School of Medicine, 1800 Orleans Street, Baltimore, MD 21287, USA
* Corresponding author. 707 North Broadway, Baltimore, MD 21205.
E-mail address: lmalone3@jhmi.edu

Phys Med Rehabil Clin N Am 34 (2023) 643–655
https://doi.org/10.1016/j.pmr.2023.03.004
1047-9651/23/© 2023 Elsevier Inc. All rights reserved.

pediatric COVID-19 cases result in hospitalization, and death is rare (0%–0.02%).[1] Although most pediatric COVID-19 patients are asymptomatic or have mild symptoms in the acute period, some children present with severe and debilitating manifestations, such as multisystem inflammatory syndrome in children (MIS-C) and post-acute sequelae of SARS-CoV-2 (PASC), also known as post-COVID conditions or "long COVID."[2–4] For the purposes of this review, the authors use the term PASC. MIS-C is a multisystemic hyperinflammatory syndrome in children and adolescents that usually occurs 2 to 6 weeks after SARS-CoV-2 infection.[3,5] There have been 8862 cases of MIS-C in the United States reported to the Center for Disease Control and Prevention (CDC) as of August 29, 2022, with an incidence of less than 0.1%. Although rare, MIS-C carries significant morbidity and mortality; 72 of the cases resulted in death.[6]

PASC is the presence of symptoms that interfere with daily activities in individuals with a history of confirmed or probable SARS-CoV-2 infection that cannot be explained by an alternate diagnosis. The diagnostic criteria and time frame vary regarding when postinfectious symptoms are considered PASC. Although some (eg, World Health Organization) define PASC as symptoms lasting at least 3 months, the CDC defines PASC as symptoms (new, recurring, or persistent) present at least 4 weeks after initial infection.[7] Adult studies estimate that approximately 30% of patients develop PASC after SARS-CoV-2 infection.[8] In children, the prevalence is less well-known and challenging to study with individual studies reporting rates between 4% and 66%,[4,8–10] but larger estimates are around 5% to 25%.[9,11,12] One concern is that pediatric PASC (pPASC) is underrecognized. Children generally have mild acute illness which can result in a lack of testing for SAR-CoV-2. The lack of confirmed COVID-19 diagnosis combined with developmental limitations of children to recognize and describe nonspecific, and indolent PASC symptoms may result in underrecognition or a delay in diagnosis of PASC in children. However, PASC can be debilitating and negatively affect children's ability to attend school and participate in daily activities[8]; therefore, the importance of awareness and screening by pediatric providers cannot be understated. More information, research, and guidance are needed to improve the diagnosis and care of children with PASC. In this review, the authors consolidate what has been observed so far about pPASC.

SYMPTOMS AND PRESENTATION OF PEDIATRIC POST-ACUTE SEQUELAE OF SEVERE ACUTE RESPIRATORY SYNDROME CORONAVIRUS 2 (SARS-CoV-2)

pPASC patients display a broad spectrum of multisystemic symptoms with variable presentations, time course, and severity. pPASC symptoms can exist in children with mild or no symptoms and in both hospitalized and nonhospitalized patients.[2,8,13–16] However, some studies suggest that potential risk factors for pPASC include severity and duration of SARS-CoV-2 infection, older age, being female, allergic disease, underlying chronic disease, and higher body mass index (BMI).[8,13,16] Although adolescents have been shown to have a greater risk of PASC, it has been observed that younger children have a higher risk for respiratory symptoms and complications.[16] Multiple time courses and symptoms have been reported. PASC symptoms can linger and remain persistent after the acute infection, or the patient can fully recover after the acute infection only to later relapse or develop new postinfectious symptoms. Alternatively, the symptoms can wax and wane throughout the disease course.[2,7,8,13,14,16]

pPASC does not affect just one organ system; symptoms can occur in the cardiorespiratory, dermatologic, gastrointestinal, otolaryngologic, musculoskeletal, neurologic, psychiatric, renal, and general systems.[8,13] The most common symptoms include fatigue (3%–87%), cognitive difficulties (2%–81%), headaches (3%–80%), abdominal pain (1%–76%), muscle and joint pain (1%–68%), sleep disturbance (2%–63%), post-exertional malaise (53%), rash (2%–52%), dizziness and lightheadedness (19%–48%), heart palpitations (4%–40%), and mood disorders (5%–59%) such as anxiety and depression.[2,8,14,16–18] Other notable symptoms include school performance decline, anosmia, ageusia, respiratory symptoms (eg, dyspnea, cough), persistent chest pain, nausea, vomiting, and diarrhea.[4,8,16,18] The extensive scope of clinical manifestations observed suggests that pPASC may be a multifactorial disease.[15]

MULTISYSTEM INFLAMMATORY SYNDROME IN CHILDREN

Although rare, MIS-C is a life-threatening post-acute complication of SARS-CoV-2 infection and early identification and treatment are critical.[3] The CDC defines MIS-C as the presence of clinically severe illness requiring hospitalization, fever for over 24 hours, laboratory evidence of systemic inflammation, and multisystemic organ involvement within 4 weeks of acute SARS-CoV-2 infection, all of which cannot be explained by another diagnosis.[3,19] Organ systems affected by MIS-C include cardiovascular (66.7%–86.5%), gastrointestinal (80%–90%), neurologic (12.2%), respiratory (36.5%), hematologic (47.5%), and mucocutaneous systems (74%–83%).[3,19,20]

Common symptoms include erythematous rashes, persistent fever, diarrhea, abdominal pain, and mucocutaneous lesions. Some children present with more severe manifestations such as hypotension, vasogenic shock, myocarditis, coronary artery aneurysm, cardiac dysfunction, and acute kidney injury.[3,19,21] Of note, MIS-C presents similarly to Kawasaki disease (KD) and toxic shock syndrome, and some studies show that MIS-C and KD may share the same host immune response.[22] The most common age of onset is between 6 and 12 years, and MIS-C often affects previously healthy children (70%–80%).[3,20,23,24] One theory on why school-age children are more affected is that MIS-C may be underreported in older age groups because those patients tend to be seen at adult hospitals, and many of the MIS-C statistics are reported from children's hospitals.[24] Another theory is that KD is more prevalent in school-age children, and if MIS-C does have a similar pathogenesis to KD, then this may give insight into why MIS-C is present more commonly in younger children.[23] Some studies show that obesity and previous genetic disposition to hyperinflammation may be risk factors for MIS-C.[3,20] In addition, the gastrointestinal microbiome in children differs in composition from adults, and it has been hypothesized to play a role in not only the development of MIS-C in this population but also as a potential factor for the more mild initial COVID-19 disease in pediatric patients in general.[25,26]

Optimal treatment of MIS-C is still being studied due to MIS-Cs low incidence. However, early and aggressive treatment regimens have been recommended to prevent potential long-term cardiovascular sequelae.[3,19] Current treatment is similar to KD protocols, focusing on immunomodulation, such as intravenous immune globulin (IVIG) and corticosteroids, and supportive care.[3] Despite the potential severity of MIS-C, the outcomes for children affected by MIS-C are overall very good.[3,6,19] Studies have shown that most children completely recover after treatment, and the mortality rate has been less than 1%.[3,6,19] One study showed that by 6 months, most of the symptoms from patients' initial acute illness resolved. However, some sequelae have been reported to linger, including muscle fatigue, reduced functional exercise capacity, proximal myopathy, dysmetria, abnormal saccades, anxiety, and emotional lability.[27] In particular, when tested 6 months after hospitalization on the 6-minute-walk test, 45% of the patients scored below the third percentile for age, demonstrating functional impairment. Ninety-eight percent of the children returned to full-time education, but formal neuropsychological testing was not done to assess school performance.[27] More research needs to be done to characterize the potential long-term effects of MIS-C.

POTENTIAL MECHANISMS OF POST-ACUTE SEQUELAE OF SARS-CoV-2

Our understanding of the mechanisms underlying the pathophysiology of PASC is constantly evolving. Although much has been published describing reputed causes, few studies include broadly generalizable clinical data.[28] In addition, it is unknown if the pathophysiology behind PASC in children differs from adults. The heterogeneity of the clinical spectrum suggests that multiple mechanisms may be at play; literature demonstrating phenotypic symptomatic clustering of patients with PASC further suggests a multifactorial process.[29] Persistent symptoms may be due to virus-driven tissue damage from acute infection in certain cases, such as acute lung damage following respiratory infection or anosmia/parosmia following direct upper respiratory infection. However, alternative explanations are needed to understand persistent or late-onset symptoms in individuals lacking evidence of direct viral tissue invasion. The proposed mechanisms for the latter include immune dysregulation and inflammation in response to a restricted or persistent viral reservoir potentially leading to autoimmunity/molecular mimicry, micro-clots and endothelial damage, metabolic and gastrointestinal microbiome alterations, or autonomic nervous system dysfunction.[30–36]

TREATMENT OF PEDIATRIC POST-ACUTE SEQUELAE OF SARS-CoV-2
Current Treatment Approaches for Overall Systems

Currently, treatment of pPASC targets symptom management, rehabilitative support, and a patient/family-centered, goal-directed return to baseline physical, cognitive, academic, and social activity. pPASC management includes a healthy diet and sleep hygiene, along with environmental supports that promote healthy adjustment.

Management begins with validation of symptoms and the diagnosis, along with education about treatment options and prognosis. For most patients and families, this starts with the primary care provider, but referral to a multidisciplinary pPASC clinic may be needed in some cases. Management is then tailored to the patient's symptoms. There are a few red flag symptoms that necessitate precautions or restrictions on treatment. For example, patients with cardiac warning signs (eg., cardiac chest pain, dyspnea, or exertional desaturation) may necessitate evaluation or discussion with a cardiologist before the initiation of any physical rehabilitation program.

Lifestyle Interventions: Lifestyle interventions can be helpful for symptomatic management and to promote overall well-being. Normalizing daytime routine and optimizing sleep are important in developing a consistent schedule. Sleep should be consolidated to the evenings with limited or no napping during the day. For those with insomnia or difficulty falling asleep, sleep hygiene strategies should be discussed, including establishing a regular bedtime, maintaining a dark and quiet environment, avoiding screen time before bed, and relaxation techniques.[37] Brain fog and other cognitive symptoms should be managed with a gradual return to cognitive activity and school accommodations when indicated. Priority should be made for children to return to school and accommodations via a medical 504 plan may be needed to work up to tolerating a full school day, such as increased time for tests and homework assignments, limiting nonessential work, and scheduled rest breaks.[15]

Maintaining adequate nutrition and hydration is also important, especially for those with weight loss due to gastrointestinal symptoms and/or altered taste/smell as well as for headache prevention.[38] Olfactory training is commonplace in patients with altered smell and/or taste. This training is being studied in patients with COVID-19 post-viral olfactory dysfunction.[39,40]

For those with orthostatic intolerance, treatments such as increased salt-fluid intake, reconditioning, sleeping in an upright position, physical countermeasure maneuvers, and compression garments are additional lifestyle interventions that can help with symptom management.[41,42]

Pursed lip breathing and other breathing exercises may be recommended for respiratory symptoms and may help augment the aerobic exercise program. By focusing on slow, deep breaths with inhalation typically through the nose and exhalation through the mouth, breathing exercises can serve to strengthen respiratory muscles—particularly the diaphragm.[43]

Physical Therapies and Specific Considerations: Fatigue and exercise intolerance are commonly reported in children with PASC.[44] There are several known benefits of physical activity in overall health and well-being,[45] and recent suggestions that individualized exercise plans may help symptom management in PASC[46] with a combination of aerobic exercise and energy conservation strategies. Premorbid and current levels of physical activity should be assessed in all children with PASC, and specific goals should be determined. Some patients report a "push and crash" cycle, where they participate in an activity when they feel more able and then end up depleting their energy level to a point that leads to a period of worsened fatigue for several hours or even days.[47] In those with post-exertional malaise, pacing and energy conservation strategies should be discussed to avoid exacerbation of fatigue and other symptoms following exercise.[48] Physical activity and exercise should be slowly progressed over time based on individual tolerance. Standardized scales, such as the Borg Rating of Perceived Exertion scale, can be used to estimate the level of exertion in children.[49] In those with orthostatic intolerance, activity can be initiated in more recumbent positions with advancement to upright positions as able.[42] Physical therapy is often helpful to guide patients in exercise progression while understanding symptom limitations.[15] Modifications may be helpful to allow children to participate in preferred sports activities such as limiting time spent in practice/games, focusing on drills that require less aerobic work, incorporating more frequent rest breaks into their schedule, and allowing children frequent access to water and snacks.

Mental Health: Mood symptoms (eg, anxiety, depression, irritability) are commonly reported in children and adolescents with PASC, which has been seen in other diagnoses that are similar and may overlap with PASC (eg, myalgic encephalomyelitis/chronic fatigue syndrome, orthostatic intolerance/postural orthostatic tachycardia syndrome (OI/POTS), and concussion).[50–52] The degree to which mental health symptoms of anxiety and depression is the consequence of PASC pathogenesis itself, secondary to patients' physical symptoms, or due to the general effects of the pandemic (eg, social isolation, loss of loved ones, disruption to routine) is still unknown.[53] Although multiple, if not all, of these effects likely contribute to mood symptoms, a recent study in adults demonstrated that patients with PASC had worse mood and cognitive functioning after SARS-CoV-2 infection, even when compared with controls that had similar pandemic experiences.[54]

Given the potential impact physical symptoms may have on daily functioning and emotional well-being, it is important to screen and address any mood symptoms in children with PASC with an assessment of functioning across a variety of domains. This clinical interview may include questions regarding adjustment to medical changes, health-related behaviors (eg, sleep, appetite, hydration, physical activity), physical symptom management, premorbid mental health concerns, behavioral concerns, and school concerns. A biopsychosocial framework[55] for assessment and intervention, which recognizes the multiple biological, psychological, and social aspects that contribute to the experience of illness, has been used in pPASC clinics[15] and can be beneficial for patients. As the symptoms of PASC can significantly impact the quality of life and daily activities of children and adolescents, many children benefit from psychotherapy. Identifying a provider who has experience working with individuals with chronic illnesses, such as chronic pain, is advantageous.[15,56]

Case Example: This case is a compilation of multiple patients with PASC designed to represent the most common symptoms and treatments. The patient is a 15-year-old boy who was diagnosed with COVID-19 in December 2021. Previously, the patient had an unremarkable medical history with only a diagnosis of mild intermittent asthma as a younger child. His family reported that he was a competitive athlete, participating in basketball and track practices five to six times a week, and had a robust social life. He earned above-average grades and did not require school accommodations. He self-reported some anxiety about the pressure of school and sports performance before his COVID-19 infection, but it did not reach a clinical level, and he described himself as well-adjusted and passionate about school, his future career, and his athletic activities.

The patient's initial COVID-19 diagnosis was characterized by mild fatigue, sore throat, congestion, and fever (T_{max} 101°F) for one day. He was not hospitalized and did not seek SARS-CoV-2-specific treatment. His acute symptoms resolved within 5 days, but fatigue remained. However, approximately 2 weeks after his initial COVID-19 diagnosis, his fatigue noticeably worsened and started to experience new daily headaches, orthostatic dizziness, nausea, and palpitations.

The patient presented to his PASC clinic approximately 6 months after his COVID-19 diagnosis. At the time of his appointment, he reported ongoing fatigue and headaches that were interfering with full-time school attendance and participation in extracurricular activities. He reported sleeping 10 to 11 hours every night and napping for 1 to 2 hours after school most days of the week and still feeling tired. He was unable to eat more than one meal per day plus snacks due to nausea as well as an ongoing abnormal sense of taste, indicating "everything tastes rotten." He frequently felt as though he was going to "pass out" when making transitions and noticed that his heart races at random times throughout the day. On physical examination, he was pale and tired appearing but otherwise in no acute distress. He had a moderate increase in heart rate when standing (118 bpm from 70 bpm while sitting) during orthostatic vital signs, and the remainder of his examination (cardiac, respiratory, musculoskeletal, skin, abdominal, and neurologic) was unremarkable. On a 6-minute walk test, he ambulated 430 m. For a healthy 15-year-old boy, the average ambulation is 697 ± 74 meters.[57] During psychological consultation, he reported that he was also experiencing significant cognitive dysfunction, noting that it was harder to remember things after he read them and to attend school when there were distractions around him. He also reported headaches that sometimes were exacerbated by reading on electronic screens. As a result, he has been doing school virtually from home for the past 3 months but was still struggling to keep up with coursework. He self-reported anxiety about his performance in school, sometimes resulting in significant difficulty falling asleep or getting started on school assignments. He also vocalized frustration with not being able to perform "at his level" in his sports and questioned if he even wanted to continue competitive sports. He was especially worried about experiencing more episodes of heart palpitations during practices and in the school setting. The patient also noted frequent anxiety and distress about when he would start to "feel back to normal." On the PROMIS Pediatric Profile-37, both the patient and his mother (via parent proxy) reported clinically elevated fatigue and anxiety scores (scores >1 standard deviation [SD] above the mean) and a clinically low physical functioning/mobility score (>1 SD below the mean).

Case Example Management: Initial recommendations for the patient included increasing fluid intake to a minimum of 80oz of non-caffeinated fluid per day, daily magnesium supplementation (400 mg per day), coenzyme q10 supplementation (initially 100 mg twice daily), as well as twice daily olfactory retraining using four scent groups for a minimum of 12 weeks. He also had not previously been vaccinated against COVID-19, so it was recommended that he receive two doses of mRNA vaccine and a booster to minimize the risk of additional SARS-CoV-2 infection and potential symptom exacerbation in the future. He was also referred to a cardiology/POTS specialist for additional evaluation for POTS/dysautonomia.

The patient received an aerobic exercise prescription that started with 10 minutes of supine exercises activity per day with a titration plan of increasing the total time by 5 minutes per week, and adding walking and aquatic exercises, to a goal of 60 minutes per day, as tolerated without symptom exacerbation the following day. Energy conservation strategies including pacing during routine activities and daily schedule prioritization were discussed.

Providers also identified school accommodations that would permit the patient to return to in-person school while also reducing expectations. He had scheduled rest periods in school, reduced classwork and homework assignments as well as extended deadlines, and was able to work in a quiet/low-light room when needed for examinations. When possible, he was given the option to have printed materials rather than need to use electronic devices to complete assignments. He practiced relaxation and grounding techniques and identified times to practice and use them at home with a psychologist. The psychologist facilitated a discussion about his priorities and helped identify small steps he could take to start engaging in more of the activities that were important to him. Given his clinically elevated anxiety score, a referral for a community therapist was also provided.

Multidisciplinary Care Approach

Given the complex and wide-ranging nature of PASC symptoms and the impact on functioning, a multidisciplinary care team (MDT) approach to evaluation and management of PASC is preferred.[58,59] The MDT model, which has been most widely used and studied in the setting of cancer care, incorporates multiple stakeholders.[60] Beyond anecdotes and logic that support the benefits of streamlined, centralized communication and plan development that is achieved by an MDT, there is some evidence in the literature that supports improved outcomes and patient experiences with complex or rare diagnoses under the care of MDTs.[61–63] However, specialized multidisciplinary clinics for pPASC are not always available to patients; currently, there are fewer than 15 pediatric post-COVID clinics in the United States.[64] It is important to not only expand access to multidisciplinary care clinics for pPASC but also to provide guidance on the multifaceted treatment approaches that can be used by individual providers.

DISCUSSION AND LIMITATIONS

It is important to note that most studies so far have had significant limitations, and it has been difficult to determine the prevalence of different pPASC symptoms, resulting in a wide range of data reported.[4,12] Many studies have no control groups, low response rates, inconsistent follow-up times, and ill-defined inclusion criteria.[4,12] Large-scale studies, which tend to rely on online surveys, have low response rates and select for patients from higher socioeconomic backgrounds, as they have better access to online technology.[4,12,65] Of note, many of these larger studies omit a portion of patients—some protocols exclude patients when they recover from COVID-19, which can be problematic, as there are numerous cases of pPASC where children recover only to relapse with symptoms in the future.[2] This could lead to an underreporting of prevalence. Conversely, it has been observed that in smaller cohort studies, there may be an overreporting of prevalence, as patients who are referred to or seek out pPASC clinics tend to present with more severe symptoms.[14] Different methods of gathering symptoms can also lead to variation; studies that provide patients with a predetermined list of symptoms to choose from are more likely to have a higher percentage of reported symptoms than, for example, those who have patients self-describe their clinical manifestations.[2,14] More studies need to be done to ascertain a more precise prevalence of pPASC symptoms.

There can be variability in the severity, time course, and individual symptoms that children experience with PASC, making the diagnosis and treatment challenging and possibly underreported in pediatric populations. pPASC symptoms are often missed due to numerous reasons. The symptoms are often nonspecific and encompass a broad differential, leading to misdiagnosis. Sometimes, PASC is not suspected if the patient showed complete recovery from acute illness, therefore leading to overlooking relapsed PASC symptoms. Identifying symptoms in children can be challenging in comparison to adults as well. Children are often not able to articulate or advocate for themselves due to developmental limitations, making it more challenging to interpret their symptoms.[66]

However, studies have found that children are distressed by these symptoms and that PASC can negatively impact children's quality of life and functioning.[15,67] Academic or school performance has been shown to decline in children with PASC.[68] Therefore, it is important to remain vigilant and appropriately screen children for symptoms of PASC after SARS-COV-2 infection. Primary care clinicians should obtain a history of SARS-CoV-2 infection and screen for symptoms of PASC. Although many children will be able to be managed in a primary care setting, those with more severe or refractory disease may benefit from coordinated, multidisciplinary subspecialty care to address multisystem organ involvement and to provide comprehensive functional rehabilitation.

CLINICS CARE POINTS

- Post-acute sequelae of SARS-CoV-2 (PASC) can occur in children with mild/asymptomatic acute symptoms; primary care physicians should screen for PASC symptoms in children with a history of SARS-CoV-2 infection.

- PASC is a complex multisystemic disease that affects the physical, mental, and social well-being of patients' lives; a multifaceted treatment approach is important in improving the quality of life of patients.

- Lifestyle interventions are key methods for managing pPASC, as there is not yet known curative treatment. Providers should prioritize helping patients develop daily routines and advocate for school accommodations. Other symptom-specific interventions, such as establishing good nutrition habits, olfactory training, orthostatic intolerance interventions, and breathing exercises may be beneficial.

- Physical rehabilitation and therapy are essential in improving the overall health and well-being of PASC patients. Treatment plans based on individualized tolerance are critical to avoid "push and crash," where patients experience prolonged worsened fatigue or other symptoms after activity.
- Mood symptoms and physical symptoms in tandem impact the experience of illness in PASC patients—screening for mood symptoms in all PASC patients is important in developing tailored treatment approaches to improve patients' quality of life.

DISCLOSURE

Authors have no conflict of interest to declare. This research received no specific grant from any funding agency.

ACKNOWLEDGMENTS

The authors would like to thank Linda Herbert, PhD, and their multidisciplinary clinical staff teams.

REFERENCES

1. American Academy of Pediatrics. Children and COVID-19: State-level data report. American Academy of Pediatrics Web site. Available at: https://www.aap.org/en/pages/2019-novel-coronavirus-covid-19-infections/children-and-covid-19-state-level-data-report/. Updated 2022. Accessed September 5, 2022.
2. Molteni E, Sudre CH, Canas LS, et al. Illness duration and symptom profile in symptomatic UK school-aged children tested for SARS-CoV-2. Lancet Child Adolesc Health 2021;5(10):708.
3. Blatz AM, Randolph AG. Severe COVID-19 and multisystem inflammatory syndrome in children in children and adolescents. Crit Care Clin 2022;38(3):571–86.
4. Zimmermann P, Pittet LF, Curtis N. How common is long COVID in children and adolescents? Pediatr Infect Dis J 2021;40(12):e482.
5. Miller AD, Yousaf AR, Bornstein E, et al. Multisystem inflammatory syndrome in children (MIS-C) during SARS-CoV-2 delta and omicron variant circulation—United States, July 2021–January 2022. Clin Infect Dis 2022. https://doi.org/10.1093/cid/ciac471.
6. Centers for Disease Control and Prevention. Health department-reported cases of multisystem inflammatory syndrome in children (MIS-C) in the United States. Available at: https://covid.cdc.gov/covid-data-tracker Web site. https://covid.cdc.gov/covid-data-tracker/#mis-national-surveillance. Updated 2022. Accessed September 5, 2022.
7. Morrow AK, Malone LA, Kokorelis C, et al. Long-term COVID 19 sequelae in adolescents: The overlap with orthostatic intolerance and ME/CFS. Curr Pediatr Rep. 2022;10(2):31-44. Available at: https://link.springer.com/article/10.1007/s40124-022-00261-4.
8. Buonsenso D, Espuny Pujol F, Munblit D, et al. Clinical characteristics, activity levels and mental health problems in children with long COVID: A survey of 510 children. Future Microbiol 2021. https://doi.org/10.20944/preprints202103.0271.v1.
9. Kikkenborg Berg S, Dam Nielsen S, Nygaard U, et al. Long COVID symptoms in SARS-CoV-2-positive adolescents and matched controls (LongCOVIDKidsDK): A national, cross-sectional study. Lancet Child Adolesc Health 2022;6(4):240-8.

10. Ludvigsson JF. Systematic review of COVID-19 in children shows milder cases and a better prognosis than adults. Acta Paediatr 2020;109(6):1088.

11. Ayoubkhani D, King S, Pawelek P. Prevalence of ongoing symptoms following coronavirus (COVID-19) infection in the UK: 7 July 2022. Office for National Statistics Web site. Available at: https://www.ons.gov.uk/peoplepopulationandcommunity/healthandsocialcare/conditionsanddiseases/bulletins/prevalenceofongoingsymptomsfollowingcoronaviruscovid19infectionintheuk/7july2022. Updated 2022. Accessed July 11, 2022.

12. Zimmermann P, Pittet LF, Curtis N. The challenge of studying long COVID: An updated review. Pediatr Infect Dis J 2022;41(5):424.

13. Esposito S, Principi N, Azzari C, et al. Italian intersociety consensus on management of long covid in children. Ital J Pediatr 2022;48(1):42. https://www.ncbi.nlm.nih.gov/pubmed/35264214.

14. Brackel CLH, Lap CR, Buddingh EP, et al. Pediatric long-COVID: An overlooked phenomenon? Pediatr Pulmonol 2021;56(8):2495–502. https://www.narcis.nl/publication/RecordID/oai:pure.amc.nl:publications%2F71b18f95-d2f1-4243-af61-b0e309053b73.

15. Morrow AK, Ng R, Vargas G, et al. Postacute/long COVID in pediatrics: Development of a multidisciplinary rehabilitation clinic and preliminary case series. American journal of physical medicine & rehabilitation. 2021;100(12):1140-1147. Available at: https://www.ncbi.nlm.nih.gov/pubmed/34793374.

16. Bloise S, Isoldi S, Marcellino A, et al. Clinical picture and long-term symptoms of SARS-CoV-2 infection in an Italian pediatric population. Italian Journal of Pediatrics. 2022;48(1):79. Available at: https://www.ncbi.nlm.nih.gov/pubmed/35598023.

17. Ashkenazi-Hoffnung L, Shmueli E, Ehrlich S, et al. Long COVID in children. Pediatr Infect Dis J 2021;40(12):e509.

18. Fainardi V, Meoli A, Chiopris G, et al. Long COVID in children and adolescents. Life (Basel, Switzerland). 2022;12(2):285. Available at: https://www.ncbi.nlm.nih.gov/pubmed/35207572.

19. CDC. Information for healthcare providers about multisystem inflammatory syndrome in children (MIS-C). Available at: https://www.cdc.gov/mis/mis-c/hcp/index.html?CDC_AA_refVal=https%3A%2F%2Fwww.cdc.gov%2Fmis%2Fhcp%2Findex.html Web site. . Updated 2021. Accessed July 25, 2022.

20. Feldstein LR, Tenforde MW, Friedman KG, et al. Characteristics and outcomes of US children and adolescents with multisystem inflammatory syndrome in children (MIS-C) compared with severe acute COVID-19. JAMA 2021;325(11):1074–87.

21. Mamishi S, Pourakbari B, Mehdizadeh M, et al. Children with SARS-CoV-2 infection during the novel coronaviral disease (COVID-19) outbreak in Iran: An alarming concern for severity and mortality of the disease. BMC Infect Dis 2022;22(1). https://doi.org/10.1186/s12879-022-07200-0.

22. Ghosh P, Katkar GD, Shimizu C, et al. An artificial intelligence-guided signature reveals the shared host immune response in MIS-C and Kawasaki disease. Nat Commun 2022;13(1). https://doi.org/10.1038/s41467-022-30357-w.

23. Dufort EM, Koumans EH, Chow EJ, et al. Multisystem inflammatory syndrome in children in New York State. New England Journal of Medicine. 2020;383(4):347-358. Available at: https://nejm.org/doi/full/10.1056/NEJMoa2021756.

24. Payne AB, Gilani Z, Godfred-Cato S, et al. Incidence of multisystem inflammatory syndrome in children among US persons infected with SARS-CoV-2. JAMA Netw Open 2021;4(6). e2116420.

25. Rivas Magali Noval, Rivas Magali Noval, Porritt Rebecca A, et al. Multisystem inflammatory syndrome in children and long COVID: The SARS-CoV-2 viral superantigen hypothesis. Front Immunol 2022;13. https://doi.org/10.3389/fimmu.2022. 941009. https://doaj.org/article/9d2a1635c46e42da826cee9dd68e7261.

26. Lorenza Romani, Federica Del Chierico, Gabriele Macari, et al. The relationship between pediatric gut microbiota and SARS-CoV-2 infection. Front Cell Infect Microbiol. 2022;12. Available at: https://doaj.org/article/459dbe94de494285a6cb4a18d6b52cdf. doi: 10.3389/fcimb.2022.908492.

27. Penner J, Abdel-Mannan O, Grant K, et al. 6-month multidisciplinary follow-up and outcomes of patients with paediatric inflammatory multisystem syndrome (PIMS-TS) at a UK tertiary paediatric hospital: A retrospective cohort study. Lancet Child Adolesc Health 2021;5:473.

28. Castanares-Zapatero D, Chalon P, Kohn L, et al. Pathophysiology and mechanism of long COVID: A comprehensive review. Annals of medicine (Helsinki). 2022;54(1):1473-1487. Available at: https://www.tandfonline.com/doi/abs/10. 1080/07853890.2022.2076901.

29. Kenny G, McCann K, O'Brien C, et al. Identification of distinct long COVID clinical phenotypes through cluster analysis of self-reported symptoms. Open Forum Infect Dis 2022;9(4):ofac060.

30. Peluso MJ, Deeks SG. Early clues regarding the pathogenesis of long-COVID. Trends Immunol 2022;43(4):268–70.

31. Chertow D, Stein S, Ramelli S, et al. SARS-CoV-2 infection and persistence throughout the human body and brain. Nature 2022;612(7941):758–63.

32. Goh D, Lim JCT, Fernández SB, et al. Persistence of residual SARS-CoV-2 viral antigen and RNA in tissues of patients with long COVID-19. Front Immunol 2022;13:939989.

33. Pretorius E, Vlok M, Venter C, et al. Persistent clotting protein pathology in long COVID/post-acute sequelae of COVID-19 (PASC) is accompanied by increased levels of antiplasmin. Cardiovascular Diabetology. 2021;20(1):1-172. Available at: https://search.proquest.com/docview/2574487375.

34. Liu Q, Mak JWY, Su Q, et al. Gut microbiota dynamics in a prospective cohort of patients with post-acute COVID-19 syndrome. Gut 2022;71(3):544.

35. Barizien N, Le Guen M, Russel S, et al. Clinical characterization of dysautonomia in long COVID-19 patients. Scientific reports. 2021;11(1):14042. Available at: https://search.proquest.com/docview/2549013995.

36. Nashed L, Mani J, Hazrati S, et al. Gut microbiota changes are detected in asymptomatic very young children with SARS-CoV-2 infection. Gut. 2022:gutjnl-326599. Available at: http://gut.bmj.com/content/early/2022/02/14/gutjnl-2021-326599.abstract. doi: 10.1136/gutjnl-2021-326599.

37. Chung K, Lee C, Yeung W, et al. Sleep hygiene education as a treatment of insomnia: A systematic review and meta-analysis. Family practice. 2018;35(4):365-375. Available at: https://www.ncbi.nlm.nih.gov/pubmed/29194467.

38. Gelfand A. Pediatric and adolescent headache. Continuum (Minneapolis, Minn.). 2018;24(4, Headache):1108-1136. Available at: http://ovidsp.ovid.com/ovidweb. cgi?T=JS&NEWS=n&CSC=Y&PAGE=fulltext&D=ovft&AN=00132979-201808000-00011.

39. Jafar A, Lasso A, Shorr R, et al. Olfactory recovery following infection with COVID-19: A systematic review. PloS one. 2021;16(11):e0259321. Available at: https://search.proquest.com/docview/2595526266.

40. Kattar N, Do TM, Unis GD, et al. Olfactory training for postviral olfactory dysfunction: Systematic review and meta-analysis. Otolaryngol Head Neck Surg 2021;164(2): 244–54. https://journals.sagepub.com/doi/full/10.1177/0194599820943550.

41. Stewart JM, Boris JR, Chelimsky G, et al. Pediatric disorders of orthostatic intolerance. Pediatrics 2018;141(1):e20171673.

42. Fu Q, Levine BD. Exercise and non-pharmacological treatment of POTS. Auton Neurosci 2018;215:20–7.

43. Yong SJ. Long COVID or post-COVID-19 syndrome: Putative pathophysiology, risk factors, and treatments. Infectious diseases (London, England). 2021;53(10):737-754. Available at: https://www.tandfonline.com/doi/abs/10. 1080/23744235.2021.1924397.

44. Lopez-Leon S, Wegman-Ostrosky T, Ayuzo del Valle, Norma Cipatli, et al. Long-COVID in children and adolescents: A systematic review and meta-analyses. Scientific reports. 2022;12(1):9950. Available at: https://search.proquest.com/docview/2679973518.

45. Warburton DER, Bredin SSD. Health benefits of physical activity: A systematic review of current systematic reviews. Curr Opin Cardiol 2017;32(5):541–56.

46. Jimeno-Almazán A, Pallarés JG, Buendía-Romero Á, et al. Post-COVID-19 syndrome and the potential benefits of exercise. Int J Environ Res Public Health 2021;18(10):5329.

47. Herrera JE, Niehaus WN, Whiteson J, et al. Multidisciplinary collaborative consensus guidance statement on the assessment and treatment of fatigue in postacute sequelae of SARS-CoV-2 infection (PASC) patients. PM & R. 2021;13(9):1027-1043. Available at: https://onlinelibrary.wiley.com/doi/abs/10. 1002/pmrj.12684.

48. Rowe PC, Underhill RA, Friedman KJ, et al. Myalgic encephalomyelitis/chronic fatigue syndrome diagnosis and management in young people: A primer. Frontiers in pediatrics. 2017;5:121. Available at: https://www.ncbi.nlm.nih.gov/pubmed/28674681.

49. Pianosi PT, Huebner M, Zhang Z, et al. Dalhousie dyspnea and perceived exertion scales: Psychophysical properties in children and adolescents. Respiratory physiology & neurobiology. 2014;199:34-40. Available at: https://www.clinicalkey.es/playcontent/1-s2.0-S1569904814001013.

50. Bould H, Lewis G, Emond A, et al. Depression and anxiety in children with CFS/ME: Cause or effect? Arch Dis Child 2011;96(3):211–4.

51. Anderson JW, Lambert EA, Sari CI, et al. Cognitive function, health-related quality of life, and symptoms of depression and anxiety sensitivity are impaired in patients with the postural orthostatic tachycardia syndrome (POTS). Front Physiol. 2014;5:230. Available at: https://www.ncbi.nlm.nih.gov/pubmed/25009504.

52. Yrondi A, Brauge D, LeMen J, et al. Depression and sports-related concussion: A systematic review. Presse Med 2017;46(10):890–902.

53. Uzunova G, Pallanti S, Hollander E. Presentation and management of anxiety in individuals with acute symptomatic or asymptomatic COVID-19 infection, and in the post-COVID-19 recovery phase. Int J Psychiatry Clin Pract 2021;25(2): 115–31.

54. Lamontagne SJ, Winters MF, Pizzagalli DA, et al. Post-acute sequelae of COVID-19: Evidence of mood & cognitive impairment. Brain Behav Immun Health 2021; 17:100347.

55. Engel GL. The clinical application of the biopsychosocial model. Am J Psychiatry 1980;137(5):535–44.

56. Fisher E, Heathcote L, Palermo TM, et al. Systematic review and meta-analysis of psychological therapies for children with chronic pain. Journal of pediatric psychology. 2014;39(8):763-782. Available at: https://www.ncbi.nlm.nih.gov/pubmed/24602890.

57. Geiger R, Strasak A, Treml B, et al. Six-minute walk test in children and adolescents. J Pediatr 2007;150(4):395–9.

58. Parkin A, Davison J, Tarrant R, et al. A multidisciplinary NHS COVID-19 service to manage post-COVID-19 syndrome in the community. J Prim Care Community Health 2021;12. 21501327211010994.

59. Nurek M, Rayner C, Freyer A, et al. Recommendations for the recognition, diagnosis, and management of long COVID: A Delphi study. Br J Gen Pract 2021; 71(712):e815.

60. Selby P, Popescu R, Lawler M, et al. The value and future developments of multidisciplinary team cancer care. Am Soc Clin Oncol Educ Book 2019;39:332–40.

61. Lamb BW, Brown KF, Nagpal K, et al. Quality of care management decisions by multidisciplinary cancer teams: A systematic review. Ann Surg Oncol 2011;18(8): 2116–25. https://link.springer.com/article/10.1245/s10434-011-1675-6.

62. Kesson EM, Allardice GM, George WD, et al. Effects of multidisciplinary team working on breast cancer survival: Retrospective, comparative, interventional cohort study of 13 722 women. BMJ 2012;344(apr26 1):e2718.

63. Taplin SH, Weaver S, Salas E, et al. Reviewing cancer care team effectiveness. Journal of oncology practice. 2015;11(3):239-246. Available at: https://www.ncbi.nlm.nih.gov/pubmed/25873056.

64. Long Covid Families. Pediatric covid clinics. Available at: www.longcovidfamilies.org Web site. https://longcovidfamilies.org/healthcare/pediatric-covid-clinics/. Accessed September 5, 2022.

65. Stephenson T, Stephenson T, Pereira SP, et al. Long COVID - the physical and mental health of children and non-hospitalised young people 3 months after SARS-CoV-2 infection; a national matched cohort study (the CLoCk) study. Lancet Child Adolesc Health 2022;6(4):230–9.

66. Srinath S, Jacob P, Sharma E, et al. Clinical practice guidelines for assessment of children and adolescents. Indian J Psychiatry 2019;61(Suppl 2):158–75.

67. Buonsenso D, Munblit D, De Rose C, et al. Preliminary evidence on long COVID in children. Acta Paediatr 2021;110(7):2208.

68. Ng R, Vargas G, Jashar DT, et al. Neurocognitive and psychosocial characteristics of pediatric patients with post-acute/long-COVID: A retrospective clinical case series. Arch Clin Neuropsychol 2022. https://doi.org/10.1093/arclin/acac056.

Addressing Rehabilitation Health Care Disparities During the Coronavirus Disease-2019 Pandemic and Beyond

Nicole B. Katz, MD[a,b,*], Tracey L. Hunter, MD[a,b],
Laura E. Flores, PhD[c], Julie K. Silver, MD[a,b]

KEYWORDS

- Rehabilitation • Disability • Disparities • Race • Ethnicity • Women • COVID-19
- Long COVID

KEY POINTS

- There are disproportionately higher rates of infection, severe illness, and hospitalization from acute coronavirus disease-2019 (COVID-19) infection in people who identify with racial/ethnic minority groups as compared with White/Caucasian individuals, which likely attributes to inequitable post-acute sequelae severe acute respiratory syndrome coronavirus 2 and rehabilitation needs.
- Individuals with disabilities have been adversely impacted by the COVID-19 pandemic and require specialized rehabilitation treatment plans.
- Telemedicine should be further explored as a modality to increase accessibility of health care to historically and socially marginalized and underrepresented populations (eg, individuals with disabilities, people who identify with race/ethnic minority groups, and pediatric, elderly, pregnant people).

INTRODUCTION

The coronavirus disease-2019 (COVID-19) global pandemic exposed and increased countless health disparities among historically marginalized and underrepresented populations in the United States and worldwide. These health and social disparities include higher rates of infection, severe illness, hospitalization, and death from acute

[a] Department of Physical Medicine and Rehabilitation, Harvard Medical School, Boston, MA, USA; [b] Spaulding Rehabilitation Hospital, 300 First Avenue, Charlestown, MA 02129, USA; [c] College of Allied Health Professions, University of Nebraska Medical Center, 42nd & Emile Street, Omaha, NE 68198, USA
* Corresponding author. Department of Physical Medicine and Rehabilitation, Harvard Medical School, Boston, MA; Spaulding Rehabilitation Hospital, 300 First Avenue, Charlestown, MA 02129, USA
E-mail address: NKatz@mgh.harvard.edu
Twitter: @NicoleBKatzMD (N.B.K.); @TraceyHunterMD (T.L.H.); @LauraFlowersE (L.E.F.); @JulieSilverMD (J.K.S.)

Phys Med Rehabil Clin N Am 34 (2023) 657–675
https://doi.org/10.1016/j.pmr.2023.03.005

infection in Pacific Islander, American Indian and Alaska Native, Latino/Hispanic, and Black/African American individuals, compared with White/Caucasian and non-Latino/Hispanic individuals.[1–10] These inequities exist in access to testing and treatment of COVID-19 as well.[11,12] The aforementioned disparities of outcomes among marginalized populations are multifactorial with significant contribution likely from historical health inequities, including lower rates of vaccine uptake and lower rates of vaccine clinical trial participation.[13] Among children, trends mirror that of adults, with children belonging to marginalized populations experiencing disproportionately higher rates of hospitalization and serious illness compared with their White/Caucasian counterparts.[14]

Another marginalized population impacted includes individuals with disabilities (IWD). In this population, including both intellectual, developmental, and physical disabilities, COVID-19 has demonstrated disparate harm,[15] resulting in higher fatality rates,[16] particularly among those living in residential settings, and suggesting that impaired cognitive and physical function may be independently associated with COVID-19 mortality.[17] Evidence supports that comorbid conditions more prevalent in individuals with intellectual disability, together with ableism, may play a role in this inequity.[18]

In addition to overt health care disparities, COVID-19 has had far-reaching consequences in terms of furthering gender inequities through significant job losses more heavily impacting women. These losses have pushed more women worldwide into extreme poverty.[19] This trend may extend to IWD, as they are already at an increased risk for low socioeconomic status (SES) compared with those without disabilities.[20] This is significant as low income individuals have an increased risk for severe illness and intensive care unit admission for COVID-19 infection.[3]

Documented disparities in rehabilitation care for specific populations have only been heightened due to COVID-19 and its unique impact on each of these populations. Thus, this review focuses on the effect that the pandemic has had and likely will continue to have on the rehabilitation care for IWD as well as those who have developed symptoms of post-acute sequelae (PASC) of SARS-CoV-2, which is also known as long COVID.

DISCUSSION

The pandemic has had incalculable effects on individuals from many marginalized and underrepresented groups. Before the pandemic, there were documented disparities in rehabilitation care for women,[21,22] children,[23] people who identify with racial/ethnic minority groups,[24–26] and IWD.[27] Rehabilitation care is not well studied in people who identify with sexual orientation or gender minority groups; nevertheless, it is reasonable to assume that they may face similar types of disparities in access to care that other marginalized groups face. For IWD or those with low SES, access to care may be affected by a host of factors related to social determinants of health such as lack of transportation to medical appointments or being uninsured/underinsured.

Importantly, the pandemic occurred at the same time as a number of other major issues affecting people living in the United States. These included, but were not limited to, the opioid crisis, historic and current racial justice concerns, and a rise in mental health symptoms and diagnoses. During the pandemic many people left their jobs (which became known as The Great Resignation) or reduced their hours, and these changes in the workforce exacerbated existing shortages of clinical personnel (eg, physicians, nurses, mental health professionals, rehabilitation therapists) as well as medical staff workers. Together these issues created a *syndemic*–which is generally defined as a set of linked problems that negatively affect the health of various populations.

The next sections will describe how the pandemic has affected access to medical and rehabilitation care for IWD, the diagnosis of PASC and rehabilitation issues as they relate to disparities for marginalized and underrepresented groups of people, as well as future directions for rehabilitation care.

Access to Medical Care for People with Preexisting Disabilities During the Pandemic

In the United States there are approximately 61 million adults living with a disability.[28,29] When considering the various marginalized groups impacted by disparities during the COVID-19 pandemic, IWD are expected to be among those most adversely impacted. Populations with preexisting disabilities, including those with intellectual challenges and debilitating comorbid conditions are likely to be at a disproportionately higher risk for experiencing poorer medical outcomes and quality of life than the general population.[18,21,28,29] Profiles of IWD have a greater likelihood to include advanced age, low SES, obesity, diabetes, and cardiovascular disease, and therefore require regular health care management.[30] This marginalized community may have been disproportionately subjected to inadequate conditions and health care access during the pandemic, which resulted in baseline health decline secondary to factors such as weight gain, lack of exercise, poor glucose control, increased mental health symptoms, and limited access to routine care and elective surgeries.[28,29,31–33] The impact on overall health may heighten long-term health issues and PASC symptoms.

IWD, including but not limited to people with spinal cord injury and stroke, are known to be at greater risk for contracting severe acute infections and diseases, including COVID-19.[34] Despite this, during the pandemic, IWD had lower rates of COVID-19 vaccination than populations without disabilities, even though IWD had reportedly less vaccination hesitancy.[35] One reason for this is likely that IWD experienced greater difficulty accessing vaccines secondary to accessibility of scheduling and vaccination sites.[35] Beyond equitable access to preventative care, these populations require specialized management and treatment of acute infection and PASC-related symptoms.

The insufficient understanding of disparaging health outcomes for IWD in circumstances such as the pandemic is largely rooted in a paucity of data, consistent findings, and clinical guidelines that are needed to adequately guide medical care.[34,36] Much remains unknown due to the lack of information about IWD with rehabilitation needs. Current medical research has not fully explored the detrimental experiences that perpetuate pandemic disparities for IWD nor is there sufficient guidance to assist clinicians to effectively treat this population.[34] However, it is important to note that the American Academy of Physical Medicine and Rehabilitation (AAPM&R) has developed a consortium of interdisciplinary experts, and they have followed a modified Delphi approach with published PASC guidance statements that include key recommendations as well as information regarding health disparities (**Table 1**).

Highlighting provisions that impact health care access for IWD aids the reallocation of resources and eradication of harmful medical protocols. During the early pandemic in 2020, the Department of Health and Human Services Office of Civil Rights removed guidelines that enforced solely objective assessments of IWD without direct treatment based on their diagnosis.[29] Furthermore, some state laws excluded certain populations, such as persons with spinal muscular atrophy, from receiving ventilator support

Table 1
Healthy equity clinical recommendations and considerations included in American Academy of Physical Medicine and Rehabilitation post-acute sequelae of severe acute respiratory syndrome coronavirus 2 guidelines

Health Equity Category	Autonomic Dysfunction (Blitshteyn et al.,[54] 2022)	Breathing Discomfort (Maley et al.,[2] 2021)	Cardiovascular Symptoms (Whiteson et al.,[34] 2022)	Cognitive Symptoms (Fine et al.,[51] 2021)	Fatigue (Herrera et al.,[52] 2021)
Age		For children, clear clinical guidance should be given regarding return to sport following established protocols.	Athletes may require ECG, echocardiogram, cardiac MRI, and/or 23-h Holter ECG before return to sport.	Cognitive testing should be conducted by clinicians experienced with older individuals and all medications should be reviewed.	Patients of older age may have diminished activity tolerance preceding PASC and testing/symptoms should be interpreted in context.
Biologic sex	Clinicians should be aware of sex-related bias, which may add to diagnostic delays faced by female patients.	Pregnant people may have baseline respiratory discomfort exacerbated by COVID-19/PASC; Alternative diagnostic testing and treatment may be required.	Clinicians should be aware that females may be underdiagnosed and undertreated for cardiac conditions (including referrals to cardiac rehabilitation) and should work to ensure equitable care.	Pregnant/postpartum people may experience cognitive dysfunction difficult to differentiate from PASC; Alternative diagnostic testing and treatment may be needed.	Pregnant people may experience pregnancy-related fatigue and require alternative diagnostic testing and treatment to differentiate from PASC.

Disability	Autonomic dysfunction may be present at baseline for IWD, and determining PASC-related autonomic dysfunction may require testing modifications.	Patients with cervical spinal cord injuries should be given priority for diagnostic/treatment intervention for sleep-related breathing disorders and pneumonia.	Cardiac assessments may need to be modified to accommodate certain disabilities and interpretation of modified tests should be done in context.	PASC cognitive symptoms may increase difficulty with primary disability and recommendations should be individualized to specific impairments.	An understanding of the Americans with Disabilities Care Act should be used to advocate for patients.
Environmental Exposure		Patients may be limited in seeking care by community exposure from mass transportation/ride sharing.		Patients' natural and psychosocial environmental-related stressors may impact PASC cognitive recovery and interventions should be enacted when possible.	
Gender				Women may report PASC cognitive dysfunction more than men.	Gender affirming care should be considered regarding impact on fatigue (eg.; exogenous hormone use, sleep, mental health).
Immigration				Treatments should be customized to accommodate language and cultural preferences.	Efforts should be made to communicate in patients' native language and to provide assistive resources.

(continued on next page)

Table 1
(continued)

Health Equity Category	Autonomic Dysfunction (Blitshteyn et al.,[54] 2022)	Breathing Discomfort (Maley et al.,[2] 2021)	Cardiovascular Symptoms (Whiteson et al.,[34] 2022)	Cognitive Symptoms (Fine et al.,[51] 2021)	Fatigue (Herrera et al.,[52] 2021)
Insurance	Patients may require referrals to autonomic specialty clinics, which may be limited by cost.	Low-cost diagnostic tests (eg.: chest X-ray) and interventions (generic brands) should be considered.	Consideration should be given to necessity/ benefit of expensive testing/treatments for patients with no insurance or high copayments/ deductibles.		Those immigrating, of low SES, and/or of racial/ethnic minority groups may have higher rates of uninsured and care and resources should be tailored.
Justice (prison/ detention centers)			Cardiovascular disease is the leading cause of death among incarcerated individuals and appropriate testing/ treatment should be made available.		Public health measures should include access to social distancing, quarantining, and telehealth.
Obesity	Patients with autonomic dysfunction and obesity may require specialized rehabilitation including tailored weight loss strategies and sleep apnea assessments.		Obesity may increase risk of PASC cardiac complications and weight loss recommendations should be made with considerations for patients' social determinants of heath.		Care should be provided with an understanding of patients' SES/ability to follow recommendations such as consuming a healthier diet.

Religion				Encouragement may be provided for patients to return to/pursue involvement in religious/spiritual practices to aid social connection and community support.	Clinical recommendations should be made, when possible, in accordance with religious preferences/ observations.
People of Racial/ethnic minority groups	Race may be a variable impacting heart rate variability and POTS should not be missed in those of racial minority groups.	People of racial/ethnic minority groups may be predisposed to working conditions that worsen respiratory health; Specialized respiratory-related rehabilitation should be considered.	Those from racial/ethnic minority groups have been under-referred to cardiac rehabilitation; All individuals with cardiac disease should be considered for cardiac rehabilitation.	Clinicians administering tests should be aware of stereotype threat and other factors that may affect test scores and clinical recommendations.	An awareness of systemic racism in medicine and an anti-racist multidisciplinary approach should be used to decrease compounded fatigue from racial/ethnic injustices.

Abbreviations: ECG, electrocardiogram; IWD, individuals with disabilities; PASC, post-acute sequelae of SARS-CoV-2; POTS, postural orthostatic tachycardia syndrome; SES, socioeconomic status.

or critical care resources.[28] Public disagreement has helped abolish discriminatory legislature and practices.[28]

Incorporating the specific personal and situational needs of IWD into public health policy could improve treatment options and health outcomes for this patient population.[34] Use of technology-based platforms (eg,: videoconferences, other computer and smartphone applications) has grown substantially during the pandemic years, but understanding the benefits for IWD remains complex.[29,37] The Americans with Disabilities Act was designed to protect IWD against discriminatory circumstances such as employment and transportation, which includes access to physical spaces.[29] Virtual platforms are technologies that have not been fully addressed in regulatory health care matters for IWD.[28,29] In-person physical exams are often essential for individuals with physical impairments (eg,: spasticity, contractures), which are commonly treated to minimize pain and optimize daily functionality.[29,38] However, using telemedicine during the pandemic often restricted adequate medical assessment of IWD, especially those without caretaker assistance or use of assistive equipment or devices that may enhance the performance of virtual exams.[29] Telehealth has the potential to provide high-quality, accessible health care for IWD and could be beneficial in assessing if patients with IWD have physical and mental health conditions that require further medical attention through in-person appointments.[29,39–41]

There is great potential for virtual health care platforms for IWD, especially during a pandemic from a highly contagious airborne virus. Benefits include minimizing infection exposures by staying home and reducing accessibility challenges, costs, and time-consuming factors of travel for in-person health care visits.[36,37,42] Data have shown that incorporating mobile health applications may be adventitious for certain groups, such as individuals participating in cardiac rehabilitation or orthopedic surgery prehabilitation.[21,32] Varnfield and colleagues[43] found that remote home-based group cardiac rehabilitation, in comparison to traditional facility-based cardiac rehabilitation, revealed greater program adherence and completion along with improvements in the 6-min walk test after a 6-week period. Other positive outcomes included improved emotional health and health-related quality of life after 6 weeks. Tele-prehabilitation may also have promising outcomes for total hip and knee arthroscopy candidates, with patients reporting high compliance and satisfaction.[32] Considering prolonged periods awaiting elective surgery can be detrimental to post-operative outcomes, remote prehabilitation programs may optimize perioperative health by prevent worsening disability.[32]

There is much unexplored territory in research around the intersectionality of race, ethnicity, and disability.[29] Many studies have revealed that people from minority groups, especially Black/African American, Latino/Hispanic American, and Native American individuals, have a higher risk of COVID-19 infection and mortality.[29,44] Similar outcomes are seen among uninsured communities, with Latino/Hispanic having the highest rate of any other racial/ethnic group in the United States.[29,45] A large multicenter study by Adepoju and colleagues[46] revealed that those from ethnic/racial minority groups, including Black/African American, Latino/Hispanic, American Indian/Alaska Native and other Pacific Islander, and Asian patients were significantly less likely than their White/Caucasian counterparts to use telehealth visits during the pandemic. Limitations of telehealth for racial/ethnic minority groups including those with disability are largely attributed to barriers of internet access and digital literacy.[29] Smart technologies can be a luxury as individuals of lower SES, including many people of racial/ethnic minority groups, often have limited, prepaid cellphone plans or no internet access at home.[29,46] When telecommunication was accessible and used by Latino/Hispanic patients, a lack of readily available instructions in Spanish or language translator services were an obstacle.[29] Language barriers also hinder access to personal online health record portals.[29] Greater research is needed to learn more about the impact of pandemic-related health outcomes and health care access for IWD who identify with racial/ethnic minority groups. Addressing systemic flaws of accessing health care involves expanding technological access and revising legislative infrastructure in public health to be more inclusive of various minority groups including IWD and those with intersectional identities (**Fig. 1**).[36]

Post-Acute Sequelae of Severe Acute Respiratory Syndrome Coronavirus 2

PASC can manifest in a multitude of debilitating intermittent or persistent symptoms. This condition has also been referred to as "long COVID," "long-haul COVID," "post-acute COVID-19," "long term effects of COVID," "post-COVID-19 conditions," and "chronic COVID."[47] The World Health Organization (WHO) defined this condition as beginning within 3 months of acute COVID-19 symptom onset and lasting for at least 2 months while being unexplained by an alternative diagnosis.[47] There is variation in the reported duration of PASC symptoms. Whereas Sudre and colleagues[48] found symptoms lasted for $\geq$ 4 weeks in 13.3%, $\geq$ 8 weeks in 4.5%, and $\geq$ 12 weeks in 2.38% patients, in a study by Davis and colleagues,[49] it took greater than 35 weeks to reach recovery for 91% of the participants. More than 100 clinical manifestations of PASC have been reported with some of the most common and detrimental to quality of life being fatigue, cognitive symptoms, respiratory symptoms, cardiovascular complications, and autonomic dysfunction.[2,34,47,50–55] Adult and pediatric patients

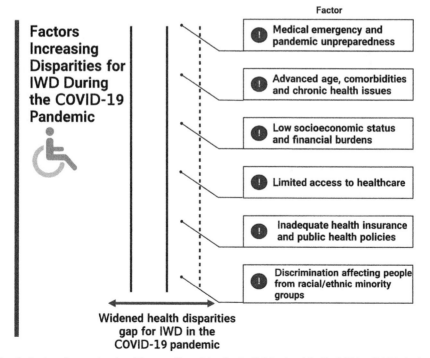

Fig. 1. Factors increasing health care disparities for individuals with disabilities (IWD) during the SARS-CoV-2 pandemic. (Figure created with BioRender.com.)

of racial/ethnic minority groups, female sex, and older ages face have well-documented health care inequities with regards to acute COVID-19 infection, which has translated to inequities in severity and duration of PASC and subsequent rehabilitation needs (**Fig. 2**).[48,53,56–61] Even within a cohort that had similar incidence of PASC symptoms, Black/African American individuals were found to use outpatient rehabilitation services significantly less than White/Caucasian individuals.[62]

Fatigue may adversely impact quality of life by impeding energy, motivation, and/or concentration. This symptom, defined as intermittent or persistent mild to severe physical or mental tiredness, lack of energy, or weariness likely improves over time, but can last for months following acute COVID-19.[52,63–65] Huang and colleagues[53] found that 59% to 81% patients experienced fatigue or muscle weakness 6 months after acute infection. Although fatigue is experienced differently by all individuals, the impact on those with certain identities is disproportionate and requires specific consideration. Whereas some data illustrated that Latino/Hispanic individuals had a significantly higher incidence of PASC fatigue compared with non-Latino/Hispanic individuals,[62] alternative data found that in non-hospitalized patients, compared with non-Latino/Hispanic White/Caucasian individuals, Black/African American (OR: 0.76, 95% CI: 0.66 to 0.88, $q < 0.001$) and Latino/Hispanic individuals (OR: 0.83, 95% CI: 0.74 to 0.94, $q = 0.009$) had lower odds of PASC malaise or fatigue[10] Pregnant people already have an increased risk of feeling fatigued and are at higher risk of more severe COVID-19 infections, which raises their susceptibility to more intense PASC fatigue. Moreover, the diagnostic and treatment options are limited in this population to due to fetal health concerns.[52,66] Fatigue may also be more common in older

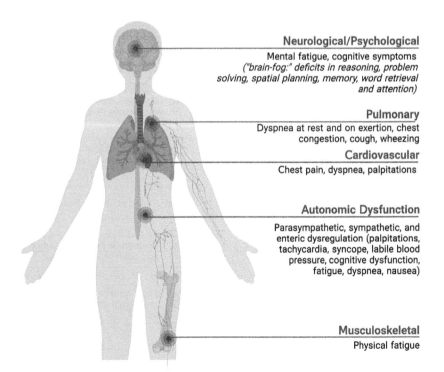

Fig. 2. Post-acute sequelae of SARS-CoV-2 (PASC) by system. Examples of post-acute sequelae of SARS-CoV-2, not intended to be an exhaustive list of all reported sequelae.

adults who similarly to pregnant individuals, may be limited in pharmacologic intervention given established comorbidities and medications.[67] Beyond anthropomorphic variables of race, sex, and age, SES is also impactful. Patients of lower SES are at greater risk for obesity, which has been associated with more severe PASC[68] and fatigue.[69] Additionally, these individuals may be limited in their ability to adhere to current treatment guidelines including healthier diet and slow, paced return to work given financial limitations.

PASC may also present with cognitive symptoms commonly referred to as "brain fog," which can largely impact quality of life. "Brain fog" may be the most frequent neurologic PASC symptom (81%)[70] and can include deficits in reasoning, problem solving, spatial planning, memory, word retrieval, and attention.[71–74] Non-hospitalized Latino/Hispanic individuals were found to have higher odds of PASC dementia diagnosis (OR: 1.75, 95% CI: 1.19 to 2.59, $q = 0.01$) compared with non-hospitalized non-Latino/Hispanic White/Caucasian individuals.[10] However, the constellation of PASC cognitive symptoms holds unique risks for individuals from racial/ethnic minority groups, such as those who identify as Black/African American, American-Indian/Alaska Native, Pacific Islander, Asian-American, and Mixed Race, and/or Latino/Hispanic in regards to the common diagnostic screening tools used (Montreal Cognitive Assessment, Mini-Mental State Exam, Saint Louis University Mental Status Examination, Mini-cog, Short Test of Mental Status).[51] Baseline and PASC-related cognitive testing may be inaccurate secondary to bias, stereotype threat (when concern for negative stereotype about one's own group impacts performance),[75] and testing not inclusive of those with variable primary languages and educational backgrounds.[76] IWD, including those with hearing and vision impairments, may also have inaccurate cognitive testing,[51] which would interfere with appropriate medical diagnosis and management. Regardless of race, ethnicity or ability, older individuals are at greater risk for preexisting cognitive conditions that compounded with PASC-related cognitive decline, may result in more significant impairment than PASC-related "brain fog" alone. In children, the most reported PASC-related neuropsychiatric symptoms between 90 and 150 days after initial positive test include headache (2.4%), cognitive symptoms (2.3%), and fatigue (1.1%) with symptoms most common in children of older age, female sex, Latino/Hispanic ethnicity, and with public insurance.[55,77]

Continued respiratory symptoms following acute COVID-19 infection have also been reported with the most common being shortness of breath at rest and with activity, exercise intolerance, cough, and chest pain as well as discomfort.[53,63,78–81] Moreover, the severity of PASC respiratory symptoms is suggested to be positively associated with the severity of acute infection, and given individuals of racial/ethnic minority groups as well as low income groups have higher rates of infection, hospitalization, and death from the acute illness, these inequities have been continued and then expanded upon with PASC.[1–5] Incidence of PASC dyspnea was significantly higher in Latino/Hispanic individuals compared with non-Latino/Hispanic individuals[62] and odds of PASC-related pulmonary embolism in non-hospitalized patients was higher for Black/African American individuals compared with non-hospitalized White/Caucasian individuals (OR: 1.68, 95% CI: 1.20 to 2.36, $q = 0.009$).[10] Hypoxemia may also be underdiagnosed, and therefore, under reported and treated in Black/African America patients given known discordance in hypoxemia measured by arterial blood gas versus pulse oximetry compared with White/Caucasian patients.[82]

Cardiac manifestations of PASC can vary drastically between and within individuals. Structures involved may include the heart, peripheral vasculature, and/or central vasculature,[83] and reported pathology include myocarditis, pericarditis, venous thrombosis, persistent dysrhythmias, heart failure and late effects of venous thrombo-embolism.[34,84] Clinically, individuals may experience shortness of breath, fatigue, chest pain, palpitation, dizziness, abdominal bloating, leg swelling, and impaired activity tolerance. Huang and colleagues[53] found that 6 months after acute infection, 5% to 9% patients reported chest pain and 9% to 11% reported palpitations. At baseline, females are undertreated and underdiagnosed for cardiac conditions,[85] which directly impacts PASC cardiac care,[34] as an unknown cardiac medical history or misdiagnosed current symptoms delays or even prevents appropriate care for PASC cardiac manifestations. Inequities exist beyond sex to include those who identify as IWD and with racial/ethnic minority groups. IWD are at a greater risk for developing cardiovascular disease such as myocardial infarction, myocarditis, and thromboembolism, with chances being amplified by a history of COVID-19.[34,36,86] Furthermore, a common modality used in the cardiac assessment is the exercise stress test, which would need to be adapted for certain IWD and could result in variable cardiopulmonary outcomes and subsequent inaccurate interpretation of results.[34] The odds of PASC-related chest pain was higher for non-hospitalized Black/African American patients compared with non-hospitalized White/Caucasian patients (OR: 1.34, 95% CI: 1.18 to 1.51, $q < 0.001$).[10] The North American COVID-19 and ST-segment Elevation Myocardial Infarction (STEMI) registry found that STEMIs in COVID-19 patients disproportionately included patients that were Latino/Hispanic or Black/African American.[87] This, in consequence with individuals in these racial/ethnic groups having lower referral rates to cardiac rehabilitation, further increases care and treatment disparities.[34]

Autonomic dysfunction is a PASC-related condition that overlaps with the aforementioned symptoms, and poses diagnostic/treatment complexities. This condition may involve systems and symptoms such as cardiovascular (palpitations, tachycardia [resting and postural], syncope, labile blood pressure, exercise intolerance, dizziness), neurologic (fatigue, cognitive dysfunction, headache, anxiety, insomnia, neuropathic pain), respiratory (dyspnea), and gastrointestinal (nausea, dysmotility). Collectively, some presentations may be due to diagnoses of neurocardiogenic syncope, orthostatic hypotension/intolerance, inappropriate sinus tachycardia, or postural orthostatic tachycardia syndrome (POTS).[54,88,89] The prevalence of autonomic dysfunction in specific marginalized and underrepresented populations is largely unexplored; however, disparities have been reported in diagnostic delays (eg, female adults may experience time to POTS diagnosis of 2 years longer compared with male counterparts, with their symptoms misattributed to psychological/psychiatric conditions).[54,90] Clinicians should be cognizant of sex-related biases regarding autonomic dysfunction, especially POTS, which is likely more prevalent in those of female sex and during childbearing years.[90] Race has also been suggested to be a confounder for heart rate variability,[91] and timely diagnosis of POTS in those from racial/ethnic minority groups should be a priority.

Future Directions

Greater research and clinical understanding of the impacts of acute COVID-19 and PASC on historically marginalized and underrepresented populations including, but not limited to IWD and those from racial/ethnic minority groups, is needed. With this increased knowledge, clinicians may provide more effective care. Assessing future research directions via the Plan-Act-Do-Check model[92] can provide organized insight around objectives and goals of addressing rehabilitation and other health care changes for IWD and promoting disability inclusivity can help reduce health care disparities and disability stigma (**Fig. 3**).[36] This work involves decreasing the existing

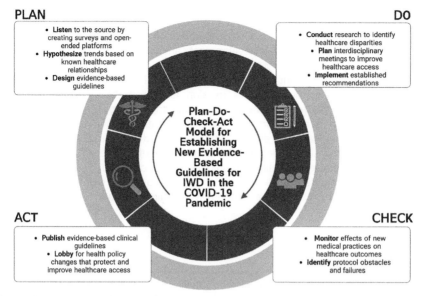

PLAN
- **Listen** to the source by creating surveys and open-ended platforms
- **Hypothesize** trends based on known healthcare relationships
- **Design** evidence-based guidelines

DO
- **Conduct** research to identify healthcare disparities
- **Plan** interdisciplinary meetings to improve healthcare access
- **Implement** established recommendations

Plan-Do-Check-Act Model for Establishing New Evidence-Based Guidelines for IWD in the COVID-19 Pandemic

ACT
- **Publish** evidence-based clinical guidelines
- **Lobby** for health policy changes that protect and improve healthcare access

CHECK
- **Monitor** effects of new medical practices on healthcare outcomes
- **Identify** protocol obstacles and failures

Fig. 3. Plan-Act-Do-Check model for increasing SARS-CoV-2 research, public policy, and clinical guidance for individuals with disabilities (IWD).

knowledge gaps by expanding data collection to include greater representation of subpopulations of disability, as most research is comprised of IWD who reside in assisted-living facilities.[93]

Interdisciplinary advocacy is also an important means to address harmful disparities and promote development of comprehensive, patient-centered health care. It is critical to reconstruct policy and provide marginalized people with administrative platforms to voice their concerns about unjust health care to help promote equitable pandemic and general emergency preparedness.[36] Beyond educating policymakers, directly educating clinicians is needed to drive public health change to benefit these populations.[29,36]

As research expands and policies advance, clinicians should be further educated about the specific needs of these populations and available resources. As mentioned previously, the AAPM&R has published multiple guidance statements that include dedicated sections on addressing health equity and specialized treatment (see **Table 1**), a precedent to be followed in future published rehabilitation clinical recommendations. To address health inequities clinically, clinical care strategies should be appropriate for the culture and community in which they are created. One of these evolving modalities, telemedicine (phone calls, virtual visits), should be incorporated into standard care to increase accessibility. Promoting telehealth decreases financial limitations to health care as well as increases accessibility for those with occupational restrictions preventing them from taking time away for medical appointments. Telemedicine has the potential to increase delivery of prehabilitation, mental health, and routine screening and follow-up appointments to underserved populations and those most at risk from the COVID-19 pandemic.[31,32,34,36,41,42,94] Progress in research and clinical guidance on caring for historically marginalized and underrepresented populations with acute infection and PASC, may reduce the long-term disease sequelae, morbidity, and mortality.

SUMMARY

The COVID-19 pandemic exposed and expanded upon preexisting health care disparities. Individuals with intellectual, development, and physical disabilities have been disproportionately adversely impacted by this pandemic with higher fatality rates. People of racial/ethnic minority groups have also had disproportionately higher rates of acute infection, hospitalization, re-admission, and death.[1–9,15,16] These inequities are likely present in the proportions of individuals impacted by PASC infection and requiring specialized rehabilitation care. Special populations including pregnant, pediatric, and older individuals may also necessitate tailored medical care. The advancement of telemedicine should be capitalized on to benefit these populations as this modality may increase accessibility and help reduce the care gap. Dedicated research and further clinical guidance are needed to provide equitable, culturally competent, and individualized care to these historically marginalized and underrepresented populations.

CLINICS CARE POINTS

- Telemedicine can be used to increase accessibility for marginalized/underrepresented populations (individuals with disabilities, individuals from racial/ethnic minority groups, pediatric, elderly, and pregnant people). Attention should be given to ensure a translator for the necessary language is available when using a virtual platform, the same as for in-person care.

- People from racial/ethnic minority groups have disproportionately high rates of acute coronavirus disease-2019 infection, hospitalization, and death; clinicians should consider their own possible biases when assessing symptoms and providing care to help rectify these inequities.

- Individualized, culturally competent and situation-dependent treatment is needed when caring for post-acute sequelae of severe acute respiratory syndrome coronavirus 2 infection.

DISCLOSURE

The authors have nothing to disclose.

REFERENCES

1. Abdallah SJ, Voduc N, Corrales-Medina VF, et al. Symptoms, Pulmonary Function, and Functional Capacity Four Months after COVID-19. Ann Am Thorac Soc 2021;18(11):1912–7.
2. Maley JH, Alba GA, Barry JT, et al. Multi-disciplinary collaborative consensus guidance statement on the assessment and treatment of breathing discomfort and respiratory sequelae in patients with post-acute sequelae of SARS-CoV-2 infection (PASC). Journal of Injury, Function, And Rehabilitation 2022;14(1): 77–95.
3. Muñoz-Price LS, Nattinger AB, Rivera F, et al. Racial Disparities in Incidence and Outcomes Among Patients With COVID-19. JAMA Netw Open 2020;3(9): e2021892.
4. Wang AZ, Ehrman R, Bucca A, et al. Can we predict which COVID-19 patients will need transfer to intensive care within 24 hours of floor admission? Acad Emerg Med 2021;28(5):511–8.

5. Konkol SB, Ramani C, Martin DN, et al. Differences in lung function between major race/ethnicity groups following hospitalization with COVID-19. Respir Med 2022;201:106939.

6. Cha L, Le T, Ve'e T, et al. Pacific Islanders in the Era of COVID-19: an Overlooked Community in Need. J Racial Ethn Health Disparities 2022;9(4):1347–56.

7. Habibdoust A, Tatar M, Wilson FA. Estimating Excess Deaths by Race/Ethnicity in the State of California During the COVID-19 Pandemic. J Racial Ethn Health Disparities 2022;1–13.

8. Siegel M, Critchfield-Jain I, Boykin M, et al. Actual Racial/Ethnic Disparities in COVID-19 Mortality for the Non-Hispanic Black Compared to Non-Hispanic White Population in 35 US States and Their Association with Structural Racism. J Racial Ethn Health Disparities 2022;9(3):886–98.

9. Musshafen LA, El-Sadek L, Lirette ST, et al. In-Hospital Mortality Disparities Among American Indian and Alaska Native, Black, and White Patients With COVID-19. JAMA Netw Open 2022;5(3):e224822.

10. Khullar D, Zhang Y, Zang C, et al. Racial/Ethnic Disparities in Post-acute Sequelae of SARS-CoV-2 Infection in New York: an EHR-Based Cohort Study from the RECOVER Program. J Gen Intern Med 2023;1–10.

11. Pond EN, Rutkow L, Blauer B, et al. Disparities in SARS-CoV-2 Testing for Hispanic/Latino Populations: An Analysis of State-Published Demographic Data. J Public Health Manag Pract 2022;28(4):330–3.

12. Thakore N, Khazanchi R, Orav EJ, et al. Association of Social Vulnerability, COVID-19 vaccine site density, and vaccination rates in the United States. Healthc (Amst) 2021;9(4):100583.

13. Williams AM, Clayton HB, Singleton JA. Racial and Ethnic Disparities in COVID-19 Vaccination Coverage: The Contribution of Socioeconomic and Demographic Factors. Am J Prev Med 2022;62(4):473–82.

14. Smitherman LC, Golden WC, Walton JR. Health Disparities and Their Effects on Children and Their Caregivers During the Coronavirus Disease 2019 Pandemic. Pediatr Clin North Am 2021;68(5):1133–45.

15. Bosworth ML, Ayoubkhani D, Nafilyan V, et al. Deaths involving COVID-19 by self-reported disability status during the first two waves of the COVID-19 pandemic in England: a retrospective, population-based cohort study. Lancet Public Health 2021;6(11):e817–25.

16. Landes SD, Turk MA, Ervin DA. COVID-19 case-fatality disparities among people with intellectual and developmental disabilities: Evidence from 12 US jurisdictions. Disabil Health J 2021;14(4):101116.

17. Panagiotou OA, Kosar CM, White EM, et al. Risk Factors Associated With All-Cause 30-Day Mortality in Nursing Home Residents With COVID-19. JAMA Intern Med 2021;181(4):439–48.

18. Chicoine C, Hickey EE, Kirschner KL, et al. Ableism at the Bedside: People with Intellectual Disabilities and COVID-19. J Am Board Fam Med 2022;35(2):390–3.

19. Su Z, Cheshmehzangi A, McDonnell D, et al. Gender inequality and health disparity amid COVID-19. Nurs Outlook 2022;70(1):89–95.

20. Banks LM, Davey C, Shakespeare T, et al. Disability-inclusive responses to COVID-19: Lessons learnt from research on social protection in low- and middle-income countries. World Dev 2021;137:105178.

21. Sawan MA, Calhoun AE, Fatade YA, et al. Cardiac rehabilitation in women, challenges and opportunities. Prog Cardiovasc Dis 2022;70:111–8.

22. Parsons JL, Coen SE, Bekker S. Anterior cruciate ligament injury: towards a gendered environmental approach. Br J Sports Med 2021;55(17):984–90.

23. Flanagan D, Gaebler D, Bart-Plange EB, et al. Addressing disparities among children with cerebral palsy: Optimizing enablement, functioning, and participation. J Pediatr Rehabil Med 2021;14(2):153–9.

24. Odonkor CA, Esparza R, Flores LE, et al. Disparities in Health Care for Black Patients in Physical Medicine and Rehabilitation in the United States: A Narrative Review. PM&R 2021;13(2):180–203.

25. Flores LE, Verduzco-Gutierrez M, Molinares D, et al. Disparities in Health Care for Hispanic Patients in Physical Medicine and Rehabilitation in the United States: A Narrative Review. Am J Phys Med Rehabil 2020;99(4):338–47.

26. Mathews L, Brewer LC. A Review of Disparities in Cardiac Rehabilitation: EVIDENCE, DRIVERS, AND SOLUTIONS. J Cardiopulm Rehabil Prev 2021;41(6):375–82.

27. Medeiros AA, Galvão MHR, Barbosa IR, et al. Use of rehabilitation services by persons with disabilities in Brazil: A multivariate analysis from Andersen's behavioral model. PLoS One 2021;16(4):e0250615.

28. McQuillen M, Terry SF. Genetic and Disability Discrimination During COVID-19. Genet Test Mol Biomarkers 2020;24(12):759–60.

29. Verduzco-Gutierrez M, Lara AM, Annaswamy TM. When Disparities and Disabilities Collide: Inequities during the COVID-19 Pandemic. Journal Of Injury, Function, And Rehabilitation 2021;13(4):412–4.

30. Annaswamy TM, Verduzco-Gutierrez M, Frieden L. Telemedicine barriers and challenges for persons with disabilities: COVID-19 and beyond. Disabil Health J 2020;13(4):100973.

31. Aragaki D, Luo J, Weiner E, et al. Cardiopulmonary Telerehabilitation. Phys Med Rehabil Clin N Am 2021;32(2):263–76.

32. Doiron-Cadrin P, Kairy D, Vendittoli PA, et al. Feasibility and preliminary effects of a tele-prehabilitation program and an in-person prehablitation program compared to usual care for total hip or knee arthroplasty candidates: a pilot randomized controlled trial. Disabil Rehabil 2020;42(7):989–98.

33. Silver JK, Santa Mina D, Bates A, et al. Physical and Psychological Health Behavior Changes During the COVID-19 Pandemic that May Inform Surgical Prehabilitation: a Narrative Review. Curr Anesthesiol Rep 2022;12(1):109–24.

34. Whiteson JH, Azola A, Barry JT, et al. Multi-disciplinary collaborative consensus guidance statement on the assessment and treatment of cardiovascular complications in patients with post-acute sequelae of SARS-CoV-2 infection (PASC). Journal Of Injury, Function, And Rehabilitation 2022;14(7):855–78.

35. Ryerson AB, Rice CE, Hung MC, et al. Disparities in COVID-19 Vaccination Status, Intent, and Perceived Access for Noninstitutionalized Adults, by Disability Status - National Immunization Survey Adult COVID Module, United States, May 30-June 26, 2021. MMWR Morbidity and mortality weekly report 2021;70(39):1365–71.

36. Jesus TS, Kamalakannan S, Bhattacharjya S, et al. PREparedness, REsponse and SySTemic transformation (PRE-RE-SyST): a model for disability-inclusive pandemic responses and systemic disparities reduction derived from a scoping review and thematic analysis. Int J Equity Health 2021;20(1):204.

37. Colbert GB, Venegas-Vera AV, Lerma EV. Utility of telemedicine in the COVID-19 era. Rev Cardiovasc Med 2020;21(4):583–7.

38. Chang E, Ghosh N, Yanni D, et al. A Review of Spasticity Treatments: Pharmacological and Interventional Approaches. Crit Rev Phys Rehabil Med 2013;25(1–2):11–22.

39. Benziger CP, Huffman MD, Sweis RN, et al. The Telehealth Ten: A Guide for a Patient-Assisted Virtual Physical Examination. Am J Med 2021;134(1):48–51.

40. Phuphanich ME, Sinha KR, Truong M, et al. Telemedicine for Musculoskeletal Rehabilitation and Orthopedic Postoperative Rehabilitation. Phys Med Rehabil Clin N Am 2021;32(2):319–53.

41. Zhou X, Snoswell CL, Harding LE, et al. The Role of Telehealth in Reducing the Mental Health Burden from COVID-19. Telemed J e Health 2020;26(4):377–9.

42. Kim EJ, Kaminecki I, Gaid EA, et al. Development of a Telemedicine Screening Program During the COVID-19 Pandemic. Telemed J e Health 2022;28(8):1199–205.

43. Varnfield M, Karunanithi M, Lee CK, et al. Smartphone-based home care model improved use of cardiac rehabilitation in postmyocardial infarction patients: results from a randomised controlled trial. Heart 2014;100(22):1770–9.

44. Odonkor CA, Sholas MG, Verduzco-Gutierrez M, et al. African American Patient Disparities in COVID-19 Outcomes: A Call to Action for Physiatrists to Provide Rehabilitation Care to Black Survivors. Am J Phys Med Rehabil 2020;99(11):986–7.

45. Lee DC, Liang H, Shi L. The convergence of racial and income disparities in health insurance coverage in the United States. Int J Equity Health 2021;20(1):96.

46. Adepoju OE, Chae M, Ojinnaka CO, et al. Utilization Gaps During the COVID-19 Pandemic: Racial and Ethnic Disparities in Telemedicine Uptake in Federally Qualified Health Center Clinics. J Gen Intern Med 2022;37(5):1191–7.

47. Center for Disease Control and Prevention. Post-COVID Conditions: Overview for Healthcare Providers. https://www.cdc.gov/coronavirus/2019-ncov/hcp/clinical-care/post-covid-conditions.html?CDC_AA_refVal=https%3A%2F%2Fwww.cdc.gov%2Fcoronavirus%2F2019-ncov%2Fhcp%2Fclinical-care%2Flate-sequelae.html. Published 2021. Accessed 14 September, 2022.

48. Sudre CH, Murray B, Varsavsky T, et al. Attributes and predictors of long COVID. Nat Med 2021;27(4):626–31.

49. Davis HE, Assaf GS, McCorkell L, et al. Characterizing long COVID in an international cohort: 7 months of symptoms and their impact. EClinicalMedicine 2021;38:101019.

50. Hayes LD, Ingram J, Sculthorpe NF. More Than 100 Persistent Symptoms of SARS-CoV-2 (Long COVID): A Scoping Review. Front Med 2021;8:750378.

51. Fine JS, Ambrose AF, Didehbani N, et al. Multi-disciplinary collaborative consensus guidance statement on the assessment and treatment of cognitive symptoms in patients with post-acute sequelae of SARS-CoV-2 infection (PASC). PM&R 2022;14(1):96–111.

52. Herrera JE, Niehaus WN, Whiteson J, et al. Multidisciplinary collaborative consensus guidance statement on the assessment and treatment of fatigue in postacute sequelae of SARS-CoV-2 infection (PASC) patients. PM&R 2021;13(9):1027–43.

53. Huang C, Huang L, Wang Y, et al. 6-month consequences of COVID-19 in patients discharged from hospital: a cohort study. Lancet 2021;397(10270):220–32.

54. Blitshteyn S, Whiteson J, Abramoff B, et al. Multi-Disciplinary Collaborative Consensus Guidance Statement on the Assessment and Treatment of Autonomic Dysfunction in Patients with Post-Acute Sequelae of SARS-CoV-2 Infection (PASC). PM&R 2022;14(10):1270–91.

55. Malone LA, Morrow A, Chen Y, et al. Multi-Disciplinary Collaborative Consensus Guidance Statement on the Assessment and Treatment of Post-Acute Sequelae

of SARS-CoV-2 Infection (PASC) in Children and Adolescents. *PM&R* 2022; 14(10):1241–69.

56. Poudel AN, Zhu S, Cooper N, et al. Impact of Covid-19 on health-related quality of life of patients: A structured review. PLoS One 2021;16(10):e0259164.

57. Bucciarelli V, Nasi M, Bianco F, et al. Depression pandemic and cardiovascular risk in the COVID-19 era and long COVID syndrome: Gender makes a difference. Trends Cardiovasc Med 2022;32(1):12–7.

58. Bechmann N, Barthel A, Schedl A, et al. Sexual dimorphism in COVID-19: potential clinical and public health implications. Lancet Diabetes Endocrinol 2022; 10(3):221–30.

59. Sylvester SV, Rusu R, Chan B, et al. Sex differences in sequelae from COVID-19 infection and in long COVID syndrome: a review. Curr Med Res Opin 2022;38(8): 1391–9.

60. Centers for Disease Control and Prevention. Assessing Risk Factors. https://www.cdc.gov/coronavirus/2019-ncov/covid-data/investigations-discovery/assessing-risk-factors.html. Published 2020. Accessed 14 Septemer, 2022.

61. Kim L, Whitaker M, O'Halloran A, et al. Hospitalization Rates and Characteristics of Children Aged <18 Years Hospitalized with Laboratory-Confirmed COVID-19 - COVID-NET, 14 States, March 1-July 25, 2020. MMWR Morbidity and mortality weekly report 2020;69(32):1081–8.

62. Hentschel CB, Abramoff BA, Dillingham TR, et al. Race, ethnicity, and utilization of outpatient rehabilitation for treatment of post COVID-19 condition, P&MR 2022; 14(11):1315–24.

63. Havervall S, Rosell A, Phillipson M, et al. Symptoms and Functional Impairment Assessed 8 Months After Mild COVID-19 Among Health Care Workers. JAMA 2021;325(19):2015–6.

64. Logue JK, Franko NM, McCulloch DJ, et al. Sequelae in Adults at 6 Months After COVID-19 Infection. JAMA Netw Open 2021;4(2):e210830.

65. Nalbandian A, Sehgal K, Gupta A, et al. Post-acute COVID-19 syndrome. Nat Med 2021;27(4):601–15.

66. Lassi ZS, Ana A, Das JK, et al. A systematic review and meta-analysis of data on pregnant women with confirmed COVID-19: Clinical presentation, and pregnancy and perinatal outcomes based on COVID-19 severity. J Glob Health 2021;11:05018.

67. Torossian M, Jacelon CS. Chronic Illness and Fatigue in Older Individuals: A Systematic Review. Rehabil Nurs 2021;46(3):125–36.

68. Stefan N, Birkenfeld AL, Schulze MB. Global pandemics interconnected - obesity, impaired metabolic health and COVID-19. Nat Rev Endocrinol 2021;17(3):135–49.

69. Vgontzas AN, Bixler EO, Chrousos GP. Obesity-related sleepiness and fatigue: the role of the stress system and cytokines. Ann N Y Acad Sci 2006;1083:329–44.

70. Graham EL, Clark JR, Orban ZS, et al. Persistent neurologic symptoms and cognitive dysfunction in non-hospitalized Covid-19 "long haulers. Ann Clin Transl Neurol 2021;8(5):1073–85.

71. Ritchie K, Chan D. The emergence of cognitive COVID. World Psychiatr 2021; 20(1):52–3.

72. Jaywant A, Vanderlind WM, Alexopoulos GS, et al. Frequency and profile of objective cognitive deficits in hospitalized patients recovering from COVID-19. Neuropsychopharmacology 2021;46(13):2235–40.

73. Zhou H, Lu S, Chen J, et al. The landscape of cognitive function in recovered COVID-19 patients. J Psychiatr Res 2020;129:98–102.

74. Hampshire A, Trender W, Chamberlain SR, et al. Cognitive deficits in people who have recovered from COVID-19. EClinicalMedicine 2021;39:101044.

75. Moritz S, Spirandelli K, Happach I, et al. Dysfunction by Disclosure? Stereotype Threat as a Source of Secondary Neurocognitive Malperformance in Obsessive-Compulsive Disorder. J Int Neuropsychol Soc 2018;24(6):584–92.

76. VanLandingham H, Ellison RL, Laique A, et al. A scoping review of stereotype threat for BIPOC: Cognitive effects and intervention strategies for the field of neuropsychology. Clin Neuropsychol 2022;36(2):503–22.

77. Castro VM, Gunning FM, Perlis RH. Persistence of neuropsychiatric symptoms associated with SARS-CoV-2 positivity among a cohort of children and adolescents. medRxiv 2021;21264259.

78. Halpin SJ, McIvor C, Whyatt G, et al. Postdischarge symptoms and rehabilitation needs in survivors of COVID-19 infection: A cross-sectional evaluation. J Med Virol 2021;93(2):1013–22.

79. Singh I, Joseph P, Heerdt PM, et al. Persistent Exertional Intolerance After COVID-19: Insights From Invasive Cardiopulmonary Exercise Testing. Chest 2022;161(1):54–63.

80. Torres-Castro R, Vasconcello-Castillo L, Alsina-Restoy X, et al. Respiratory function in patients post-infection by COVID-19: a systematic review and meta-analysis. Pulmonology 2021;27(4):328–37.

81. Carfì A, Bernabei R, Landi F. Persistent Symptoms in Patients After Acute COVID-19. JAMA 2020;324(6):603–5.

82. Sjoding MW, Dickson RP, Iwashyna TJ, et al. Racial Bias in Pulse Oximetry Measurement. N Engl J Med 2020;383(25):2477–8.

83. Chang WT, Toh HS, Liao CT, et al. Cardiac Involvement of COVID-19: A Comprehensive Review. Am J Med Sci 2021;361(1):14–22.

84. Xie Y, Xu E, Bowe B, et al. Long-term cardiovascular outcomes of COVID-19. Nat Med 2022;28(3):583–90.

85. Galick A, D'Arrigo-Patrick E, Knudson-Martin C. Can Anyone Hear Me? Does Anyone See Me? A Qualitative Meta-Analysis of Women's Experiences of Heart Disease. Qual Health Res 2015;25(8):1123–38.

86. Wilby ML. Physical Mobility Impairment and Risk for Cardiovascular Disease. Health Equity 2019;3(1):527–31.

87. Garcia S, Dehghani P, Grines C, et al. Initial Findings From the North American COVID-19 Myocardial Infarction Registry. J Am Coll Cardiol 2021;77(16):1994–2003.

88. Larsen NW, Stiles LE, Miglis MG. Preparing for the long-haul: Autonomic complications of COVID-19. Auton Neurosci 2021;235:102841.

89. Fedorowski A. Postural orthostatic tachycardia syndrome: clinical presentation, aetiology and management. J Intern Med 2019;285(4):352–66.

90. Shaw BH, Stiles LE, Bourne K, et al. The face of postural tachycardia syndrome - insights from a large cross-sectional online community-based survey. J Intern Med 2019;286(4):438–48.

91. Swai J, Hu Z, Zhao X, et al. Heart rate and heart rate variability comparison between postural orthostatic tachycardia syndrome versus healthy participants; a systematic review and meta-analysis. BMC Cardiovasc Disord 2019;19(1):320.

92. Plan-Do-Study-Act (PDSA) Directions and Examples. 2020. https://www.ahrq.gov/health-literacy/improve/precautions/tool2b.html. Accessed September 18, 2022. Accessed September 2020.

93. Reed NS, Meeks LM, Swenor BK. Disability and COVID-19: who counts depends on who is counted. Lancet Public Health 2020;5(8):e423.

94. Mayston M. Telehealth for disability management: what really matters? Dev Med Child Neurol 2021;63(2):124.

Integrative Medicine in Long COVID

Irene M. Estores, MD[a],*, Paula Ackerman, DO[b]

KEYWORDS

- COVID-19 • Long COVID • Integrative medicine • Osteopathic manipulation
- Acupuncture • Mind–body medicine • Dietary supplements • Nutrition

KEY POINTS

- Based on plausible mechanisms to explain persistent symptoms following COVID infection, previous use in other viral illnesses, and current preliminary data, physiatrists can include complementary and integrative therapies in a comprehensive plan that supports recovery and optimal function for persons living with long COVID.
- Biomedical makers and functional outcomes can be used to track clinical course and recovery.
- If ongoing trials on several complementary modalities demonstrate safety and efficacy, the next steps should include implementation and utilization in different health settings.
- An integrative approach is not an eclectic use of complementary and conventional therapies. It is a patient and relationship-centered approach grounded in empathy, respect, open-mindedness, inquiry, and professional humility, an approach that enhances the care for persons living with long COVID.

INTRODUCTION

Physical Medicine and Rehabilitation Medicine at its core is an integrative practice. Physiatrists work with patients, their families, and an interdisciplinary team of rehabilitation professionals to address the physical, emotional, medical, social, and emotional needs of persons with functional limitations due to disease or injury. The philosophy and practice of Physiatry and Integrative Medicine share similar aims of optimizing health and function and the use of non-drug treatment modalities such as exercise and physical agents. Physiatrists provide care to patients with chronic musculoskeletal and neurologic conditions, such as chronic low back and neck pain, fibromyalgia, stroke, multiple sclerosis, and arthritis, who also seek complementary and integrative health (CIH) treatments.

a Department of Physical Medicine and Rehabilitation, Integrative Medicine Program, University of Florida College of Medicine, 3450 Hull Road, Gainesville, FL 32611, USA;
b Department of Physical Medicine and Rehabilitation, University of Florida College of Medicine, 3450 Hull Road, Gainesville, FL 32611, USA
* Corresponding author.
E-mail address: ime@ufl.edu
Twitter: imestoresmd (I.M.E.)

Phys Med Rehabil Clin N Am 34 (2023) 677–688
https://doi.org/10.1016/j.pmr.2023.03.006
1047-9651/23/© 2023 Elsevier Inc. All rights reserved.

pmr.theclinics.com

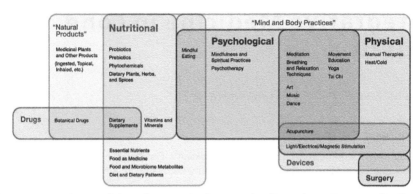

Fig. 1. Integrative medicine therapeutic framework. (*From* https://www.nccih.nih.gov/about/nccih-strategic-plan-2021-2025/introduction/reframing-how-we-think-about-natural-products-and-mindand-body-practices, with permission.)

Although the implementation of vaccination programs has been effective in preventing serious morbidity and mortality from severe acute respiratory syndrome- coronavirus-2 (SARS-CoV-2) infection, vaccination only reduces the risk of developing long COVID in modest and varying degrees.[1] The current lack of knowledge on proven treatments for long COVID has resulted in a surge of both demand and use of CIH treatments, especially in low- and middle-income countries whose populations utilize these modalities for health care.[2] Complementary, alternative, and non-specific treatments are also being used by physicians in "therapeutically indeterminate situations", as has occurred with the treatment of long COVID at this time. Currently, two situations are occurring where CIH can be leveraged: (1) when there is a desire for treatment by the physician, patient, or both; and (2) when there is no need for treatment, no accepted treatment is available, or existing effective treatments are not acceptable to the patient.[3]

The National Center for Complementary and Integrative Health divides CIH treatments into four main groups based on how these therapies are delivered. These categories are nutritional, psychological, physical, and combinations of these categories as illustrated in **Fig. 1**. Examples of nutritional therapies include dietary modifications, natural products, herbs, and supplements. Psychological therapies include psychotherapy, meditation, guided imagery, and spiritual practices. Physical treatments include osteopathic manipulative therapy, massage, cryotherapy, and electrical stimulation. Whole systems of medicine such as Traditional Chinese, Ayurvedic, Naturopathic, and Functional Medicine typically have nutritional, psychological, and physical components. Representative therapies from each category are reviewed in this article. The selection is based on the availability of published and ongoing research on its use specifically for post-COVID conditions.

We start with a composite case of a patient seen in our post-COVID clinic. Acknowledging that the clinical presentation is mixed in complexity and symptomatology, this composite is purposefully developed to illustrate an integrative approach to the management of long COVID.

CASE COMPOSITE
Physical Treatments

Osteopathic manipulative treatment
Osteopathic medicine developed as a philosophy of medicine in 1974, pioneered by AT Still, an allopathic trained physician and civil war surgeon in Kirksville, MO (**Box 1**).

Box 1
Case Composite

PM, a 52-year old man
- *Past Medical History*: GERD
- *Functional History*: Recently retired from job as warehouse supervisor, enjoyed hiking, gardening, and yard work
- *COVID History*: Date of infection—January 2021, no prior vaccination, PCR+
  - Acute symptoms of low-grade fever, fatigue, chest tightness, cough, generalized arthralgia and myalgia, and dyspnea
  - Symptomatic management
  - No antiviral or monoclonal antibody therapy or hospital admission with symptom improvement after 1 week.
  - Persistent exertional dyspnea, dizziness, lightheadedness, tachycardia, and palpitation with minimal physical exertion and bending forward.
  - Seen at post-COVID clinic 8 months after initial infection.
- Initial Clinic Visit:
  - Normal vital signs, non-orthostatic
  - Normal cardiopulmonary and musculoskeletal examination except for
    - L shoulder tenderness, pain, restricted motion
  - Normal laboratory data, but no testing for inflammatory markers
  - PROMIS-29 scores: moderate limitation—fatigue, pain, physical function, sleep
  - GAD-7 score: 5
  - PHQ-9 score: 5
  - Plan:
    - Education on long COVID, pacing, sleep, anti-inflammatory diet
    - Labs: D-dimer, hs-CRP, ferritin, vitamin D
    - Referrals to PT for shoulder rehab program, osteopathic physician for OMT, instruction on daily relaxation breathing
- Four subsequent telemedicine visits in a span of 8 months
  - Laboratory testing showed elevated D-dimer and hs-CRP. Enteric-coated ASA 81 mg/day prescribed, advised to monitor GERD symptoms
  - Improvements noted with OMT, PT for shoulder rehab, shoulder pain resolved, mobility normal
  - Downward trend for both D-dimer and hs-CRP
  - PROMIS-29 score—minimal limitation in fatigue
  - GAD-7 score: 2
  - PHQ-9 score: 2

After the death of his three children from spinal meningitis, Dr Still developed manual techniques to optimize the body's facilitation for self-healing and modification[4] During the influenza pandemic of 1918, Smith reported that of the 6258 pandemic influenza pneumonia patients, the group receiving osteopathic manipulative treatment (OMT) had a 0.25% mortality rate, lower than the non-OMT group.[5] Osteopathic manual techniques support the respiratory system, influence the circulatory, lymphatic and autonomic nervous systems, impact the activity of endocrine and metabolic systems[6] and are used as adjuvant care in the SARS-CoV-2 global pandemic. The osteopathic approach to each patient is individualized, however, there are generalized examples of OMT techniques commonly used to facilitate the respiratory system for a patient with a history of pneumonia that focus on the diaphragm, ribs, vertebra, and associated facial attachments that can impact circulatory, lymphatic, and nervous structures.[7] OMT utilizes the interconnectedness between the musculoskeletal and organ systems to affect the tissue texture changes manifested in the organ system by viscero-somatic reflex and treatment of the associated musculoskeletal structures to influence the nervous, lymphatic, and autonomic system via somato-visceral reflexes.

Improvements in lymphatic motility have demonstrated in vivo cytokine modulation and in vitro reduction of tumor necrosis factor - alpha (TNF-α).[8]

OMT has been used to treat several respiratory conditions and has been studied in comparison to conventional care and other manual techniques. Noll and colleagues published the results of a randomized controlled study of 406 hospitalized subjects aged 50 years or older comparing conventional care only, light touch treatment, and OMT groups following specified protocols. Reduced length of stay compared to conventional care was demonstrated, but no difference was observed between light touch and OMT groups.[9] In a retrospective observational cohort matched review of patients hospitalized with COVID-19-related respiratory distress, patients receiving daily OMT reported high satisfaction and greater ease of breathing, but no significant difference in secondary outcomes such as length of stay (6.9 days OMT versus 8.6 days control; P =.053) or discharge status compared to a control group.[10] Importantly, OMT provided patients a personal management options and relief from isolation.

Similar to other complementary therapies and modalities, clinical trials investigating the effect of OMT on long COVID symptoms are in progress. **Table 1** provides a summary of OMT and other therapies discussed in this article.

WHOLE SYSTEMS
Acupuncture and Traditional Chinese Medicine

Classical Traditional Chinese Medicine (TCM) theory of health posits that this is maintained by a normal flow of and balance of Qi, blood, and body fluids. External factors such as toxins, infectious agents, environmental extremes, and internal factors such as unmitigated stress, poor sleep, and nutrition can cause a disruption of this healthy flow. Treatment is aimed at restoring this balance or "homeostasis" by modifying these internal and external factors and with the use of selected acupuncture points to correct imbalances. The specific imbalance is identified using information from the person's clinical history, presentation, disease timeline, general examination, and specific examination of the tongue and pulses.

Acupuncture research has demonstrated peripheral, central, immune, and neuroendocrine biologic effects to explain its effects on animals and humans. This included peripheral release of adenosine,[11] and changes in cortical and spinal cord dorsal column activity, endogenous opioids, autonomic tone, and connective tissue,[12] that extend beyond non-specific or placebo effects. Some investigators propose that long COVID provokes a strong general protective response, a synchronized reaction involving the autonomic nervous system, hypothalamus-pituitary-adrenal axis, and the inflammatory and immune systems in an effort to restore homeostasis.[13] Although this is a normal physiologic response to any internal or external stressor, and it is not unique to COVID, if this response is not effective, this can lead to a prolong cell danger response.[14] If not reversed, regenerative processes cannot begin. This framework ties in traditional TCM and modern medical theory to explain persistent multi-system symptoms following COVID-19 infection.

Interventional evidence for the use of acupuncture in long COVID management is very sparse. Two case studies describing the improvement of long COVID symptoms, either alone [15] or as part of a multidisciplinary program,[16] have been published. Improvement in chest pressure and heart palpitations, followed by complete resolution of symptoms occurred with seven sessions of scalp, auricular, and body acupuncture when coupled with physical activity.[16] Larger clinical trials are underway to rigorously investigate its effects on olfactory dysfunction (NCT04952389) and fatigue (NCT05212688, NCT05289154). Details are found in **Table 1**.

Table 1
Active research studies on effect of complementary modalities on long COVID symptoms

Study Name And/Or ID Number	Intervention/Study Design	Outcome Measures	Study Site	Estimated Study Completion Date
NCT05012826 Osteopathy and Physiotherapy Compared to Physiotherapy Alone on Fatigue and Functional Status in Long COVID	OMT + PT vs PT alone Controlled, assessor-blinded, pragmatic RCT 2 months intervention 3-month follow-up	Fatigue Severity Scale, Post-COVID Functional Scale Perceived Change Scale-Patient	Centro Universitário Augusto Motta	Currently Recruiting July 2023
NCT05112887 Osteopathic Manipulative Therapy Effects on Prolonged Post-COVID Olfactory Dysfunction	True vs sham OMT	0–10 NRS of smell intensity Smell identification (four substances) Quantitative smell experience	Ohio University	Completed September 2021 Data not yet published
NCT05212688 Randomized Study to Investigate the Effectiveness of Acupuncture for the Relief of Long COVID-19-Related Fatigue (ACU-COVID)	Weekly acupuncture vs weekly semi-structured phone consultation RCT 6-week intervention	Multidimensional Fatigue Inventory (MFI)	Royal Marsden Trust	Recruiting July 2025
NCT05356936 Pilot Study of Vitamin K2 (MK-7) and Vitamin D3 Supplementation and the Effects on PASC Symptomatology and Inflammatory Biomarkers	Daily oral vitamin K2 (MK7) and D-3 vs no treatment Randomized 24-week intervention	Vit K-2 and D3 level Hs-CRP, IL-6, Ifab, sTNF-RII	University Hospitals Cleveland Medical Center	Recruiting June 2022
NCT04960215 Coenzyme Q10 (COQ-10) as	Daily oral ubiquinone 100 mg 5 times a day vs placebo RCT, cross-over design	EQ-5D-5L Long-term COVID-specific questionnaire	Aarhus University Hospital, Denmark	Completed February 2022 No data published

(continued on next page)

Table 1
(continued)

Study Name And/Or ID Number	Intervention/Study Design	Outcome Measures	Study Site	Estimated Study Completion Date
Treatment of Long-Term COVID-19 (QVID)		COQ-10 plasma and PBMC levels Cytokines, metabolites in kynurenic pathway	VA Salt Lake City Health Care System, Utah	
NCT05373043 Long-term COVID and Rehabilitation	Exercise + placebo vs Exercise + mitoquinone (Mito-Q) RCT, double-blinded			
NCT04952389 Acupuncture and Olfactory Dysfunction	10 sessions of acupuncture + standard of care vs standard of care (budesonide and olfactory training) Randomized, open	UPSIT SNOT	Mayo Clinic, Rochester	Recruiting
NCT05212688 Acupressure and QiGong in Chronic Fatigue Post-COVID-19	Self-applied acupressure and online Qigong course vs advice literature RCT	SF-36PFS EuroQol5D, Chalder Fatigue Scale	Charité Universitätsmedizin Campus Mitte Berlin, Germany	Recruiting
NCT04813718 Post-COVID-19 syndrome and the Gut-Lung Axis	Omni-Biotic Pro Vi 5 Pre- and probiotic vs placebo RCT, triple-masked	Measure of microbiome composition, intestinal barrier function, endotoxins, interleukins, neutrophil and monocyte function, spirometry, lung volumes, gas diffusion	Medical University of Graz	Active, not recruiting

NCT05121766 Feasibility Pilot Clinical Trial of Omega-3 Supplement vs Placebo for Post-COVID-19 Recovery Among Health Care Workers	Drug: Omega-3 (EPA + DHA) Drug: Placebo RCT, blinded	Self-reported improvement of symptoms	Hackensack Meridian Health Edison, New Jersey, United States	Recruiting
NCT04809974 Clinical Trial of Niagen to Examine Recovery in People with Persistent Cognitive and Physical Symptoms After COVID-19 Illness (long COVID)	Niagen vs placebo	Beck Depression Inventory, Beck Anxiety Inventory, Self-reported physical symptoms, Neuropsychological test scores	Clinical Translational Research Unit Boston, Massachusetts, United States	Recruiting
NCT05371288 The Role of Glutathione Deficiency and MSIDS Variables in Long COVID-19	NAC (N-acetyl cysteine), Alpha-lipoic acid (ALA), liposomal glutathione (GSH) for 28 days vs multivitamin + magnesium for 14 days followed by study supplement	Self-reported symptoms, time to clinical recovery, COVID Severity of Symptoms Questionnaire, SF-36	University of California Irvine Medical Center Orange, California, United States	Active, not yet recruiting

Abbreviations: EQ-5D-5L, EuroQol Five-dimension Five-Level scale; hs-CRP, high-sensitivity C-reactive protein; Ifab, intestinal fatty acid binding protein; IL-6, inter-leukin-6; RCT, randomized controlled trial; SNOT, Sino-Nasal Outcome Test; sTNF-RII, soluble tumor necrosis factor receptor II; UPSIT, University of Pittsburgh Smell Identification Test.

MIND–BODY INTERVENTIONS

These interventions encompass a wide range of practices such as meditation, yoga, Tai'Chi, Qigong, breathing, and biofeedback. These have the same effect of activating the parasympathetic nervous system, the so-called relaxation response. This programmed physiologic response, the opposite of the sympathetic or "fight or flight" response can induce several health benefits including reduction of anxiety, menopausal symptoms, blood pressure, and the number of clinic visits for chronic pain management.[17] Learning a skill that is relatively low risk and low cost enhances self-efficacy and healthy behaviors in persons who live with a chronic illness.[17] Teaching and learning these practices can be done in telemedicine/telehealth-based visits, thus, enhancing access and reducing travel burden and exposure. Patients can choose to learn a practice based on their preferences and beliefs and implement these practices in conjunction with other modalities.

One randomized controlled trial (RCT) compared the effect of a 6-week telerehabilitation program consisting of breathing exercises, thoracic expansion, and aerobic and strengthening exercises versus no rehabilitation in COVID-19 survivors with dyspnea. The intervention group demonstrated superior gains in walking distance (15.5% vs 3.4%), wall sit muscle endurance time (83.6% vs 20.7%), and the physical component of the Short Health Form Survey-12 (20.0% vs 9.7%) compared to the no rehabilitation group.[18]

NUTRITION AND DIETARY SUPPLEMENTS

Optimizing nutrition can reduce chronic inflammation and susceptibility to several infectious agents and improve clinical outcomes of persons with various chronic diseases such as obesity, diabetes, cancer, and hypertension.[19] Dietary practices minimize intake of processed food, simple carbohydrates, sugar-sweetened beverage, saturated and trans-fat, and emphasize the intake of whole-food, plant-based food consumption (rich in monounsaturated and polyunsaturated fat, vegetables, lean protein, and complex carbohydrates). This provides the necessary macronutrients, micronutrients, and phytochemicals to support convalescence from disease or injury.[20] There are no available data or current trials investigating its benefit for persons with long COVID. However, based on the positive effects of this diet on weight, mood, sleep, and pain,[21] it is an essential component of an integrative health plan.

Dietary supplements and natural products that modulate systemic inflammation, immunity, gut microbiota composition, and mitochondrial function are being used based on the current understanding of the role of these pathophysiologic mechanisms in long COVID. Most of the data available on the effect of these supplements on long COVID come from pilot observational studies using a combination of different compounds such as vitamin C, acetyl-L-carnitine, hydroxytyrosol/olive polyphenols, thiamine, vitamin B6, folic acid, vitamin D-3, and vitamin B-12.[22] A different proprietary formulation (Apportal), consisting of group B vitamins, minerals in sucrosomial forms such as iron, magnesium, zinc and selenium, arginine and carnitine, Panax ginseng and Eleutherococcus senticosus taken for 28 consecutive days, was also observed in a pilot uncontrolled study to improve symptoms of fatigue, health status, and quality of life as measured by the Functional Assessment of Chronic Illness Therapy—Fatigue and the EQ-5D scales.[23]

COVID-19 infection has been associated with gastrointestinal symptoms ranging from mild to severe. Alterations in the composition of gut microbiota have been demonstrated in both acute[24] and chronic COVID infection.[25] The gut–lung axis is a potential link between dysbiosis, translocation of bacterial products and hyperinflammation has been proposed.[26] The gut microbiome is being explored as a potential therapeutic target because of its extensive connections with the autonomic and central nervous systems. Rigorously designed trials, such as the use of probiotics (post-COVID-19 syndrome and the gut–lung Axis NCT04813718), will provide information on both relevant biomarkers and effects of clinical course and symptoms.

There is an active feasibility double-blind placebo-controlled trial investigating the effect of omega-3 fatty acid supplement (total of 4200 mg/day—504 mg of eicosapentaenoic acid [EPA] and 204 mg of docosahexaenoic acid [DHA]) taken for 12 weeks (NCT05121766) on the feasibility of use and COVID symptoms compared to a placebo. The study participants are health care workers who were not hospitalized and have one or more of the following persistent symptoms: dyspnea, cough, loss of smell/taste, and fatigue. This dose is on the high end of typical dosing but is still considered safe.

Nicotinamide riboside (vitamin B3; Niagen) at a dose of 2000 mg/day is being studied in a randomized, parallel, placebo-controlled trial (NCT04809974) specifically examining effects on cognitive function and mood compared to a placebo over 22 weeks. Executive function, memory, and composite scores (representative of 'brain fog') are primary outcomes, and depression, anxiety, and physical symptoms are secondary outcomes.

Compounds with antioxidant properties, specifically vitamin C, are used as an adjunct therapy in viral illnesses, including COVID-19. However, a meta-analysis of six RCTs (N = 592 patients) found no significant benefit on intensive care length of stay, need for mechanical ventilation, and mortality in COVID-19 treatment irrespective of the route of administration in the acute care setting.[27] It remains unclear if patients with vitamin C deficiencies may obtain better effects with administration, or have protection against development of long COVID.[28] Using a specifically-designed survey of symptoms associated with long COVID, Izzo and colleagues[29] observed a beneficial effect of combination of L-arginine (1.66 g) and liposomal vitamin C (500 mg) taken daily for 30 consecutive days compared to an 'alternative treatment' (vitamin B multivitamin combination; vitamin B1: 388 mg; vitamin B2: 443 mg; nicotinamide: 18 mg; folic acid: 200 μg; pantothenic acid: 2493 g; vitamin B6: 831 mg; vitamin B12: 416 μg). Benefits of L-arginine + vitamin C included lower severities or absence of COVID-19 symptoms such as headaches, dizziness, dyspnea, gastrointestinal disorders, concentration difficulty, anosmia, and sleeplessness compared to the alternative treatment.

Low levels of glutathione in the anterior cingulate cortex have been reported in COVID-19 survivors with depressive symptoms and cerebral white matter hypodensities and hyperintensities.[30] A phase 1 RCT comparing the use of liposomal glutathione, acetyl-L- cysteine, and alpha-lipoic acid (NCT05371288) is registered.

SUMMARY AND FUTURE DIRECTIONS

Physiatrists possess the skill set and mindset to work with persons living with chronic illness to optimize recovery and function. Persons living with long COVID present with several disabling symptoms, experience unpredictable and mixed clinical experiences, and have minimal information on definitive treatments. It is indeed imperative that we practice evidence-informed medicine. However, with the current paucity of data from clinical trials, it is reasonable to use an approach that addresses underlying pathophysiologic mechanisms, optimizing lifestyle modifications to manage symptoms, improve metabolic and mental health, and promote recovery and function. Integrative practice involves more than a combination of conventional and complementary therapies. In the face of medical uncertainty and suffering brought about by COVID-19 and long COVID, integrative physicians must ground their practice with empathy, respect, and professional humility. The ongoing trials on several complementary modalities may yield information to guide future treatments and health policy. The next step should involve phase 3 trials based on phase 2 results and the development of protocols that integrate effective modalities into current treatments. These should be implemented in cost-effective ways and in different health care settings to ensure access for all.

CLINICS CARE POINTS

- Based on plausible mechanisms to explain persistent symptoms following COVID-19 infection, previous use in other viral illnesses, and current preliminary data, physiatrists can include complementary and integrative therapies in a comprehensive plan that supports recovery and optimal function for persons living with long COVID.

- Biomedical makers and functional outcomes can be used to track clinical course and recovery.

- If ongoing trials on several complementary modalities demonstrate safety and efficacy, the next steps should include implementation and utilization in different health settings.

- An integrative approach is not an eclectic use of complementary and conventional therapies. It is a patient and relationship-centered approach grounded in empathy, respect, openmindedness, inquiry, and professional humility, an approach that enhances the care for persons living with long COVID.

DISCLOSURE

The authors have nothing to disclose.

REFERENCES

1. Al-Aly Z, Bowe B, Xie Y. Long COVID after breakthrough SARS-CoV-2 infection. Nat Med 2022;28(7):1461–7.
2. Shaikh BT, Hatcher J. Complementary and alternative medicine in pakistan: prospects and limitations. Evid-Based Complement Altern Med ECAM 2005;2(2): 139–42.
3. Ostermaier A, Barth N, Schneider A, et al. On the edges of medicine - a qualitative study on the function of complementary, alternative, and non-specific therapies in handling therapeutically indeterminate situations. BMC Fam Pract 2019; 20(1):55.
4. Chila AG. Foundations of osteopathic medicine. Philadelphia, PA, USA: Lippincott Williams & Wilkins; 2011.
5. Smith RK. One hundred thousand cases of influenza with a death rate of one-fortieth of that officially reported under conventional medical treatment. 1919. J Am Osteopath Assoc 2000;100(5):320–3.
6. Baroni F, Mancini D, Tuscano SC, et al. Osteopathic manipulative treatment and the Spanish flu: a historical literature review. J Osteopath Med 2021;121(2): 181–90.
7. Roberts A, Harris K, Outen B, et al. Osteopathic manipulative medicine: a brief review of the hands-on treatment approaches and their therapeutic uses. Medicines 2022;9(5):33.

8. Marin T, Maxel X, Robin A, et al. Evidence-based assessment of potential thera-peutic effects of adjunct osteopathic medicine for multidisciplinary care of acute and convalescent COVID-19 patients. Explore N Y N 2021;17(2):141–7.

9. Noll DR, Degenhardt BF, Morley TF, et al. Efficacy of osteopathic manipulation as an adjunctive treatment for hospitalized patients with pneumonia: a randomized controlled trial. Osteopath Med Prim Care 2010;4:2.

10. Lennon RP, Dong H, Zgierska AE, et al. Adjunctive osteopathic therapy for hos-pitalized COVID-19 patients: a feasibility-oriented chart review study with matched controls. Int J Osteopath Med 2022;44:3–8.

11. Takano T, Chen X, Luo F, et al. Traditional acupuncture triggers a local increase in adenosine in human subjects. J Pain 2012;13(12):1215–23.

12. MacPherson H, Hammerschlag R, Coeytaux RR, et al. Unanticipated insights into biomedicine from the study of acupuncture. J Altern Complement Med 2016; 22(2):101–7.

13. Calloway T, Hsiao AF, Brand M, et al. Conceptualizing a traditional chinese med-icine and pathology of arousal diagnostic and pathophysiological framework for postacute sequelae of COVID-19. Med Acupunct 2022;34(3):167–71.

14. Naviaux RK. Metabolic features of the cell danger response. Mitochondrion 2014; 16:7–17.

15. Hollifield M, Cocozza K, Calloway T, et al. Improvement in long-COVID symptoms using acupuncture: a case study. Med Acupunct 2022;34(3):172–6.

16. Trager RJ, Brewka EC, Kaiser CM, et al. Acupuncture in multidisciplinary treat-ment for post-COVID-19 syndrome. Med Acupunct 2022;34(3):177–83.

17. Stahl JE, Dossett ML, LaJoie AS, et al. Relaxation response and resiliency training and its effect on healthcare resource utilization. PLoS One 2015;10(10): e0140212.

18. Li J, Xia W, Zhan C, et al. A telerehabilitation programme in post-discharge COVID-19 patients (TERECO): a randomised controlled trial. Thorax 2022; 77(7):697–706.

19. Seifert G, Jeitler M, Stange R, et al. The relevance of complementary and integra-tive medicine in the COVID-19 pandemic: a qualitative review of the literature. Front Med 2020;7:587749.

20. Alschuler L, Chiasson AM, Horwitz R, et al. Integrative medicine considerations for convalescence from mild-to-moderate COVID-19 disease. Explore N Y N 2022;18(2):140–8.

21. Storz MA. Lifestyle adjustments in long-COVID management: potential benefits of plant-based diets. Curr Nutr Rep 2021;10(4):352–63.

22. Naureen Z, Dautaj A, Nodari S, et al. Proposal of a food supplement for the man-agement of post-COVID syndrome. Eur Rev Med Pharmacol Sci 2021;25(1 Suppl):67–73.

23. Rossato MS, Brilli E, Ferri N, et al. Observational study on the benefit of a nutri-tional supplement, supporting immune function and energy metabolism, on chronic fatigue associated with the SARS-CoV-2 post-infection progress. Clin Nutr ESPEN 2021;46:510–8.

24. Lu ZH, Zhou HW, Wu WK, et al. Alterations in the composition of intestinal DNA virome in patients with COVID-19. Front Cell Infect Microbiol 2021;11:790422.

25. Liu Q, Wing Yan Mak J, Su Q, et al. Gut microbiota dynamics in a prospective cohort of patients with post-acute COVID-19 syndrome. Gut 2022;71:544–52.

26. Gang J, Wang H, Xue X, et al. Microbiota and COVID-19: long-term and complex influencing factors. Front Microbiol 2022;13:963488.

27. Rawat D, Roy A, Maitra S, et al. Vitamin C and COVID-19 treatment: a systematic review and meta-analysis of randomized controlled trials. Diabetes Metab Syndr Clin Res Rev 2021;15(6). https://doi.org/10.1016/J.DSX.2021.102324.

28. Vollbracht C, Kraft K. Oxidative stress and hyper-inflammation as major drivers of severe COVID-19 and long COVID: implications for the benefit of high-dose intravenous vitamin C. Front Pharmacol 2022;13:899198.

29. Izzo R, Trimarco V, Mone P, et al. Combining L-Arginine with vitamin C improves long-COVID symptoms: the LINCOLN Survey. Pharmacol Res 2022;183. https://doi.org/10.1016/J.PHRS.2022.106360.

30. Poletti S, Paolini M, Mazza MG, et al. Lower levels of glutathione in the anterior cingulate cortex associate with depressive symptoms and white matter hyperintensities in COVID-19 survivors. Eur Neuropsychopharmacol 2022;61:71–7.

Integrated Care Models for Long Coronavirus Disease

Surendra Barshikar, MD, MBA*, Martin Laguerre, MD,
Patricia Gordon, MSN, MPH, APRN, FNP-BC, Marielisa Lopez, MD

KEYWORDS

- Long COVID • Post-acute sequelae of SARS CoV-2 • Models of care

KEY POINTS

- The wide range of persistent symptoms in long COVID requires a coordinated response from multiple medical specialties.
- Formalized models of care systems and multidisciplinary collaborations began in early 2021 as health care providers recognized the needs of the affected population.
- Multidisciplinary models largely exist in academic centers and larger cities; however, most care for PASC patients is provided by the primary care providers.

INTRODUCTION

As of July 2022, there have been more than 540 million confirmed cases of coronavirus disease (severe acute respiratory syndrome coronavirus 2 [SARS CoV-2], coronavirus disease 2019 [COVID-19]) during the global pandemic.[1] Severe acute cases of SARS-CoV-2 respiratory illness continue to strain communities, health care systems, and nations. Evidence-based medical treatments have greatly improved patient outcomes; however, a growing population of survivors with persisting long-term complications has been recognized. This syndrome has been labeled as long COVID or the Post-Acute Sequelae of SARS CoV-2 (PASC).[2,3]

There is no single accepted definition of PASC. However, PASC is characterized by persistent and/or delayed symptoms or complications beyond 4 weeks of symptom onset or 3 months after a confirmed SARS CoV-2 infection.[3] The population that experiences PASC is extremely heterogeneous, from those initially asymptomatic with no prior comorbidities to those with preexisting respiratory conditions and prolonged intensive care unit (ICU) stays. The exact prevalence of PASC in the population is unknown with reports of patients with PASC ranging from 10% to 81% of confirmed cases.[4] Given this large population, treatment resource, health care needs, and social costs will continue to be a growing burden on already exhausted health care systems.[5]

Physical Medicine and Rehabilitation UT Southwestern Medical Center, 5161 Harry Hines Boulevard, Dallas, TX 75390-9055, USA
* Corresponding author.
E-mail address: surendra.barshikar@utsouthwestern.edu

Phys Med Rehabil Clin N Am 34 (2023) 689–700
https://doi.org/10.1016/j.pmr.2023.03.007

BACKGROUND
Models of Care Concept

The concept of models of care is not new to medicine. In the United States, multiple models of care exist for conditions such as burns, traumatic brain injury, diabetes, chronic obstructive pulmonary disease, and spinal cord injury.[6,7] These model systems standardize assessment, patient care and help formulate, and study outcomes. These efforts impact policy reform, patient and physician behaviors, and further program development.[7]

Lack of Early Models of Care

COVID-19 is a multisystem disease with factors such as inflammation, endothelial dysfunction, and hypercoagulability leading to a diversity of end-organ damage over the course of the illness.[8] The wide range of persistent symptoms requires a coordinated response from multiple medical specialties. PASC models of care were mostly unavailable until mid-2021. Many primary care providers (PCPs) have been unfamiliar with the presentation and unsure of appropriate treatment options.[9]

Early Collaboration and Academic Model Systems

Formalized models of care systems and multidisciplinary collaborations began in early 2021 as health care providers recognized the needs of the affected population as a new and separate issue. As the primary stakeholders, patient-led collaborations were some of the first to document symptoms and publish reports concerning PASC. These groups also brought advocacy to the forefront for marginalized and underserved populations lacking access to care.[10] The American Academy of Physical Medicine and Rehabilitation (AAPMR) would soon follow with a coordinated call to address this population through the Multi-disciplinary PASC Collaborative in March 2021.[11] This group brought together expert health care providers from not only the field of rehabilitation but also in pulmonology, cardiology, neurology, primary care, and patient advocates to continually develop and update clinical guidance, education, and resources in the wake of the ever-expanding knowledge about this newly recognized condition. The Centers for Disease Control (CDC) provided further guidance in June 2021 with a Clinician Outreach and Communication Activity specifically addressing PASC, providing a framework for the evaluation, management, and follow-up of these patients.[12] The initial focus was on the continued care need posthospital and emergency room care, but as the cases increased, the need for community based focus and primary care became readily apparent. Coinciding with the availability of payor-sanctioned telemedicine, the community and primary care model of care for this population began to develop its own framework for evaluation, management, and referrals.[13] Large academic medical centers with large catchment populations and a variety of clinical settings provided an excellent incubator for an integrative approach to PASC management. Early academic models initially centered on the medical specialties of physiatry (given the chronicity of symptoms and already established paradigms for traumatic brain injury, cardiac and pulmonary rehabilitation), cardiology, pulmonology, neurology, and psychiatry. As PASC became more clearly defined as a multisystem pathology, more specialties were folded into the various academic models of care. Early adopters such as University of Texas Southwestern Medical Center, University of Texas Health Science Center at San Antonio Program, and the Veterans Administration Greater Los Angeles Health Care System provided unique frameworks for their differing PASC patient populations.[14] New York-Presbyterian/Weill Cornell Medical Center established a model which included a

30-bed unit for patients preparing to transition out of the acute phase that was led by a hospital medicine physician and a physiatrist.[15] A similar unit was established at the Los Angeles VA Hospital for patients with active infection but not requiring high-acuity services.[16]

APPROACH
Long Coronavirus Disease Care Models Core Components

Every model of care has core components that form an integral part of such a model, and other disciplines are included on an as-needed basis. Depending on the condition and organ system involved, the lead for such a model may be based in a particular specialty or discipline. For PASC, as the impact is multisystemic, multiple disciplines can potentially serve as leads. A survey conducted by the AAPMR Long COVID Collaborative showed that most clinics were housed in physical medicine and rehabilitation (PM&R) (40%), pulmonology (22%), and internal medicine (16%). The most common specialties considered part of the treatment team were physical therapy, pulmonology, PM&R, neurology, cardiology, psychology, neuropsychology, speech and language pathology, occupational therapy, and psychiatry. Fifty-five percent (55%) of the survey respondents reported that the treatment team consisted of anywhere between 6 and 10 specialties, whereas 31% reported that their team consisted of over 10 specialties.[17] The numbers may be somewhat biased as the survey was carried out by the AAPMR. Of the 94 established PASC clinics, many used telemedicine visits as their standard for the initial intake visit or otherwise provided it as an option.

Role of allied health Professions

PM&R has been in the forefront of the multidisciplinary care models to date, and physical, occupational, and speech/cognitive therapies have played a vital role in these programs.[14] Targets for physical therapy include management of respiratory insufficiencies, gait and balance disorders, poor endurance, and other mobility-related issues. Occupational therapists perform activity analysis addressing the management of fatigue and post-exertional malaise. Speech and cognitive therapists address cognitive and communication deficits when needed.[18] Mental health diagnoses, both new and long-standing, are common, and recognition and treatment involve therapists, counselors, psychiatrists, and psychologists.[19] With the symptoms of PASC including cognitive difficulties often described as "brain fog," neuropsychological assessments are also used.[17] In addition, the multidisciplinary team works together to identify barriers to return to work, school, or the community as appropriate and provides potential solutions. These can include accommodations at school or work.

Last, patients with PASC often have complex social needs which present challenges to them and their families. Care coordinators, social workers, or case managers can help with patient navigation, resource identification, and patient adherence to treatment plans.[20] A number of models included advanced practice providers and nurses to increased patient accessibility.[21]

APPLICATION
Primary Care Model

The role of primary care in the management of PASC is vital. Although multidisciplinary models largely exist in academic centers and larger cities, most care for PASC patients is provided by the primary care providers (PCPs). A consensus statement using Delphi method stresses the central role of PCPs.[22] At centers where specialist availability is limited, PCPs can use standardized assessment and screening to initially triage, manage, and refer appropriate patients to specialists. A tiered model with self-management, primary care, and the multidisciplinary team as three levels was proposed by the National Health Service (NHS) in accordance with the National Institute for Health and Care Excellence (NICE) guidelines (**Fig. 1**).[23] Many other publications stress the importance of primary care and make recommendations regarding basic symptoms management.[24,25]

Examining systematic reviews of care models for PASC, a common element in the most proposed models of care is the need for and involvement of primary care into long-term care.[17,26,27] Developing a system to integrate primary care into a principal helps to supplement scare specialty long COVID clinics which usually have long waiting lists and barriers to access for patients with geographical and funding challenges.[16] Primary care-centered models offer a sustainable solution to ensuring that patients with PASC receive optimal medical care.

NYC Health Hospitals represent an innovative primary care PASC model. Given the particularly heavy and early disease burden in New York City, New York City (NYC) Health established three COVID-19 Centers of Excellence in the Bronx, Queens, and Brooklyn.[28] These centers provided comprehensive primary care services designed to provide longitudinal care for PASC patients. Onsite specialists (mental health professionals, cardiologists, and pulmonologists) and diagnostic equipment (imaging, transthoracic echocardiograms, and pulmonary function testing) are available. These centers provide a structured on-site pathway to subspecialists within NYC Health system.

Hennepin Healthcare System is another example of a primary care-based model system. An interdisciplinary team of PCPs, physiatrist, and therapy services developed assessment tools and treatment/referral algorithms to manage PASC patients. These tools and algorithms were integrated directly into Hennepin's health care community clinics.[26] The tools are modified to have versions for patients who specifically present for PASC symptom evaluation (long version) or for patients who during an unrelated visit report PASC symptoms (short version). Screening results identify possible needs that would be met by a therapy for specialty clinic referral. Patients with multiple system involvement or ongoing deficits limiting their function 4 weeks past their initial COVID infection were referred to the physiatry-led post-COVID recovery Clinic. PCPs can be a great resource to patients for validating their experience, detecting and acting on the "red-flag" symptoms and taking appropriate actions, encouraging self-management, creating realistic goals, and helping patients improve their function (**Fig. 2**).[29]

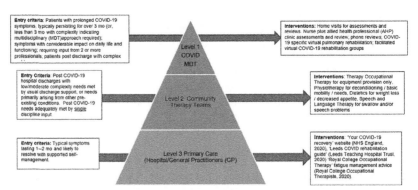

Fig. 1. Tiered pathway of input needs. (*Data from* Parkin A, Davison J, Tarrant R, Ross D, Halpin S, Simms A, Salman R, Sivan M. A Multidisciplinary NHS COVID-19 Service to Manage Post-COVID-19 Syndrome in the Community. J Prim Care Community Health. 2021 Jan-Dec;12:21501327211010994. https://doi.org/10.1177/21501327211010994. PMID: 33880955; PMCID: PMC8064663.)

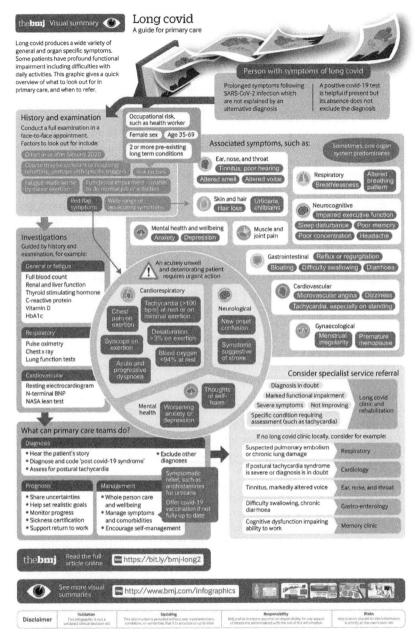

Fig. 2. Long COVID: a guide for primary care. (*Data from* Greenhalgh T, Sivam M, Delaney B, Evans R, Milne R. Long covid- an udate for primary care BMJ 2022:e072117 https://doi.org/10.1136/bmj-2033-072117.)

Home Care Models and Telehealth

For some patients with extensive needs, home care models have been developed.[30] Although home care for the management of acute COVID-19 illness was readily available, home management models of PASC were not.

Many affected by PASC were not critically ill or hospitalized at the time of infection. Persons living in residential care facilities and private homes have been affected which furthers the need to equip PCPs and long-term residence health care providers in the community setting to recognize the condition and have options for home management.[31]

PASC, to a large degree, has changed the paradigm of home care and self-management. Information, both accurate and inaccurate, has been widely available on the Internet, in Podcasts, and YouTube videos.[32] Many medical centers as well as the US Department of Health and Human Services offered information on recognizing symptoms and management of these symptoms.[33] An approach to treatment in this population is empowering the patients to self-manage with oversight and guide their own progress based on the waxing and waning nature of the disorder.

The use of home pulse oximeters, incentive spirometers, and home oxygen are common for management of acute COVID-19, but technology and wearables can also be used for monitoring symptoms and management of PASC.[34] One such proposed tool used a digital platform which monitors general health, symptom fluctuations, and potential triggers, and is linked to wearable sensors.[35] Data are collected about correlations between heart rate and heart rate variability in symptom burden all while implementing targeted rehabilitation programs. Further, in other chronic illness, home-based programs have been found to be beneficial in improving overall quality of life and functional capacity compared with the groups that did not perform the home program.[36]

Although telehealth was slowly being tested in the provision of health care in the United States, the pandemic propelled its use past all expectations. The support of the Centers for Medicare and Medicaid Services and other insurers to use telehealth during the peak of the pandemic to reduce exposure to infection has changed the provision of health care.[37]

Many models and sites use telehealth as an initial visit which can serve as a screening visit and referring patient to appropriate disciplines afterward.[27] Telehealth also expands the capacity for follow-up care after discharge from an emergency room or hospitalization. Telehealth serves as a quick and effective tool to check on patients' post-discharge and assess for medication reconciliation, symptoms, function, and difficulties that patients face after hospital discharge. If a patient with PASC has considerable post-exertional malaise, a model that offers telehealth visits offers respite from a possible crash or relapse that could occur with an in-person visit. A multidisciplinary provider evaluation can also be performed using this platform. In addition, advanced practice providers (physician associates or nurse practitioners) can conduct assessments using treatment algorithms to improve access.[38]

Salient symptoms of PASC, namely fatigue and post-exertional malaise, particularly support home management as a key element in treatment. This approach improves access to patients in rural areas or with limited transportation. Treatment plans for those with PASC-related fatigue found the most successful ones included elements of peer support, self-managed exercise programs, instructing on focus awareness of triggers and functional limit as well as home-based activities all of which can be implemented remotely.[30]

Barriers of Care in Long-Term Care Facilities

During the pandemic, it became clear that those living in long-term care facilities were particularly vulnerable to COVID-19 infections with high rates of mortality and morbidity.[31] Although there are limited data on PASC in this population, one study found a higher incidence of long COVID symptoms in the institutionalized versus those in a home setting.[39] Many of those affected in this older cohort of our population have been unable to return to their prior level of function.[40] Although the need for treatment in this population has been acknowledged, there has been very little investigation and few recommendations for programs that can be initiated in long-term care setting.[39]

Standardized assessment and minimizing duplication

As PASC involves multiple systems, multiple tests, and investigations unfortunately get ordered. There is also a duplication of such tests, and the care is not standardized. The role of such models of care is vital in minimizing redundancy. Unlike the United States, countries with connected medical records and systems minimize information duplication. The AAPMR PASC Collaborative has released multiple guidance statements which recommend certain investigations and intake questionnaires that should be considered while caring for patients with PASC.[41] Routine testing for every symptom is not recommended as most of the patients are expected to improve with proper education and symptom management, but if red flags are seen, appropriate testing and specialty referral are warranted. Please refer to **Fig. 2**.

See **Table 1** for a summary of care models and their salient features.

DISCUSSION

PASC has been better defined as a separate condition, and there is an increasing need for access to care for those affected in virtually all settings. Currently, the demand far outweighs the supply with patients often waiting months for evaluation and treatment plans. Although the rate of new hospitalization and deaths has diminished, the population of those with PASC continues to increase. It is likely to become endemic in light of the poor uptake of vaccinations in many parts of the country and a lack of tracing. Complicating the picture is the continued viral mutation with acute symptom clusters changing.

Owing to these factors, it seems that PASC surveillance and management will be needed long term, and standardization of these care models is necessary to understand trajectory and intervention efficacy. There continues to be a great need for education of health care personnel.

Currently, there are no predictors of PASC symptom severity and duration. Some find fatigue a limiting factor to exercise and leisure activities, whereas others may be unable to accomplish their daily activities. The inability to return to gainful employment and the unknown trajectory of disease lead to the recognition of PASC as a disability under the Titles II (state and local government) and III (public accommodations) of the Americans with Disabilities Act, 3 Section 504 of the Rehabilitation Act of 1973 (Section 504), 4 and Section 1557 of the Patient Protection and Affordable Care Act (Section 1557).

In the primary care-based model of care section of this article, the authors discussed how health systems have been able to create guidelines and algorithms, allow for PCPs to screen both established patients who had contracted COVID as well as new patients presenting with PASC symptoms or complaints. These algorithms allow for a consensus-based approach to symptom management, specialist referral indications, and therapy indications.

In addition to guidelines, new resources have become available for PCPs and other health care providers to better familiarize themselves with PASC. Examining one example in particular, the University of New Mexico outreach program (formed in conjunction with the CDC) named Project ECHO has been working to increase the accessibility of medical knowledge to combat health care disparities.[42] This program

Table 1
Summary of care models and their salient features

Model of Care	Example	Description	Salient Features
Specialty-based model	UTSW	Physiatry lead clinic, referrals from discharge from acute care hospital, community providers, or patient self-referrals	Comprehensive plan of care with easy access to PT/OT/SLP and neuropsychology
	John Hopkins	Physiatry and pulmonary lead clinic, referrals from discharges from acute care hospital after 48 h in ICU	Comprehensive plan of care combined with remote monitoring of vitals for high-risk patients
Primary care-based model	NYC Health	Establishment of primary-based COVID-19 Centers of Excellence	Increased catchment area as well as onsite specialists
	Hennepin	Development of screening algorithm for primary care providers	Evidence-based guideline approach for primary care for indications for referrals. Algorithms can be updated with emerging evidence
Home-based/ telehealth model	Home-based exercise therapy	Guided exercises for patients to perform without any equipment aimed at improving endurance, strength, and pulmonary function	Low barrier to entry. Does require patient motivation. Owing to lack of supervision, it would be unclear if patients are doing exercises correctly
	Telehealth services	Initial screening through virtual appointments	Wide reaching access to patients in rural areas and patients without reliable transportation

Abbreviations: OT, Occupational Therapy; PT, Physical Therapy; OT, Occupational Therapy; SLP, Speech Language Pathology; UTSW, University of Texas at Southwestern Medical Center.

currently offers self-paced online courses on emerging best practices for management of PASC patients. The program also offers ongoing online monthly didactic presentations specifically related to emerging literature for PASC lead by subject matter experts. The availability and accessibility of this information is a vital tool in the arsenal of PCPs in the face of this growing patient population.

Multiple professional or governmental agencies and organizations have developed guidelines that help with defining the problem, evaluating and management of patients with PASC. The AAPMR has been in the forefront in releasing consensus statements as a part of the PASC collaborative. Guidelines for breathing discomfort, cognitive symptoms, fatigue, cardiovascular symptoms, autonomic dysfunction, and pediatrics have been released with others upcoming. The goal of the collaborative is to foster engagement and share experiences to propel the health system toward defining standards of care for persons experiencing long COVID-19. Other organizations such as the Infectious Society of America, CDC have also been involved in organizing online lectures and educational series and conducting COVID-related research. Other countries including Australia and the United Kingdom have also published guidelines to help providers with management of PASC. There have also been other publications guiding physical activity, exercise, and therapy for post-COVID. The CDC also funds projects such as the Project ECHO, which disseminates information and educates PCPs on managing illnesses like long COVID.[42]

SUMMARY

The aftermath of the COVID-19 infection, much like the start of the pandemic has prompted health care entities to work diligently to establish and expedite diagnostic modalities and treatment approaches to care. Multiple model care systems have been implemented which include those centered on medical subspecialties such as pulmonology but primarily, a primary care model has been proposed as the most accessible and potentially sustainable long term. Physiatry has been in the forefront of long COVID care incorporating a holistic approach and using its experience with interdisciplinary collaboration. In addition, allied health disciplines often included are respiratory therapy, nursing, physical therapy, occupation therapy, speech therapy, psychology, and social work. Last, with the emergence of telehealth during the pandemic, several care models include home care and virtual visits that facilitate access to care in underserved populations.

CLINICS CARE POINTS

- Post-acute sequelae of SARS CoV-2 (PASC) surveillance and management will be needed long term, and standardization of these care models is necessary.

- Primary care providers can screen patients presenting with PASC symptoms and through established algorithms and a consensus-based approach, manage symptoms, include therapy disciplines, and facilitate specialist referrals.

- Physiatrists, being uniquely skilled at adopting a holistic approach, leading an interdisciplinary team, and collaborating with multiple specialties are well equipped to care for the long COVID population.

DISCLOSURE

The authors have nothing to disclose.

REFERENCES

1. (WHO) WHO. COVID-19 Dashboard. Secondary COVID-19 Dashboard 2020. Available at: https://covid19.who.int/.
2. Nalbandian A, Sehgal K, Gupta A, et al. Post-acute COVID-19 syndrome. Nat Med 2021;27(4):601–15.
3. Organization WH. Coronavirus disease (COVID-19): Post COVID-19 condition. Secondary Coronavirus disease (COVID-19): Post COVID-19 condition 2021. Available at: https://www.who.int/news-room/questions-and-answers/item/coronavirus-disease-(covid-19)-post-covid-19-condition.
4. Montani D, Savale L, Noel N, et al. Post-acute COVID-19 syndrome. Eur Respir Rev 2022;31(163).
5. Munblit D, Bobkova P, Spiridonova E, et al. Incidence and risk factors for persistent symptoms in adults previously hospitalized for COVID-19. Clin Exp Allergy 2021;51(9):1107–20.

6. Grover A, Joshi A. An overview of chronic disease models: a systematic literature review. Glob J Health Sci 2014;7(2):210–27.

7. (MSKTC) MSKTC. Online Knowledge Translation Toolkit. Secondary Online Knowledge Translation Toolkit 2022. Available at: https://msktc.org/.

8. Montani D, Savale L, Beurnier A, et al. Multidisciplinary approach for post-acute COVID-19 syndrome: time to break down the walls. Eur Respir J 2021;58(1). https://doi.org/10.1183/13993003.01090-2021.

9. Decary S DM, Stefan T, Langlois L, Skidmore B, Bhéreur A, and LeBlanc A. Care Models for Long COVID – A Living Systematic Review. 2021. Available at: https://sporevidencealliance.ca/wp-content/uploads/2021/12/Care-Models-for-Long-COVID_Update_2021.12.04.pdf.

10. McCorkell L, S Assaf G, E Davis H, et al. Patient-Led Research Collaborative: embedding patients in the Long COVID narrative. Pain Rep 2021;6(1):e913.

11. Herrera JE, Niehaus WN, Whiteson J, et al. Multidisciplinary collaborative consensus guidance statement on the assessment and treatment of fatigue in postacute sequelae of SARS-CoV-2 infection (PASC) patients. Pharm Manag PM R 2021;13(9):1027–43.

12. Prevention CfDCa. Evaluating and caring for patients with post-covid conditions, 2021. Available at: https://emergency.cdc.gov/coca/calls/2021/callinfo_061721.asp.

13. Lutchmansingh DD, Knauert MP, Antin-Ozerkis DE, et al. A Clinic Blueprint for Post-Coronavirus Disease 2019 RECOVERY: Learning From the Past, Looking to the Future. Chest 2021;159(3):949–58.

14. Verduzco-Gutierrez M, Estores IM, Graf MJP, et al. Models of Care for Postacute COVID-19 Clinics: Experiences and a Practical Framework for Outpatient Physiatry Settings. Am J Phys Med Rehabil 2021;100(12):1133–9.

15. Gupta R GA, Ghosh A, et al. A Paradigm for the Pandemic: A Covid-19 Recovery Unit. NEJM Catalyst 2020 May 20, Available at: https://catalyst.nejm.org/doi/full/10.1056/CAT.20.0238 Accessed August 13, 2022.

16. Sohn L, Lysaght M, Schwartzman WA, et al. Establishment of a COVID-19 Recovery Unit in a Veterans Affairs Post-Acute Facility. J Am Geriatr Soc 2020;68(10):2163–6.

17. Dundumalla S, Barshikar S, Niehaus WN, et al. A survey of dedicated PASC clinics: Characteristics, barriers and spirit of collaboration. Pharm Manag PM R 2022;14(3):348–56.

18. Hersche R, Weise A. Occupational Therapy-Based Energy Management Education in People with Post-COVID-19 Condition-Related Fatigue: Results from a Focus Group Discussion. Occup Ther Int 2022;2022:4590154.

19. Taquet M, Luciano S, Geddes JR, et al. Bidirectional associations between COVID-19 and psychiatric disorder: retrospective cohort studies of 62 354 COVID-19 cases in the USA. Lancet Psychiatr 2021;8(2):130–40.

20. Brigham E, O'Toole J, Kim SY, et al. The Johns Hopkins Post-Acute COVID-19 Team (PACT): A Multidisciplinary, Collaborative, Ambulatory Framework Supporting COVID-19 Survivors. Am J Med 2021;134(4):462–7.e1.

21. Venturelli S, Benatti SV, Casati M, et al. Surviving COVID-19 in Bergamo province: a post-acute outpatient re-evaluation. Epidemiol Infect 2021;149:e32.

22. Nurek M, Rayner C, Freyer A, et al. Recommendations for the recognition, diagnosis, and management of long COVID: a Delphi study. Br J Gen Pract 2021;71(712):e815–25.

23. Parkin A, Davison J, Tarrant R, et al. A Multidisciplinary NHS COVID-19 Service to Manage Post-COVID-19 Syndrome in the Community. J Prim Care Community Health 2021;12. https://doi.org/10.1177/21501327211010994. 21501327211010994.

24. Nalbandian A, Sehgal K, Gupta A, et al. Post-acute COVID-19 syndrome. Nat Med 2021;27(4):601–15. Accessed August 12, 2022.

25. Greenhalgh T, Knight M, A'Court C, et al. Management of post-acute covid-19 in primary care. BMJ 2020;370:m3026.

26. Beaverson L. Post-Covid Care. Secondary Post-Covid Care 2022. Available at: https://www.hennepinhealthcare.org/coronavirus-information/post-covid-care/.

27. Caldera F, Pan J, Abramoff B, et al. Post-Covid Asessment and Recovery Clinic. In: System UoPH, ed. Penn Medicine, 2021. Available at: https://www.penn medicine.org/for-health-care-professionals/for-physicians/covid-information/post-covid19-assessment-and-recovery-clinic-at-penn.

28. List JM, Long TG. Community-Based Primary Care Management of 'Long COVID': A Center of Excellence Model at NYC Health+ Hospitals. Am J Med 2021;134(10):1232–5.

29. Greenhalgh T, Sivan M, Delaney B, et al. Long covid-an update for primary care. BMJ 2022;378:e072117.

30. Kesavadev J, Basanth A, Krishnan G, et al. A new interventional home care model for COVID management: Virtual Covid IP. Diabetes Metabol Syndr 2021; 15(5):102228.

31. Benvenuti E, Rivasi G, Bulgaresi M, et al. Caring for nursing home residents with COVID-19: a "hospital-at-nursing home" intermediate care intervention. Aging Clin Exp Res 2021;33(10):2917–24.

32. Jacques ETBC, Park E, Kollia B, et al. Long Haul COVID-19 Videos on YouTube: Implications for Health Communication. Community Health 2022;47(4):610–5.

33. Services USDoHH. Topic Collection: COVID-19 Long-Term Care Resources. Secondary Topic Collection: COVID-19 Long-Term Care Resources 2022. Available at: https://asprtracie.hhs.gov/technical-resources/121/covid-19-long-term-care-resources/99.

34. Channa A, Popescu N, Skibinska J, et al. The Rise of Wearable Devices during the COVID-19 Pandemic: A Systematic Review. Sensors 2021;21(17). https://doi.org/10.3390/s21175787.

35. Sivan M, Greenhalgh T, Darbyshire JL, et al. LOng COvid Multidisciplinary consortium Optimising Treatments and servIces acrOss the NHS (LOCOMOTION): protocol for a mixed-methods study in the UK. BMJ Open 2022;12(5):e063505.

36. Longobardi I, do Prado DML, Goessler KF, et al. Benefits of Home-Based Exercise Training Following Critical SARS-CoV-2 Infection: A Case Report. Front Sports Act Living 2021;3:791703.

37. Chen K, Lodaria K, Jackson HB. Patient satisfaction with telehealth versus in-person visits during COVID-19 at a large, public healthcare system. J Eval Clin Pract 2022. https://doi.org/10.1111/jep.13770.

38. Stamenova V, Chu C, Pang A, et al. Virtual care use during the COVID-19 pandemic and its impact on healthcare utilization in patients with chronic disease: A population-based repeated cross-sectional study. PLoS One 2022; 17(4):e0267218.

39. Sorensen JM, Crooks VA, Freeman S, et al. A call to action to enhance understanding of long COVID in long-term care home residents. J Am Geriatr Soc 2022;70(7):1943–5.

40. Cohen K, Ren S, Heath K, et al. Risk of persistent and new clinical sequelae among adults aged 65 years and older during the post-acute phase of SARS-CoV-2 infection: retrospective cohort study. BMJ 2022;376:e068414.

41. Rehabilitation AAoPMa. Multidisciplinary Quality Improvement Initiative. Secondary Multidisciplinary Quality Improvement Initiative 2022. Available at: https://www.aapmr.org/members-publications/covid-19/multidisciplinary-quality-improvement-initiative?utm_source=google&utm_medium=organic&utm_campaign=AAPMR.

42. Mexico TUoN. How ECHO is Making a Difference. Secondary How ECHO is Making a Difference 2022. Available at: https://hsc.unm.edu/echo/what-we-do/.

Moving?

Make sure your subscription moves with you!

To notify us of your new address, find your **Clinics Account Number** (located on your mailing label above your name), and contact customer service at:

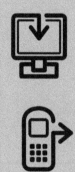

Email: **journalscustomerservice-usa@elsevier.com**

800-654-2452 (subscribers in the U.S. & Canada)
314-447-8871 (subscribers outside of the U.S. & Canada)

Fax number: 314-447-8029

Elsevier Health Sciences Division
Subscription Customer Service
3251 Riverport Lane
Maryland Heights, MO 63043

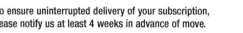

Printed and bound by CPI Group (UK) Ltd, Croydon, CR0 4YY

03/10/2024

01040465-0001